COCHLEAR IMPLANTATION FOR INFANTS AND CHILDREN

Advances

A Singular Audiology Text
Jeffrey L. Danhauer, Ph.D.
Audiology Editor

COCHLEAR IMPLANTATION FOR INFANTS AND CHILDREN
Advances

Senior Editor
Graeme M. Clark, AO, MB, BS, MS, Ph.D. (Syd.), Hon.M.D. (Hann.), Hon.M.D. (Syd.), F.R.C.S. (Lond. & Edin.), F.A.C.S.
Professor and Chairman of Otolaryngology
The University of Melbourne
Director of the Australian Research Council's Special Centre for Human Communication Research
Director of the Cooperative Research Centre for Cochlear Implant,
Speech and Hearing Research
Director of the Bionic Ear Institute
Head of the Cochlear Implant Clinic
Melbourne, Australia

Editors
Robert S. C. Cowan, B.Sc., M.Sc., Dip.Aud., Ph.D. (Melb.)
Deputy Director of the Cooperative Research Centre for Cochlear Implant,
Speech and Hearing Research
Assistant Director of the Cochlear Implant Clinic
The Royal Victorian Eye and Ear Hospital
Melbourne, Australia.

Richard C. Dowell, B.Sc., M.Sc., Dip.Aud., Ph.D. (Melb.)
Associate Professor in Audiology
Department of Otolaryngology
The University of Melbourne
Deputy Director of the Cochlear Implant Clinic,
The Royal Victorian Eye and Ear Hospital
Melbourne, Australia

SINGULAR PUBLISHING GROUP, INC.
SAN DIEGO · LONDON

COVER

Tommy, shown on the front cover, is a 4-year-old boy who received a cochlear implant at 22 months of age. He used the Multipeak speech processor strategy until 32 months of age. He then switched to the Speak strategy and is quite fluent in communicating in both English and Croatian, his mother's native tongue. He can communicate easily without the need to lipread and his voice is of normal quality.

Singular Publishing Group, Inc.
401 West A Street, Suite 325
San Diego, California 92101-7904

19 Compton Terrace
London N1 2UN, UK

e-mail: singpub©mail.cerfnet.com
Website: http://www.singpub.com

Typeset in 10/12 Bookman by So Cal Graphics
Printed in the United States of America by McNaughton & Gunn

Library of Congress Cataloging-in-Publication Data

Cochlear implantation for infants and children : Advances / senior
   editor, Graeme M. Clark : editors, Robert S.C. Cowan and Richard C. Dowell.
      p.   cm.
   Includes bibliographical references and index.
   ISBN 1-56593-727-9
      1. Cochlear implants.   2. Children, Deaf—Rehabilitation.
   I. Clark, Graeme.   II. Cowan, Robert S. C.   III. Dowell, Richard C.
   [DNLM: 1. Cochlear Implant—in infancy & childhood.   WV 274 A243
   1997}
   RF305.A38   1997
   618.92'09789—dc21
   DNLM/DLC
   for Library of Congress   96-49000
                                                                  CIP

Contents

PREFACE

The field of cochlear implantation has been expanding rapidly as research and clinical studies establish the extent of its benefits. One important frontier has been cochlear implantation in children, and moving back this frontier involves operating on younger children and infants. Clinical advances with cochlear implantation in children have now reached the point where it is timely to bring them together in a book. This book has contributions primarily from the one center, as the task of interrelating work from different centers can be difficult. Furthermore, the Center in Melbourne had the initial experience in the clinical application of multiple-channel cochlear implantation to children with the first operation in 1985 and has had a substantial involvement in the work ever since. It has also run 16 international workshops since 1991, which have helped consolidate our clinical practice. The book is aimed primarily at presenting the surgical, medical, audiological, speech and language, and habilitation aspects of cochlear implantation in infants and children. It also draws on a growing body of research that is essential in giving direction and foundation to the management of children. The book coincides with the development by Cochlear Limited in association with the Cooperative Research Centre for Cochlear Implant, Speech and Hearing Research of an advanced cochlear implant system (Nucleus-24), which makes it possible to implant infants and young children, as well as allowing improved strategies to be used on both children and adults.

Cochlear implants could be said to be one of the most complex and interdisciplinary biomedical achievements to date and for that reason have required contributions from many scientists, engineers, clinicians, and communication specialists for its success. We wish to acknowledge the contributions made by our many colleagues in Australia and overseas to this new and exciting field. There has also been close collaboration in Australia between the research and clinical activities of the Department of Otolaryngology, The University of Melbourne, the Bionic Ear Institute and the Royal Victorian Eye and Ear Hospital, and the industrial research and development of Cochlear Limited. This has led to state-of-the-art cochlear implants which are safe, effective, and reliable.

Funding for the research leading to the development and improvement of the Nucleus cochlear implant has been provided through the Australian Research Council's Special Research Centre for Human Communication Research, the U.S. National Institutes of Health, the National Health and Medical Research Council of Australia, Lions Clubs International, and more recently, the Cooperative Research Centre for Cochlear Implant Speech and Hearing Research, as well as many trusts and foundations.

We would like to thank Sue Davine, Jacky Gray, Trevor Carter, and Frank Nielsen for their organization and secretarial help and for providing high quality figures for this manuscript.

G. M. Clark
R. S. C. Cowan
R. C. Dowell

CONTRIBUTORS

Elizabeth J. Barker, B.App Sci. (Speech Pathology)
Speech Pathologist
The Royal Victorian Eye and Ear Hospital, Melbourne

Graeme M. Clark, A.O., M.B., B.S., M.S., Ph.D. (Sydney), Hon. M.D. (Hannover), Hon. M.D. (Sydney), F.R.C.S (London), F.R.C.S. (Edinburgh), F.R.A.C.S.
Professor and Chairman
The Department of Otolaryngology
The University of Melbourne
Director
The Special Research Centre for Human Communication Research
Director
The Cooperative Research Centre for Cochlear Implant, Speech and Hearing Research
Director, The Bionic Ear Institute
Head
Cochlear Implant Clinic, Royal Victorian Eye and Ear Hospital, Melbourne

Robert S. C. Cowan, B.Sc., M.Sc., Dip.Aud., Ph.D. (Melbourne)
Deputy Director
The Cooperative Research Centre for Cochlear Implant
Speech and Hearing Research
Senior Research Fellow
The Department of Otolaryngology
The University of Melbourne.
Assistant Director
Cochlear Implant Clinic
Royal Victorian Eye and Ear Hospital, Melbourne

Shani J. Dettman, B.App. Sci. (Speech Pathology)
Speech Pathologist
Cochlear Implant Clinic
The Royal Victorian Eye and Ear Hospital, Melbourne

Richard C. Dowell, B.Sc., M.Sc., Dip.Aud., Ph.D. (Melbourne)
Associate Professor
The Department of Otolaryngology
The University of Melbourne
Deputy Director
The Bionic Ear Institute
Deputy Director
Cochlear Implant Clinic
Royal Victorian Eye and Ear Hospital, Melbourne

Karyn L. Galvin, B.Sc., Dip.Aud
Research Fellow
The Bionic Ear Institute
Clinical Research Fellow
Cochlear Implant Clinic
Royal Victorian Eye and Ear Hospital, Melbourne

James F. Patrick, B.Sc., M.Sc.
Director
Research and Development
Cochlear Limited, Sydney

Brian C. Pyman, M.B., B.S., D.L.O. (Melbourne), F.R.A.C.S.
Senior Surgeon
and Deputy Director
Cochlear Implant Clinic
Royal Victorian Eye and Ear Hospital, Melbourne

Gary Rance, B.Ed., Dip.Aud.
Audiologist,
Cochlear Implant Clinic
Royal Victorian Eye and Ear Hospital,
Melbourne

Julia Z. Sarant, BSc, Dip.Aud.
Research Fellow
The Bionic Ear Institute
Clinical Research Fellow
Cochlear Implant Clinic
Royal Victorian Eye and Ear Hospital,
Melbourne

Peter M. Seligman, Ph.D. (Elec. Eng.) (Monish)
Cochlear Limited
The Royal Victorian Eye and Ear Hospital,
Melbourne

Robert K. Shepherd B.Sc., Dip.Ed., Ph.D. (Melb.)
Garnett Passe and Rodney Williams Senior
Research Fellow
The Department of Otolaryngology
The University of Melbourne,
Melbourne

Robert L. Webb M.B.B.S, F.R.A.C.S., D.L.O.
Senior Surgeon
Cochlear Implant Clinic,
The Royal Victorian Eye and Ear Hospital,
Melbourne

ACKNOWLEDGMENTS

Graeme Clark thanks his wife Margaret, children Sonya, Cecily, Roslyn, Merran, and Jonathan, and sons-in-law Ian and Peter for their unfailing support and constant encouragement, and also his grandchildren Elise, Monty, and Daniel for his renewed interest in speech and language development.

Robert Cowan thanks his wife Heather and son Dylan for their unstinting support and patience.

Richard Dowell thanks his wife Shani for support and valuable input and sons Lachlan and Tristan for providing an additional reason to be awake at 3 A.M.

1

INTRODUCTION

GRAEME M. CLARK
ROBERT S. C. COWAN
RICHARD C. DOWELL

From the time single-channel cochlear implants were first implanted in children in the early 1980s in Los Angeles (Luxford et al., 1987) closely followed in 1985 by the multiple-channel cochlear implant in Melbourne (Clark et al., 1987a, 1987b), there has been a considerable expansion in the work to apply the multiple-channel cochlear implant to infants and young children. The Nucleus multiple-channel cochlear implant systems, commercially developed by Cochlear Limited, referred to as Nucleus-22 and Nucleus-24, are shown diagramatically in Figure 1–1. The sound is picked up by a directional microphone placed above the pinna. It is transduced into electrical signals which pass via a cable to the speech processor for analysis. Two different models of speech processors are now available: one worn as an "ear level" device, and a larger, more versatile unit that can be worn in a pocket. With the speech processors, information about speech or environmental sounds is encoded as a series of electrical pulses. The encoded information, together with power to operate the implant, are transmitted by an aerial through the skin to the implanted receiver-stimulator. This receiver-stimulator decodes the signal and sends patterns of stimuli to the electrodes within the cochlea to provide stimulation of discrete groups of

auditory nerve fibers for higher auditory brain processing.

Applying the multiple-channel cochlear implant to children initially meant designing the Nucleus cochlear implant receiver-stimulator so it would be small enough to implant in children at least as young as 2 years of age, as well as creating a smaller speech processor that could be easily worn. This CI-22M receiver-stimulator and Spectra-22 speech processor are presently part of the Nucleus-22 system, which will also include an "ear level" speech processor (ESPrit™) presenting the SPEAK strategy (Figure 1–2). For infants there is a need to have a smaller implant with additional features, and this has been achieved with the new CI-24M receiver-stimulator (Figure 1–3). This implant features telemetry to enable device function to be monitored. Recording auditory nerve activity with this implant could also lead to setting thresholds and comfortable listening levels objectively. The CI-24M can be used with an "ear level" speech processor (ESPrit™) (Figure 1–4) or with the pocket-worn unit (SPrint™). The latter speech processor allows greater flexibility in the choice of speech processing strategies. These devices have been developed by Cochlear Limited with support from the Cooperative Research Centre for

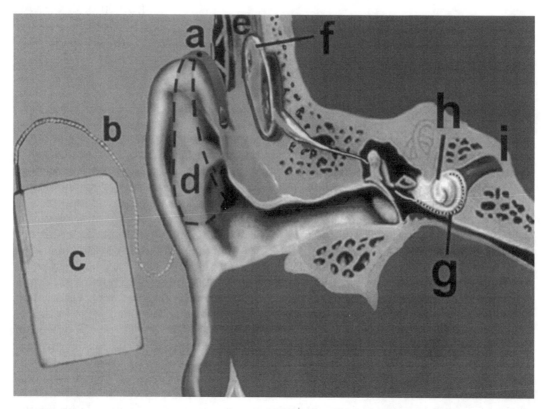

FIGURE 1-1. A diagram of the Nucleus-22 and Nucleus-24 multiple-channel cochlear implant systems. **a** = microphone; **b** = cable; **c** = body-worn speech processor; **d** = ear level speech processor; **e** = transmitter coil; **f** = receiver stimulator; **g** = electrode array; **h** = cochlea; **i** = auditory nerve. (From Clark, G. M. [1996]. Electrical stimulation of the auditory nerve: The coding of frequency, the perception of pitch, and the development of cochlear implant speech processing strategies for profoundly deaf people. *Clinical and Experimental Pharmacology and Physiology, 23*[9], 766–776. Reprinted with permission from Blackwell Science Pty. Ltd.).

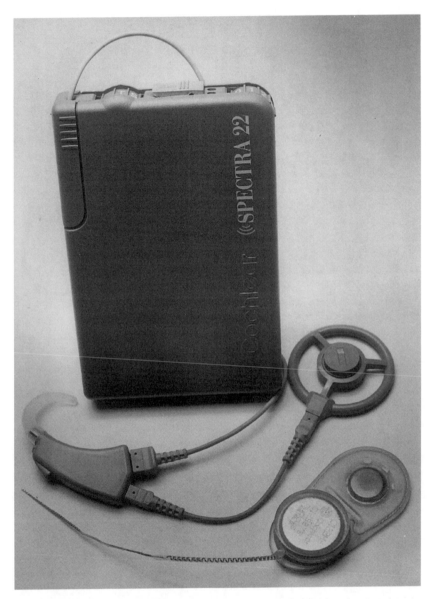

FIGURE 1–2. The CI-22M receiver-stimulator and Spectra-22 speech processor (microphone included in the behind the ear housing) for children and adults, which make up the Nucleus-22 system.

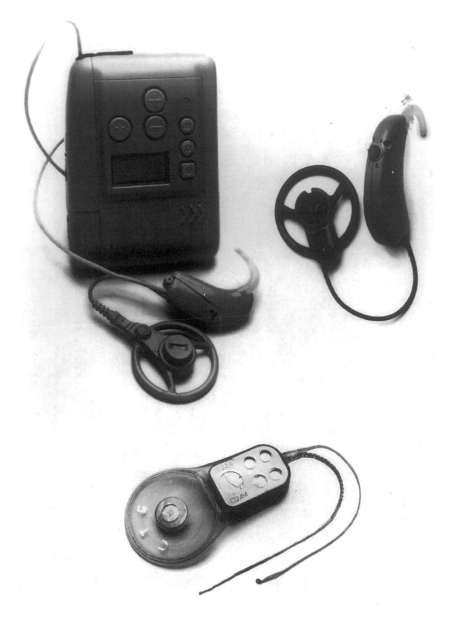

FIGURE 1–3. The CI-24M receiver-stimulator and SPrint™ and ESPrit™ speech processors for infants, children, and adults. Top left: the body-worn SPrint™ speech processor. Top right: the "ear level" ESPrit™ speech processor. Bottom: the CI-24M receiver-stimulator.

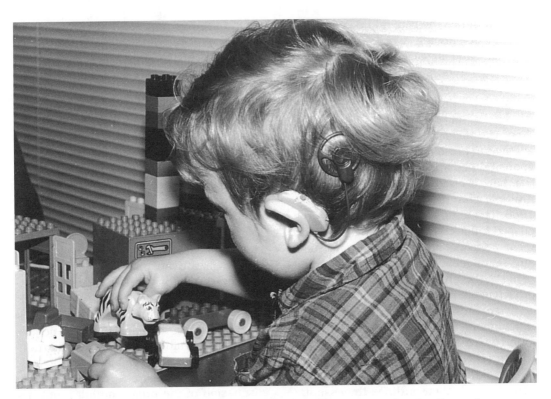

FIGURE 1–4. A photograph of a cochlear implant child with the ESPrit™ "ear level" speech processor in place.

Cochlear Implant Speech and Hearing Research, and are part of the Nucleus-24 system (Figure 1–4).

For infants, it is important that the device not affect head growth, not predispose to middle ear infections extending to the inner ear from an otitis media, and be easily explantable with another reinserted if necessary years later. Selection and evaluation procedures appropriate for preverbal infants and children have been developed. Furthermore, the surgery, although similar to that in an adult, has been modified for children.

This book gives a comprehensive description of the surgical, medical, audiological, speech and language, and habilitation aspects of cochlear implantation for infants and children. The book is written primarily by members of the Melbourne cochlear implant team, in order to provide a coordinat-

ed approach to the subject. Input on the chapter on Engineering is mainly from Cochlear Limited with whom the The University of Melbourne's Department of Otolaryngology, and the Bionic Ear Institute have an affiliation through the Cooperative Research Centre for Cochlear Implant Speech and Hearing Research.

This book is divided into 14 chapters, including the *Introduction. Historical Perspectives* provides a brief overview of the early research in cochlear implantation in the 1960s and 1970s. It then outlines the development of cochlear implants for postlinguistically deaf adults in the 1980s and 1990s, with particular reference to the Nucleus systems. It concludes with summaries of clinical studies which helped establish the value of multiple-channel implantation for severely-to-profoundly deaf children. *Biological*

Safety outlines the general questions and experimental findings required to establish the safety and efficacy of cochlear implantation on adults as well as children. It then discusses the research findings required to answer questions of specific importance when operating on infants and young children. *The Melbourne Cochlear Implant Clinic Program* presents an overview of the responsibilities and functions of the Clinic that have evolved since implanting the first multiple-channel implant on a child in 1985. The aims of the Clinic are first discussed followed by its historical development, interrelation with research, the team and management structure, the components of the program, and finally, the approach to clinical management.

Preoperative Medical Evaluation presents initially the causes of a severe-to-profound hearing loss in children likely to present to a cochlear implant clinic with a brief outline of the features of the most common conditions. It then outlines the essential aspects of the clinical history and examination, and the special investigations required. Finally, there is discussion on important preoperative management issues. *Preoperative Audiological, Speech, and Language Evaluation* discusses the general goals and problems in selection before presenting in more detail the evaluation program. This program refers in particular to establishing hearing thresholds, optimizing hearing aids, and speech and language assessment. Key issues in the selection are described, and include the factors likely to lead to good results. In conclusion, carefully selected illustrated histories are presented.

Surgery provides a description of the procedures involved. They are described under the following headings: anesthetic and preoperative prezparations, incision and creation of flaps, mastoidectomy and posterior tympanotomy, creation of a bed for the receiver-stimulator, cochleostomy and electrode insertion, and fixation of package and wound closure. Attention is also

given to the management of special problems at surgery, and postoperative complications. Particular emphasis is given to the implantation of the new CI-24M receiver-stimulator for the Nucleus-24 system.

Engineering highlights the features of the present Nucleus-22 and new Nucleus-24 systems of special relevance to the clinician and habilitationist. These include the development of speech processing strategies and device reliability. The need for a new implant system for infants and children is elaborated, and the features of the Nucleus-24 system are summarized. These include flexibility in the strategies to be used, high rate capability, telemetry, and an "ear level" speech processor. *Speech Processor Programming* provides the rationale for programming and reviews the techniques used, including the telemetry. The behavioral programming techniques are then outlined with particular emphasis on the Melbourne Clinic experience. There is also discussion of the programming problems likely to occur and their management.

Habilitation: Infants and Young Children discusses the educational approaches to communication and how the children are selected. It outlines listening and preverbal development and highlights the important principles of habilitation. The chapter covers the initial introduction to the device and then discusses how the child is helped to learn to detect and discriminate sounds. The development of auditory comprehension at home and preschool is outlined with special reference to language acquisition. *Habilitation: School-Aged Children* emphasizes habilitation issues of special relevance to school-aged children. It describes in particular the management of individual sessions, gives guidance on counseling, and discusses general issues. Counseling covers specific questions including the use of oral communication and relations with peers and the deaf community.

Evaluation of Benefit: Infants and Children first presents an analysis of the tests of speech perception presently available and their relevance to assessment of communication abilities. Special problems for measuring speech perception in children are outlined. The perception of speech in children with implants is discussed, and the factors leading to those results are considered. A comparison of the benefits of cochlear implants, hearing aids, and tactile devices is outlined, and the assessment of speech production and language is discussed. *Socioeconomic and Educational Management Issues* discusses how socioeconomic benefits can be measured, and summarizes the studies undertaken to evaluate indirect benefits from cochlear implants. In addition, the contribution of educational placement, medical costs, and device costs and reliability to the calculation of benefits are presented. *Ethical Issues* focuses primarily on how research and clinical practice for cochlear implantation in children can be viewed in the light of statements such as the Helsinki Declaration on Biomedical Research adopted by the 18th World Medical Assembly, and the Convention of the Rights of the Child adopted by the General Assembly of the United Nations, 20 November 1989.

REFERENCES

Clark, G. M. (1996). Electrical stimulation of the auditory nerve: The coding of frequency, the perception of pitch, and the development of cochlear implant speech processing strategies for profoundly deaf people. *Clinical and Experimental Pharmacology and Physiology, 23,* 766–776.

Clark, G. M., Blamey, P. J., Busby, P. A., Dowell, R. C., Franz, B. K-G., Musgrave, G. N., Nienhuys, T. G., Pyman, B. C., Roberts, S. A., Tong, Y. C., Webb, R. L., Kusma, J. A., Money, D. K., Patrick, J. F., & Seligman, P. M. (1987a). A multiple-electrode intracochlear implant for children. *Archives of Otolaryngology, 113,* 825–828.

Clark, G. M., Busby, P. A., Roberts, S. A., Dowell, R. C., Tong, Y. C., Blamey, P. J., Nienhuys, T. G., Mecklenberg, D. J., Webb, R. L., Pyman, B. C., & Franz, B. K-G. (1987b). Preliminary results for the Cochlear Corporation multi-electrode intracochlear implants on six prelingually deaf patients. *American Journal of Otology, 8,* 234–9.

Luxford, W. M., Berliner, K. I., Eisenberg, M. A., & House, W. F. (1987). Cochlear implants in children. *Annals of Otology, 96,* 136–138.

2

HISTORICAL PERSPECTIVES

GRAEME M. CLARK

INITIAL CLINICAL AND BASIC RESEARCH STUDIES

Initial attempts to help profoundly deaf people understand speech by electrically stimulating the auditory nerve commenced in the 1950s and 1960s (Djourno & Eyries, 1957; Doyle, Doyle, & Turnbull, 1964; House, Berliner, Crary, Graham, Luckey, Norton, Selters, Tobin Urban & Wexler, 1976; Simmons, Monegeon, Lewis, & Huntington, 1964). The procedures were carried out on isolated patients. Raw or filtered speech was presented to the electrodes, but no speech understanding was obtained.

To achieve speech perception with electrical stimulation there were a number of fundamental questions that needed to be answered. First, how to adequately reproduce the coding of sound frequency and intensity (a prerequisite for speech perception). Second, it was thought that people who are profoundly deaf will have lost most cochlear hair cells, in addition to a reduction in the population of spiral ganglion cells below a critical level required for speech understanding by acoustic or electrical stimulation (Kerr & Schuknecht, 1968). Third, there was also concern that placing electrodes within the cochlea would result in the loss of the auditory nerve fibers that were to be stimulated.

Basic research was required to help answer these questions before proceeding with electrical stimulation of the auditory nerve in patients who were profoundly deaf. Acute physiological studies on auditory brainstem nuclei (Clark, 1969, 1970a, 1970b) were carried out to determine whether a rate or time/period code could convey frequencies in the speech range. The animal studies showed that the sustained firing of units within the brainstem seen for all acoustic frequencies did not occur for electrical stimulation above about 500 pulses/s. This suggested that a rate or time/period code alone would not be adequate for conveying speech frequencies above 500 Hz, and that place coding of frequency would be needed. The limitations of using single-channel stimulation to provide rate coding were confirmed by behavioral studies on experimental animals to measure difference limens for rate (Clark, Nathar, Kranz, & Maritz, 1972; Clark, Kranz, & Minus, 1973; Williams, Clark, & Stanley, 1976).

With the place coding of frequency, inserting electrodes along the length of the cochlea was required for stimulating localized groups of nerve fibers arranged tono-topically (according to a frequency scale) in the speech frequency range. Localizing the current to discrete groups of nerve fibers presented a problem, as the current could spread along the low resistance pathway of the perilymph within the scala tympani of the cochlea, and away from the neural elements. The current spread could limit the place coding of frequency. Research to solve this problem was undertaken by Merzenich (1975), Black (1978), and Black and Clark (1977, 1978, 1980). The studies showed that more localized excitation of the auditory nerve fibers was produced by bipolar and common ground rather than monopolar stimulation. These results were from acute experiments in the cat, and need to be qualified when applied to the human for the following reasons: (1) the experimental animal had normal cochleas, and no fibrous tissue or bone in the scalae to alter the current spread; (2) the neurons had peripheral processes, which is not usually seen with a profound hearing loss in humans; (3) the spiral ganglion cells in the cat are located higher in the scala tympani, and closer to the organ of Corti (Clark, 1995).

Before undertaking our first cochlear implant operation on a postlinguistically deaf patient, it was also necessary to be sure the surgery would not lead to the loss of the residual spiral ganglion cells it was planned to excite. Studies by Simmons (1967), Clark (1973), Schindler and Merzenich (1974), and Clark, Tong, Black, Forster, Patrick, and Dewhurst (1977) showed that electrodes could be inserted into the cochlea and especially along the scala tympani without marked loss of the neurons, providing there was no perforation of the basilar membrane, no fracture of the spiral lamina, and no resulting labyrinthitis. A timeline for the basic and clinical research leading to the development of the multiple–channel cochlear implant for children is shown in Table 2–1.

TABLE 2–1. Timeline for development of cochlear implant systems with special relevance to the Nucleus systems for children. (Events in italics are of direct relevance to cochlear implantation in children.)

1967	January	Commencement of experimental animal studies to determine if electrical stimulation could simulate brainstem neuron responses to sound (G.M. Clark, University of Sydney).
1970	January	Commencement of behavioral studies on the experimental animal to compare electrical and acoustic stimulation (The University of Melbourne).
1974	June	Commencement of the development of The University of Melbourne's prototype fully implantable multiple-channel receiver-stimulator.
1978	August	First postlinguistically deaf adult implanted with The University of Melbourne's prototype multiple-channel receiver-stimulator at the Royal Victorian Eye and Ear Hospital, Melbourne.
1978–79		Formant-based speech processing strategy (F0/F2) devised by the Department of Otolaryngology, University of Melbourne team.
1980		*3M House single-channel device implanted in first child at House Ear Institute, Los Angeles.*
1982		Nucleus developed first multiple-channel receiver-stimulator for FDA clinical trial in adults.

1982	September	The University of Melbourne team at the Royal Victorian Eye and Ear Hospital implanted first Nucleus clinical trial receiver-stimulator in postlinguistically deaf adult.
1984	November	The US Food and Drug Administration (FDA) approves 3M-House single-channel implant for use in postlinguistically deaf adults.
1985	September	*The University of Melbourne team, Royal Victorian Eye and Ear Hospital, implants first Nucleus CI–22M receiver–stimulator in a child.*
1985	October	FDA approves the Nucleus F0/F2–WSPII strategy and processor as safe and effective for postlinguistically deaf adults.
1986	November	*Multi-center FDA clinical trial of the CI-22M receiver-stimulator, and the F0/F1/F2–WSP III strategy and processor commences on children from 2 to 18 years of age.*
1986	May	FDA approves the Nucleus F0/F1/F2–WSPIII strategy and processor for postlinguistically deaf adults
1987	May	*Department of Otolaryngology University of Melbourne commenced NIH 5-year contract No 1-NS-7-2342 on Studies on Pediatric Auditory Pros-thesis Implants to examine biological safety issues of special importance for cochlear implants in infants.*
1987	May	*Coleman and Epstein laboratories, University of California, San Francisco, commenced NIH 5-year contract DC-7-2391 on Studies on Pediatric Auditory Prosthesis Implants.*
1988	January	*First child to receive the Nucleus multiple-channel system in mainland Europe (Oslo).*
1989	March	*First child to receive the Nucleus multiple-channel system in U.K. (Nottingham).*
1989	October	FDA approves the Nucleus Multipeak–MSP strategy and processor for postlinguistically deaf adults.
1990	June	*FDA approves the Nucleus F0/F1/F2–WSP III and Multipeak–MSP strategies and processors for use in profoundly deaf children from 2 years of age and older.*
1994	March	FDA approves the Nucleus SPEAK–Spectra-22 strategy and processor for postlinguistically deaf adults and deaf children.
1995	August	FDA approves Nucleus Multipeak SPEAK strategies for severely deaf adults.
1996	April	FDA approves Clarion system for adults.
1996	September	FDA approves clinical trial of Nucleus-24 system in adults.

IMPLANTS IN ADULTS

Our first postlinguistically deaf adult was implanted in 1978 (Clark, Pyman, & Bailey, 1979) (Table 2–1). Initial psychophysical research examined the perception of rate and place pitch perception as well as loudness (Tong, Black, Clark, Forster, Millar, O'Loughlin, & Patrick, 1979). It was found that rate discrimination for stimuli at 100 and 200 pulses/s was limited, but comparable to that seen in the experimental animal (Clark et al., 1972; Clark et al., 1973; Tong, Clark, Blamey, Busby, & Dowell, 1982). Rate pitch had a different quality from that of place pitch, the latter being better described as timbre. With place of stimulation, the patient was able to rank the timbre as sharp to dull when electrodes were stimulated from base to apex (Tong et al., 1982).

Our first speech processing strategy to be evaluated was one that filtered the sound as occurs with basilar membrane motion (Laird, 1979). The processor, which used fixed filters, also modeled auditory nerve firing patterns. However, the patient's understanding of running speech was poor, as unpredictable variations in loudness occurred due to the interaction of electric fields from simultaneous stimulation. This emphasized the importance for cochlear implant speech processing of not allowing simultaneous stimulation to occur.

F0/F2–WSPII Strategy and Processor

The first clue to developing a speech processor that helped profoundly deaf people understand running speech, especially for electrical stimulation alone, came when it was observed that electrical stimulation at individual sites within the cochlea produced vowel-like sounds, and that the vowel sounds corresponded to the single formant vowels heard by a person with normal hearing when corresponding areas in the cochlea were excited (Clark, 1995).

As a result of this discovery, we developed a speech processing strategy (Clark, Tong, Bailey, Black, Martin, Millar, O'Loughlin, Patrick, & Pyman, 1978) that allowed our first patient and subsequently others to understand running speech, both with and without assistance from lipreading. This inaugural strategy extracted the second formant frequency (F2), and presented it to an appropriate electrode in the cochlea on a place coding basis. The amplitude of the sound energy of the second formant (A2) was used to set the current level of the stimulating electrode. The voicing or fundamental frequency (F0) was

presented to each electrode being stimulated as a rate code. The speech perception results with this strategy were good enough for the patients to be evaluated using standard audiological tests. These tests showed there was considerable improvement in understanding running speech when the strategy was used in combination with lipreading, and significant understanding for electrical stimulation alone when tested with open-sets of monosyllabic words and CID sentences (Clark, Tong, Martin, & Busby, 1981a; Clark, Tong, & Martin, 1981b). The mean sentence scores in quiet for unselected patients presenting at the Cochlear Implant Clinic of the Royal Victorian Eye and Ear Hospital are shown in Figure 2–1. The clinical trial of the F0/F2–WSP II strategy and processor was commenced in 1983 on 40 postlinguistically deaf adults at nine centers worldwide and approved by the U.S. Food and Drug Administration (FDA) as safe and effective in October, 1985.

In the late 1970s and early 1980s studies on profoundly deaf adults also took place in other centers to see whether speech perception could be achieved with a multiple-electrode cochlear implant. Fixed filter schemes with minimal processing of speech were mainly assessed. The outputs from up to six filters were used to stimulate electrodes on a place coding basis. The studies at Stanford (Atlas, Herndon, Simmons, Dent, & White, 1983), Salt Lake City (Eddington, 1980), San Francisco (Michelson & Schindler, 1981), and Paris (Chouard, 1980) showed no open-set speech understanding except for one patient in San Francisco. Single-channel electrical stimulation on adults was carried out in Los Angeles (House, Luetje, & Campos, 1981), London (Fourcin, Rosen, & Moore, 1979), and Vienna (Burian, Hochmair, & Hochmair-Desoyer, 1979), and was found to provide some closed-set but no open-set speech perception with electrical stimulation alone (Clark, 1996).

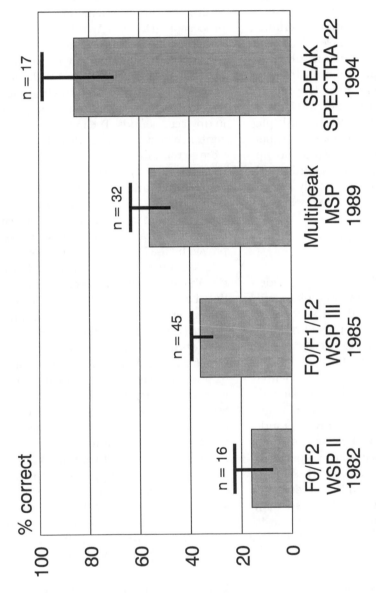

FIGURE 2–1. Mean open-set CID sentence scores for the F0/F2, F0/F1/F2, Multipeak, and SPEAK University of Melbourne/Nucleus speech processing strategies in quiet for electrical stimulation alone on unselected patients presenting at the Cochlear Implant Clinic of the Royal Victorian Eye and Ear Hospital. The speech processor which presents the strategies is shown following the strategy. (From Clark, G. M. [1997]. Cochlear implants. In H. Ludman & A. Wright [Eds.], *Diseases of the ear*. London: Edward Arnold. Reprinted with permission from Professor A. Wright, London.)

A more detailed review of the results of these systems is provided by Millar, Tong, and Clark, (1984).

A well-controlled comparative study of the Los Angeles (3M) and Vienna single-channel and the Salt Lake City (Ineraid) and University of Melbourne (Nucleus) multiple-channel systems was undertaken at Iowa (Gantz, McCabe, Tyler, & Preece, 1987). The speech perception results were better for the multiple-channel than for the single-channel systems. The results for the Salt Lake City (Ineraid) and University of Melbourne (Nucleus) multiple-channel systems were the same in quiet, but in noise the Salt Lake City (Ineraid) appeared to provide more information, although there was no statistically significant difference between the two systems.

F0/F1/F2–WSP III Strategy and Processor

It was next found that when we added more formant information on a place coding basis, in this case the first formant (F1), speech perception improved not only in quiet but also in noise. The results for this speech feature extraction (F0/F1/F2) speech-processing strategy, implemented in the WSP III speech processor (Dowell, Seligman, Blamey, & Clark, 1987), are shown in Figure 2–1. These findings indicate the importance of F1 as well as F2 information in the perception of speech in quiet. The improvement over the F0/F2 strategy was also seen in the presence of noise. This F0/F1/F2–WSP III strategy and processor was approved for use in postlinguistically deaf adults by the FDA in May 1986.

Multipeak–MSP Strategy and Processor

Further improvements in speech perception were obtained by extracting high frequency spectral information, and present-ing this information on a place coding basis. With voiced sounds the energy in the frequency bands 2.0–2.8 kHz; 2.8–4.0 kHz; and above 4.0 kHz, as well as the energy of F1 and F2 was presented to appropriate electrodes by a strategy called Multipeak, and implemented in the MSP processor (Dowell, Whitford, Seligman, Franz, & Clark, 1990). For unvoiced sounds, the energy in the frequency bands 2.0–2.8 kHz; 2.8–4.0 kHz; and above 4.0 kHz together with only F2 was used to stimulate the cochlea, as F1 is not normally emphasized in unvoiced sounds. The mean open-set CID sentence tests results with this strategy were significantly better than those obtained with the F0/F1/F2 strategy, as shown in Figure 2–1 (Clark, Dowell, Cowan, Pyman, & Webb, 1996). The improvement was also seen in quiet and in noise. The Multipeak–MSP strategy and processor was approved by the FDA in October 1989.

When the Multipeak–MSP and F0/F1/F2–WSP III systems were compared with the Salt Lake City (Ineraid) system in a controlled study by Cohen, Waltzman, and Fisher (1993), the mean open-set monosyllabic word and sentence score with the Symbion (or Ineraid) system was approximately 42% as compared with approximately 75% with the Multipeak–MSP system. On the other hand, there was no significant difference between the F0/F1/F2–WSP III and Symbion or Ineraid systems.

The data suggest that, if one looks at the place coding of spectral information alone, the preprocessing of speech into two stimulus channels with the F0/F1/F2 strategy gives comparable results to the presentation of the outputs from four band-pass filters with the Symbion (Ineraid).

SPEAK–Spectra-22 Strategy and Processor

In 1990 (Tong, van Hoesel, Lai, Vandali, Harrison, & Clark, 1990) the Multipeak–MSP system was compared with a filter bank strategy which selected the four highest spectral peaks and coded these on a place basis. Electrical stimulation occurred at a constant rate of 166 Hz. There was a significant improvement in the perception of vowels and consonants in one of two patients using the filter bank strategy. The research that led to this study is presented in more detail by Clark et al. (1996). This encouraging finding caused us to decide whether to assess a strategy which extracted six spectral maxima or six spectral peaks and presented the outputs of the filters on a place coding basis, both at a constant stimulus rate. As preliminary investigations did not show six peaks made a significant difference it was decided to proceed with a strategy that extracted the six spectral maxima instead. In 1990 the scheme that extracted six spectral maxima (Spectral Maxima Sound Processing–SMSP) was implemented on a digital signal processor (DSP), tested on an initial patient (PS), and found to give significant benefit. For this reason, in 1990 a pilot study was carried out on two other patients who used the F0/F1/F2–MSP system (McKay, McDermott, & Clark, 1991) to compare this system with the SMSP strategy implemented as an Analogue processor (McKay, McDermott, Vandali, & Clark, 1992). The patients alternated in the use of the F0/F1/F2–MSP and SMSP–Analogue systems. There were very significant improvements in the consonant, open–set CNC word, and CID sentence scores with the SMSP–Analogue scheme. The Multipeak–MSP was evaluated on one of these patients, and the results for electrical stimulation alone were not as good as those for the SMSP–Analogue scheme (Clark et al., 1996).

The SMSP strategy was implemented by Cochlear Limited as a strategy called SPEAK in a speech processor referred to as Spectra-22. The only differences between the two strategies being that SMSP selected six maxima from a bank of 16 filters and stimulated at a constant rate of 250 Hz, whereas SPEAK selected up to eight spectral maxima from the outputs of 20 analog filters and stimulated at a rate which varies randomly from 180 Hz to 250 Hz (average 230 Hz). The SPEAK–Spectra-22 strategy and processor was compared with Multipeak–MSP in our Clinic on unselected patients and in a multicenter trial for the FDA in the United States and Australia. Results from the multicenter trial of 68 postlinguistically deaf adults (Skinner, Clark, Whitford, Seligman, Staller, Shipp, Shallop, Everingham, Menapace, Arndt, Antogenelli, Brimacombe, Pijl, Daniels, George, McDermott, & Beiter, 1994) showed significant improvements in speech perception for SPEAK–Spectra-22, particularly for open-sets of words and open-sets of words in sentences when presented by electrical stimu-lation alone. For open-sets of words in sentences the scores were 76% for SPEAK–Spectra-22 and 67% for Multipeak–MSP (Skinner et al., 1994). Patients also performed significantly better with SPEAK–Spectra-22 in the presence of background noise. SPEAK–Spectra-22 was approved by the FDA for postlinguistically deaf adults in March 1994.

It is of interest to compare the published results for both SPEAK and an alternative speech processor called CIS (Continuous Interleaved Sampler). This system, like SPEAK, stimulates at a constant rate to reduce channel interaction. It differs from SPEAK by taking the outputs from six or more fixed filters rather than the spectral maxima from 20 band pass filters. It also stimulates at a rate of approximately 800 pulses/s rather than 250 pulses/s with SPEAK. The published mean open-set sentence score for the CIS strategy on 68 patients using the Clarion speech processor was 60% (Kessler, Loeb, & Barker, 1995). These data were presented by the Advanced Bionics Corporation to the FDA in July 1995. In comparison, the mean open-set sentence score on 51 profoundly deaf adults using the SPEAK strategy was 70%. These data were presented by Cochlear

Corporation to the FDA in January 1996. The data from Kessler et al. (1995) also showed that with the CIS strategy and Clarion speech processor there was a bimodal distribution of results, with at least a quarter of adult patients having scores poorer than 20%. This high proportion of patients with poor scores for the CIS strategy was not seen for SPEAK and could explain the differences in the results.

IMPLANTS IN CHILDREN

In the 1980s the 3M single-channel implant was first implanted in a child in Los Angeles. The results for this device on 49 children, ranging in age from 2 to 17 years, were reported by Luxford, Berliner, Eisenberg, and House (1987), and showed the children could discriminate syllable patterns, but that only two could obtain any open-set understanding. The single-channel device permitted speech and syllabic pattern discrimination, but did not give sufficient auditory information for most children to identify or comprehend significant amounts of speech information.

Our first multiple-channel implant on children was not carried out until after it had been first implanted and evaluated in postlinguistically deaf adults who used the F0/F2 and later the F0/F1/F2 strategy. Prior to implanting children it was also implanted in two prelinguistically deaf adults; one on 20 September 1983, and the other on 15 November 1983 (Clark, Blamey, Busby, et al., 1987; Clark, Busby, et al., 1987) to see if they could obtain similar results to those for postlinguistically deaf adults. The two patients were educated in both signed English and sign language of the deaf. Their speech perception performances, however, were poor when using the F0/F2 speech processing strategy, and this was associated with inadequate place pitch discrimination. It was concluded that not only was signing a possible detrimental

factor, but the loss of hearing before speech and language acquisition and the long period of time before implantation were also significant negative factors. It was therefore decided to operate on younger people, and preferably those with an auditory-oral education. For this reason, a 14-year-old boy who had been taught by cued speech next had the operation on 8 January 1985. Subsequently, a 22-year-old woman who was thought to be severely deaf at birth, and had progressively lost her hearing and been taught by auditory/oral methods, was operated on 17 September 1985. The results for both patients were encouraging. In the case of the 14-year-old boy, electrode place and stimulus rate identification and the ability to understand running speech in combination with lipreading were better than the results obtained with the two prelinguistically deaf adults. The 22-year-old prelinguistically deaf woman had an 87% improvement in the perception of CNC words when electrical stimulation was used in combination with lipreading compared with lipreading alone, and an 86% improvement for CID sentences. Although she obtained limited open-set speech understanding for electrical stimulation alone, her results approached those for postlinguistically deaf adults.

Prior to implanting young children it must be appreciated how important it was to obtain good results on older children, and to see a trend for performances to improve at younger ages. It was also realized that a smaller (flatter) receiver-stimulator was required so that it would not protrude above the surface of the thinner skulls of the children to such an extent that it became unsightly. Our anatomical and surgical studies had shown in the adult that the maximum depth a bed could be drilled in the mastoid and occipital and/or parietal bones for the receiver-stimulator was 6mm, 3–4 mm being more usual (Clark, Blamey, Brown, et al., 1987). In young children the bone could be as thin as 1 mm. The maximum height superficial to the bone that is cosmetically acceptable in an adult is about 5–6 mm. The initial Cochlear Limited receiver-stimulator had a thickness of 9.5 mm due in large part to a connector incorporated on the under surface, and making up the "stalk" of the package (Clark, Pyman, Webb, Bailey, & Shepherd, 1984). The connector was there to allow the receiver-stimulator to be separated from the electrode array and replaced with another should it fail.

When explanting The University of Melbourne's smooth free-fitting banded electrode array in experimental animal studies, as well as replacing it in patients who had the University's prototype package and electrode replaced with the Cochlear clinical trial device, we found that the electrode slipped out easily, and another could be reinserted without difficulty for the same or greater distance. This indicated that a connector was not necessary, and we advised that its use could be discontinued. This opened the way for a package to be constructed with a thickness of about 5 mm.

It was also considered important to use a receiver-stimulator incorporating a rare earth magnet (Dormer, Richard, Hough, & Hewett, 1980) that would attract a magnet in the transmitting coil on the head set, so the coil could be easily aligned by a child. The fabrication of this implant commenced early in 1985. It was completed for implantation in children at about the time the first clinical trial receiver-stimulator, the F0/F2 strategy, and WSP II processor were approved by the U.S. FDA for use in postlinguistically deaf adults in October 1985.

Prior to implanting children with the receiver–stimulator (named the "Mini"; Figure 2–2) The University of Melbourne's research team developed an appropriate clinical evaluation and training program. It was considered important to not only understand how the children perceived

speech, as was the case with adults, but whether the implant led to improved speech production as well as receptive and expressive language. The program, first established at The University of Melbourne, and reported in 1985 at the International Cochlear Implant Symposium in Melbourne by Nienhuys, Musgrave, Busby, Blamey, Nott, Tong, Dowell, Brown, and Clark (1987), recommended that the procedure for evaluating the benefits of the implant would be through a single subject AB design to take into consideration the influence of training and education. This approach using repeated behavioral observations would be made in the preimplant phase to establish a base line of behavior. In the postimplant phase multiple observations would be repeated allowing changes in the dependent variable to be observed. In particular, changes in the baseline slope both before and after surgery were important to determine whether there was improved learning as a result of the implantation of the device.

The speech perception tests for children included the Monosyllable-Spondee-Trochee-Polysyllable (MSTP) test (Erber & Alencewicz, 1976; Plant, 1984) which was used to determine syllable pattern recognition. The Picture Vocabulary test measured vowel discrimination (Plant, 1984). The Northwestern University Children's Perception of Speech (NU-CHIPS; Elliott & Katz, 1980) test assessed their ability to identify consonants from a closed-set of words. Older children were assessed using open-sets of BKB sentences (Bench & Bamford, 1979) to measure speech comprehension.

Speech production assessments included using the Phonetic Level Evaluation (PLE; Ling, 1976) for a range of suprasegmental and segmental skills. The test of Articulation Competence (Fisher & Logemann, 1971) assessed the production of vowels and consonants using simple words presented as pictures. The McGarr

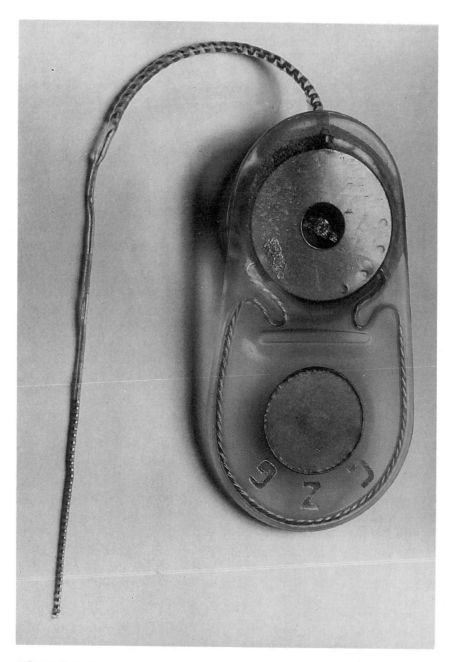

FIGURE 2–2. The receiver–stimulator named the "Mini" (CI-22M) with rare earth magnet for aligning and attaching the external transmitter coil. This was developed by Cochlear Limited particularly with children in mind.

(1983) Intelligibility test measured the intelligibility of key words in sentences, presented in written form.

Language and communication assessment included the Peabody Picture Vocabulary Test (PPVT; Dunn & Dunn, 1981) to measure receptive vocabulary, and the Preschool Language Scale (PLS) for receptive and expressive language (Zimmerman, Steiner, & Pond, 1979). The Grammatical Analysis of Elicited Language tests (GAEL; Moog & Geers, 1979, 1980) determined the prompted and imitative expressive language skills. The Language Assessment Remediation and Screening Procedure (LARSP) assessed spontaneous expressive language used in conversations.

The preoperative assessment program also required that the child had an adequate trial with a hearing aid as well as a tactile vocoder. At this stage in the history of cochlear implants there was insufficient evidence to say that an implant would give better results than tactile representation of speech. For this reason, to err on the side of conservatism, we not only required the child have experience with a single-channel vibrator, but also use the multiple-channel electrotactile aid or "Tickle Talker" so the benefits of a multiple-channel device (Blamey & Clark, 1985) could be assessed. The trial with a tactile aid was subsequently eliminated when the benefits of the implant were experienced.

The University of Melbourne program was then modified, following discussions with staff from Cochlear Corporation, to establish the protocol for the multi-center FDA clinical trial on children in the United States.

To implement our management and evaluation program it became necessary to enlarge the numbers and expertise of the staff in the Cochlear Implant Clinic at the Royal Victorian Eye and Ear Hospital, which until then had been managing adults. As a result, pediatric audiologists, speech pathologists, and educators of the deaf were appointed.

When The University of Melbourne's clinical program had been organized and the new receiver-stimulator engineered and made compatible with the wearable F0/F2 speech processor, we proceeded to implant the first child (Figure 2–3) to receive this Nucleus multiple-channel device in September 1985. He was a 10-year-old who lost hearing at the age of 3 years 6 months due to meningitis. He was fitted with a hearing aid soon afterward and educated by total communication. His speech production was at a 0% level on the McGarr Intelligibility test, and his speech reception vocabulary at a 5 year 11 month level. This child was also an initial subject with an electrotactile aid or "Tickle Talker." To complicate the preoperative assessment he had experienced episodes of Jacksonian epilepsy approximately 1 week after an introductory session using the "Tickle–Talker." Although there was no direct relationship between these events, to be sure that electrotactile stimulation could not have indirectly produced or triggered an epileptic focus, a series of safety studies of electrotactile stimulation were carried out with this child and a group of 10 normally hearing subjects and 4 hearing-impaired adults. The study included monitoring the EEGs during the presentation of stimuli, but no abnormalites in the EEG were seen. Although stimulating an epileptogenic focus had been seen as a possibility if we proceeded to implant this child the risk was considered small in view of the negative results from the electrotactile safety studies. The child then had the implant and the management was relatively straightforward.

With the more encouraging results with this 10-year-old child, it was decided to operate on even younger children. At the same time Cochlear Limited proceeded to seek FDA approval to carry out an extended clinical trial at multicenters in the United States. The protocol for this evaluation was based on the one established at The University of Melbourne.

We next operated on a 5-year-old child (Figure 2–4) in April 1986. This child had become profoundly deaf at the age of 3

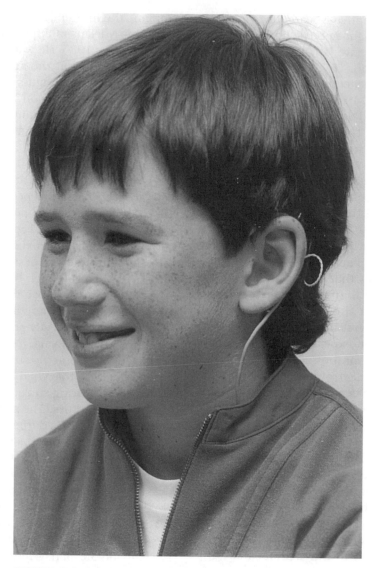

FIGURE 2–3. The 10-year-old boy (SS) who was the first child to have the multiple-channel implant "Mini" system incorporating a rare earth magnet in September 1985.

years due to meningitis and had binaural hearing aids fitted one month after recovery. He commenced his education in a cued speech environment. Six months prior to implantation he used a single-channel vibrator and preferred this to his hearing aid. He had a speech reception level of 2 years on the PPVT test, and his speech intelligibility was poor. Prior to implantation he had cross modality training in scaling the intensity of light and the electrotactile stimuli as we were not sure how easy it would be to set thresholds and comfort and discomfort levels (Clark, Blamey, Busby, et al., 1987; Clark, Busby, et al., 1987). It had been said that difficul-

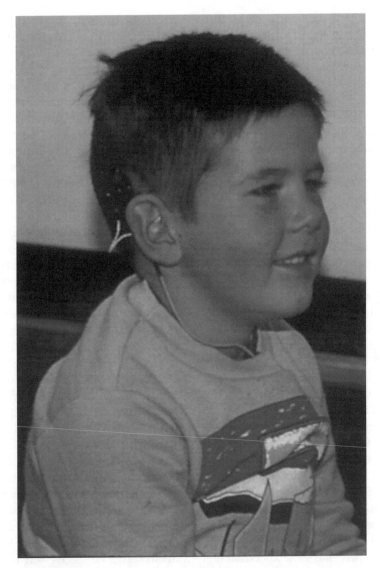

FIGURE 2–4. Our first young child (BD) aged 5 years to have the "Mini" receiver-stimulator in April 1986.

ty in setting these levels for each electrode would be one of the disadvantages of using a multiple versus a single-channel device. Postoperatively, however, no difficulties in setting behavioral levels were experienced. This was accomplished through getting him to relate the intensity of the stimulus to block size. Over some months the perception and production skills of this child improved, and after 10 years of implant experience, he now attends a normal school along with hearing peers, with minimal intervention at that school. He scores 100% on any closed-set word tests and can understand approximately 40% of sentence material presented listening alone. Additionally, that score becomes 96% using lipreading and listening of sentence material.

Although the above child was perilinguistically deaf, his good results were encouraging for both congenitally and postlinguistically deaf children. As a result, we proceeded to operate on younger children, including those who were congenitally deaf. This also applied to the other centers in the FDA trial. When this trial had been initiated and was in progress, a conference was held in Durango in November 1986 to assess further aspects of the children's implant program. The areas to be assessed were the selection of children for cochlear implantation, pre- and postoperative evaluation, cochlear implant surgery, developmental factors influencing implantation and rehabilitation, psychosocial issues, speech production, auditory skill development, clinical objectives, and research design. This symposium confirmed the procedures that had been adopted for the FDA clinical trial.

The clinical trial for the FDA was undertaken on 142 children using the F0/F1/F2–WSP III system. The results were presented to the U.S. FDA, and on 27 June 1990 the receiver-stimulator and F0/F1/F2 strategy were appproved as safe and effective for use in children. The results showed that 51% of the children had significant open-set performance with their cochlear prosthesis compared with 6% preoperatively. In addition, 68% of the children could perceive some spectral cues for speech perception with their cochlear prosthesis compared with 23% preoperatively. Performance also improved over time with significant increases in open-set and closed-set speech perception between 1 and 3 years postoperatively. When the test results on 91 prelinguistically deaf children in the study were examined separately it was found that improvements were comparable with the postlinguistic group in many areas, however, performance was poorer on the open-set measures for the prelinguistic group (Clark et al., 1996).

Ten children with the F0/F1/F2–WSP III system were changed over to the Multipeak–MSP system in 1989. Apart from an initial decrement of response in one child, performance continued to improve in five and was similar for the other children. As a controlled trial was not carried out, it was not clear whether the improvements were due to learning or to the new strategy and processor. The Multipeak–MSP system was also approved by the FDA for use in children on 27 June 1990 on the basis of the F0/F1/F2–WSP III approval for children and the Multipeak–MSP approval for adults.

The approval by the FDA took into consideration the biological safety issues that had been applicable to postlinguistically deaf adults. This was relevant and appropriate as there were no especially different issues for children from 2 years and older.

The latest Nucleus speech processing strategy SPEAK has been compared with Multipeak on 12 children from centers in Melbourne and Sydney. The children in the trial all had more than 1 year's experience with Multipeak–MSP, and had some open-set speech understanding using electrical stimulation alone. The results of the study (Cowan, Brown, Whitford, Galvin, Sarant, Barker, Shaw, King, Skok, Seligman, Dowell, Everingham, Gibson, & Clark, 1995) showed that in quiet their mean sentence scores were 60% for SPEAK and 53% for Multipeak. At a 15 dB signal-to-noise ratio the scores were 58% SPEAK and 48% Multipeak. These results indicate that childrens' central auditory nervous systems are adaptable or plastic enough to process new patterns of stimulation. It is also important to know that the new SPEAK strategy provides better speech comprehension in the presence of background noise compared to Multipeak as this ability is needed in everyday situations, including the classroom.

The above strategies have been used for children age 2 years and older. Children under 2 years of age had specific biological concerns. These were (a) the effect of head growth on the electrode and lead wire assembly, (b) the effect of the package itself on head growth, (c) the effect of electrical stimulation per se on a young cochlea and maturing auditory pathways, and (d) the problem of otitis media and the possibility that infection could extend around the electrode track into the inner ear and cause labyrinthitis and even meningitis. To establish the biological safety for children under age 2 in anticipation of subsequent operations on this age group, the U.S. National Institutes of Health awarded two safety contracts to study biological safety, one to The University of Melbourne and the other to the Coleman laboratories.

The studies by The University of Melbourne showed that implantation, even if over a cranial suture, did not affect head growth. However, head growth could affect the electrode and lead wire assembly and cause the electrode to be withdrawn from the cochlea if it was not fixed close to the cochlea, and a U-shaped redundancy made in the lead wire of an appropriate length. Electrical stimulation of the young cochlea with stimuli used with the Nucleus device had no significant effect on the spiral ganglion cell population. Furthermore, it was found that, with middle ear infection, implantation did not lead to any greater chance of the infection tracking to the inner ear and causing labyrinthitis than in the normal unimplanted ear.

Until the results of this study were known, The University of Melbourne's Cochlear Implant Clinic did not operate on children under 2 years of age. Children under 2 are now receiving the multiple-channel cochlear implant, and Cochlear Limited has developed a new receiver-stimulator (CI–24M) that is smaller and flatter, allowing it to be implanted in a 6-month-old infant. It also has telemetry so that the compound action potentials for electrical stimuli can be transmitted externally and so help set the thresholds and comfortable levels. This receiver-stimulator is part of the Nucleus-24 system, which will also include an "behind the ear" speech processor.

ACKNOWLEDGMENTS

Our cochlear implant development for infants and children has involved significant input from many scientists, engineers, surgeons, audiologists, speech pathologists, and educators of the deaf both nationally and internationally. In my 30 years of research in this field I have had valued collaboration with many colleagues. It is not possible to single them out individually, but I thank them for their contributions. There has been important and essential collaboration with the Australian firm Nucleus (subsequently, Cochlear Limited) due in particular to enlightened management and transfer of personnel from The University of Melbourne. Cochlear Limited has established an extremely high standard in biomedical engineering with the development of the Nucleus-22 and Nucleus-24 implant systems.

REFERENCES

Atlas, L. E., Herndon, M. K., Simmons, F. B., Dent, L. J., & White, R. L. (1983). Results of stimulus and speech-coding schemes applied to multichannel electrodes. Cochlear Prostheses, an International Symposium. *Annals of the New York Academy of Sciences, 405,* 377–386.

Bench, R. J., & Bamford, J. (Eds.). (1979). *Speech-hearing tests and the spoken lan-*

guage of hearing-impaired children. London: Academic Press

Black, R. C. (1978). *The cochlear prosthesis: Electrochemical and electrophysiological studies.* Doctoral dissertation, University of Melbourne.

Black, R. C., & Clark, G. M. (1977). Electrical transmission line properties in the cat cochlea. *Proceedings of the Australian Physiological and Pharmacological Society, 8,* 137P.

Black, R. C., & Clark, G. M. (1978). Electrical network properties and distribution of potentials in the cat cochlea. *Proceedings of the Australian Physiological and Pharmacological Society, 9,* 71P.

Black, R. C., & Clark, G. M. (1980). Differential electrical excitation of the auditory nerve. *Journal of the Acoustical Society of America, 67,* 868–874.

Blamey, P. J., & Clark, G. M. (1985). A wearable multiple-electrode electrotactile speech processor for the profoundly deaf. *Journal of the Acoustical Society of America, 77,* 1619–1621.

Burian, K., Hochmair, E., & Hochmair-Desoyer, I. (1979). Designing of and experience with multichannel cochlear implants. *Acta Oto-laryngologica, 87,* 190–195.

Chouard, C. H. (1980). The surgical rehabilitation of total deafness with the multichannel cochlear implant. Indications and results. *Audiology, 19,* 137–145.

Clark, G. M. (1969). Responses of cells in the superior olivary complex of the cat to electrical stimulation of the auditory nerve. *Experimental Neurology, 24,* 124–136.

Clark, G.M. (1970a). *Middle ear and neural mechanisms in hearing and the management of deafness.* Doctoral dissertation, University of Sydney.

Clark, G. M. (1970b). A neurophysiological assessment of the surgical treatment of perceptive deafness. *International Audiology, 9,* 103–109.

Clark, G. M. (1973). A hearing prosthesis for severe perceptive deafness—experimental studies. *Journal of Laryngology and Otology, 87*(10), 929–945.

Clark, G. M. (1995). Cochlear implants: Historical perspectives. In G. Plant & K.-E Spens (Eds.), *Profound deafness and speech communication.* (pp. 165–218) London: Whurr Publishers Ltd.

Clark, G. M. (1997). Cochlear implants. In H. Ludman & A. Wright (Eds.), *Diseases of the ear.* London: Edward Arnold.

Clark, G. M., Kranz, H. G., & Minas, H. J. (1973). Behavioural thresholds in the cat to frequency modulated sound and electrical stimulation of the auditory nerve. *Experimental Neurology, 41,* 190–200.

Clark, G. M., Nathar, J. M., Kranz, H. G., & Maritz, J. S. A. (1972). Behavioural study on electrical stimulation of the cochlea and central auditory pathways of the cat. *Experimental Neurology, 36*(2), 350–361.

Clark, G. M., Blamey, P. J., Brown, A. M., Busby, P. A., Dowell, R. C., Franz, B. K-G., Pyman, B. C., Shepherd, R. K., Tong, Y. C., Webb, R. L., Hirshorn, M. S., Kusma, J., Mecklenburg, D. J., Money, D. K., Patrick, J. F., & Seligman, P. M. (1987). The University of Melbourne—Nucleus Multi-Electrode Cochlear Implant. *Advances in Oto-Rhino-Laryngology, 38.*

Clark, G. M., Blamey, P. J. H., Busby, P. A., Dowell, R. C., Franz, B. K-G., Musgrave, G. N., Nienhuys, T. G., Pyman, B. C., Roberts, S. A., Tong, Y. C., Webb, R. L., Kuzma, J. A., Money, D. K., Patrick, J. F., & Seligman, P. M. (1987). A multiple-electrode intracochlear implant for children. *Archives of Otolaryngology, 113,* 825–828.

Clark, G. M., Busby, P. A., Roberts, S. A., Dowell, R. C., Tong, Y. C., Blamey, P. J., Nienhuys, T.G., Mecklenburg, D. J., Webb, R. L., Pyman, B. C., & Franz, B. K-G. (1987b). Preliminary results for the Cochlear Corporation Multi-Electrode intracochlear implants on six prelingually deaf patients. *American Journal of Otology, 8*(3), 234–239.

Clark, G. M., Dowell, R. C., Cowan, R. S., Pyman, B. C., & Webb, R. L. (1996, June). Multicentre evaluations of speech perception in adults and children with the Nucleus (Cochlear) 22-channel cochlear implant. In M. Portmann (Ed.), *Proceedings of the Third International Symposium on Transplants and Implants in Otology* (pp. 353–363). The Netherlands: Kugler Publications.

Clark, G. M., Pyman, B. C., & Bailey, Q. R. (1979). The surgery for multiple-electrode cochlear implantations. *Journal of Laryngology and Otology, 93*(3), 215–223.

Clark, G. M., Pyman, B. C., Webb, R. L., Bailey, Q. E., Shepherd, R. K. (1984). Surgery for an improved multiple-channel cochlear implant. *Annals of Otology, Rhinology and Laryngology, 93*(3), 204–207.

Clark, G. M., Tong, Y. C., Bailey, Q. R., Black, R. C., Martin, L. F., Millar, J. B., O'Loughlin, B. J., Patrick, J. F., & Pyman, B. C. (1978). A multiple electrode cochlear implant. *Journal of the Oto-Laryngological Society of Australia, 4*(3), 208–212.

Clark, G. M., Tong, Y. C., Black, R. C., Forster, I. C., Patrick, J. F., & Dewhurst, D. J. (1977). A multiple electrode cochlear implant. *Journal of Laryngology & Otology, 91*, 935–945.

Clark, G. M., Tong, Y. C., Martin, L. F. A., & Busby, P. A. (1981). A multiple-channel cochlear implant. An evaluation using an open-set word test. *Acta Otolaryngologica (Stockh.), 91*, 173–175.

Clark, G. M., Tong, Y. C., & Martin, L. F. A. (1981). A multiple-channel cochlear implant. An evaluation using open-set CID sentences. *Laryngoscope, 91*(4), 628–634.

Cohen, N. L., Waltzman, S. B., & Fisher, S. G. (1993). A prospective, randomized study of cochlear implants. *New England Journal of Medicine, 328*, 233–282.

Cowan, R. S. C., Brown, C., Whitford, L. A., Galvin, K. L., Sarant, J. Z., Barker, E. J., Shaw, S., King, A., Skok, M. C., Seligman, P. M., Dowell, R. C., Everingham, C., Gibson, W. P. R., & Clark, G. M. (1995). Speech perception in children using the advanced SPEAK speech processing strategy. *Annals of Otology, Rhinology and Laryngology, 104*(Suppl. 166), 318–321.

Djourno, A., & Eyries, C. (1957). Prothèse auditive par excitation électrique a distance du nerf sensoriel a l'aide d'un bobinage inclus a demeure. *Presse Medicale, 35*, 14–17.

Dormer, K. J., Richard, G., Hough, J. V. D., & Hewett, T. (1980). The cochlear implant (auditory prosthesis) utilizing rare earth magnets. *American Journal of Otology, 2*, 22–27.

Dowell, R. C., Seligman, P. M., Blamey, P. J., & Clark, G. M. (1987). Speech perception using a two-formant 22-electrode cochlear prosthesis in quiet and in noise. *Acta Otolaryngologica (Stockh.), 104*, 439–446.

Dowell, R. C., Whitford, L. A., Seligman, P. M., Franz, B. K-G., & Clark, G. M. (1990). Preliminary results with a miniature speech processor for the 22-electrode Melbourne/Cochlear hearing prosthesis. *Otorhinolaryngology, Head and Neck Surgery. Proceedings of the XIV Congress of Oto-Rhino-Laryngology, Head and Neck Surgery* (pp. 1167–1173). Madrid, Spain.

Doyle, J. H., Doyle, J. B., & Turnbull, F. M. (1964). Electrical stimulation of eighth cranial nerve. *Archives of Otolaryngology, 80*, 388–391.

Dunn, L. M., & Dunn, L. M. (1981). *Peabody Picture Vocabulary Test—revised.* Circle Pines, MN: American Guidance Service.

Eddington, D. K. (1980). Speech discrimination in deaf subjects with cochlear implants. *Journal of the Acoustical Society of America, 68*, 885–891.

Elliott, L. L., & Katz, D. R. (1980). *Northwestern University Children's Perception of Speech (NU-CHIPS).* St Louis: Auditec.

Erber, N. P., & Alencewicz, C. M. (1976). Audiologic evaluation of deaf children. *Journal of Speech and Hearing Disorders, 41*, 256–267.

Fisher, H. B., & Logemann, J. A. (1971). *Test of Articulation Competence.* New York: Houghton & Mifflin.

Fourcin, A. J., Rosen, S. M., & Moore, B. C. J. (1979). External electrical stimulation of the cochlea: Clinical, psychophysical, speech-perceptual and histological findings. *British Journal of Audiology, 13*, 85–107.

Gantz, B. J., McCabe, B. F., Tyler, R. S., & Preece, J. P. (1987). Evaluation of four cochlear implant designs. *Annals of Otology, 96*, 145–147.

House, W. F., Berliner, K., Crary, W., Graham, M., Luckey, R., Norton, N., Selters, W., Tobin, H., Urban, J., & Wexler, M. (1976). Cochlear implants. *Annals of Otology, 85*, (Suppl. 27), 3–6.

House, W. F., Luetje, C. M., & Campos, C. T. (1981). The cochlear implant: performance of deaf patients, practicality in clinical practice, co–investigator experience. *Hearing Instruments, 32*, 12–30.

Kerr, A., & Schuknecht, H. F. (1968). The spiral ganglion in profound deafness. *Acta Otolaryngologica, 65*, 586–598.

Kessler, D. K., Loeb, G. E., & Barker, M. J. (1995). Distribution of speech recognition results with the Clarion cochlear prosthesis. *Annals of Otology, Rhinology and Laryngology, 104*(Suppl 166), 283–285.

Laird, R. K. (1979). *The bioengineering development of a sound encoder for an implantable hearing prosthesis for the profoundly deaf.* Master of Engineering Science Thesis, The University of Melbourne.

Ling, D. (1976). *Speech and the hearing-impaired child: Theory and practice.* Washington, DC: Alexander Graham Bell Association of the Deaf.

Luxford, W. M., Berliner, K. I., Eisenberg, M. A., & House, W. F. (1987). Cochlear implants in children. *Annals of Otology, Rhinology and Laryngology, 96*, 136–138.

McKay, C. M., McDermott, H. J., Vandali, A. E., & Clark, G.M. (1992). A comparison of speech perception of Cochlear implantees using the Spectral Maxima Sound Processor (SMSP) and the MSP (MULTIPEAK) Processor. *Acta Otolaryngologica (Stockh.), 112*, 752–761.

McKay, C. M., McDermott, H. J., & Clark, G. M. (1991). Preliminary results with a six spectral maxima speech processor for The University of Melbourne/Nucleus multiple-electrode cochlear implant. *Journal of the Otolarygological Society of Australia, 6*, 354–359.

McGarr, N. S. (1983). The intelligibility of deaf speech to experienced and inexperienced listeners. *Journal of Speech and Hearing Research, 26*, 451–458.

Merzenich, M. M. (1975). Studies on electrical stimulation of the auditory nerve in animals and man: Cochlear implants. In *The nervous system. Vol. 3: human communication and its disorders* (pp. 537–548). New York: Raven Press.

Michelson, R. P., & Schindler, R. A. (1981). Multichannel cochlear implant: Preliminary results in man. *Laryngoscope, 91*, 38–42.

Millar, J. B., Tong, Y. C., & Clark, G. M. (1984). Speech processing for cochlear implant prostheses. *Journal of Speech and Hearing Research, 27*, 280–296.

Moog, J. S., Geers, A. E. (1979). *Grammatical analysis of elicited language: Simple sentence level.* St. Louis: Central Institute for the Deaf.

Moog, J. S., & Geers, A. E. (1980). *Grammatical analysis of elicited language: Complex sentence level.* St. Louis: Central Institute for the Deaf.

Nienhuys, T. G., Musgrave, G. N., Busby, P. A., Blamey, P. J., Nott, P., Tong, Y. C., Dowell, R. C., Brown, L., & Clark, G. M. (1987). Educational assessment and management of children with multichannel cochlear implants. *Annals of Otology, Rhinology and Laryngology, 128*, 80–83.

Plant, G. (1984). A diagnostic speech test for severely and profoundly hearing-impaired children. *Australian Journal of Audiology, 6*, 1–9.

Schindler, R. A., & Merzenich, M. M. (1974). Chronic intracochlear electrode implantation: Cochlear pathology and acoustic nerve survival. *Annals of Otolaryngology, 83*, 202–215.

Simmons, F. B. (1967). Permanent intracochlear electrodes in cats. Tissue tolerance and cochlear microphonics. *Laryngoscope, 77*, 171–186.

Simmons, F. B., Monegeon, C. J., Lewis, W. R., & Huntington, D. A.. (1964). Electrical stimulation of acoustical nerve and inferior colliculus. *Archives of Otolaryngology, 79*, 559–567.

Skinner, M. W., Clark, G. M, Whitford, L. A., Seligman, P. M., Staller, S. J., Shipp, D. B., Shallop, J. K., Everingham, C., Menapace, C. M., Arndt, P. L., Antogenelli, T., Brimacombe, J. A., Pijl, S., Daniels, P., George, C. R., McDermott, H. J., & Beiter, A. L. (1994). Evaluation of a new spectral peak coding strategy for the Nucleus 22 channel cochlear implant system. *The American Journal of Otology, 15*, 15–27.

Tong, Y. C., Black, R. C., Clark, G. M., Forster, I. C., Millar, J. B., O'Loughlin, B. J., & Patrick, J. F. (1979). A preliminary report on a multiple–channel cochlear implant operation. *Journal of Laryngology and Otology, 93*(7), 679–695.

Tong, Y. C., Clark, G. M., Blamey, P. J., Busby, P. A., & Dowell, R. C. (1982). Psychophysical studies for two multiple-channel cochlear implant patients. *Journal of the Acoustical Society of America, 71*(1), 153–160.

Tong, Y. C., van Hoesel, R., Lai, W. K., Vandali, A., Harrison, J. M., & Clark, G. M. (1990). *Speech processors for auditory prostheses.* Sixth quarterly progress report NIH Contract NO 1-DC-9-2400. June 1–August 31.

Williams, A. J., Clark, G. M., & Stanley, G. V. (1976). Pitch discrimination in the cat through electrical stimulation of the terminal auditory nerve fibres. *Physiological Psychology, 4,* 23–27.

Zimmerman, I. L., Steiner, V. C., & Pond, R. E. (1979). *Preschool Language Scale.* Columbus: Merrill.

3

BIOLOGICAL SAFETY

GRAEME M. CLARK
ROBERT K. SHEPHERD

Biological safety has been extensively studied at the Department of Otolaryngology, The University of Melbourne, for cochlear implantation in adults, and subsequently for specific issues in infants and young children. Many of the studies have general applicability to cochlear implantation, but some have specific relevance to the Nucleus (Cochlear Limited) multiple-channel cochlear implant systems, and have been fundamental to their approval by the U.S. Food and Drug Administration (FDA). The Nucleus system was first approved by the FDA as safe and effective for postlinguistically deaf adults in October 1985, and 5 years later, on 27 June 1990, was approved for use in children from 2 years of age and older. The general research questions studied for adults are directly relevant for children and infants, but there are also specific questions that need to be answered when operating on children under 2 years of age. The general questions of importance for cochlear implantation are the biocompatability of materials, the tissue responses of the cochlea to implantation, the electrical stimulus parameters that do not lead to adverse tissue responses, especially the loss of residual auditory neurons, and the prevention of infection entering the inner ear following surgery

or a middle ear infection. The specific questions of importance for infants and young children include the effect of the implant on head growth, the effect of head growth on the electrode and lead wire assembly, the effect of implantation and electrical stimulation on the cochlea of a young child, the ease of explanting an electrode and reinserting another at some stage during the child's lifetime, should the device fail or an improved system become available, and the spread of infection from otitis media around the electrode entry point into the inner ear.

The general questions were examined in a number of studies carried out, in particular, by the Department of Otolaryngology at The University of Melbourne. These studies were complemented by additional studies undertaken by agencies for Cochlear Limited when first seeking FDA approval, and were reported in some detail by Clark, Blamey et al. (1987) and Shepherd, Franz, and Clark, (1990). The specific issues of importance for cochlear implantation in infants and young children were studied, in particular, in a 5-year contract with the U.S. National Institutes of Health Studies "Studies on Pediatric Prosthesis Implants" NIH contract No. 1-NS-7-2342 undertaken from 1 May 1987 to 30 April 1992.

29

GENERAL QUESTIONS

Biocompatibility of Materials

All materials used for a cochlear implant should be evaluated in the experimental animal to ensure they are biocompatible, and considerable research has been done to ensure that this is so for the materials used with the Nucleus (Cochlear Limited) multiple-channel cochlear implant (Clark, Blamey, et al., 1987). The studies were needed as there had been inadequate reports in the literature on the biocompatibility of a number of the candidate materials. The procedures used for evaluation were modifications of those laid down in the U.S. Pharmacopeia (1980). The main modification was evaluating the materials after being placed subcutaneously, intramuscularly, and intracochlearly, as previous studies on the toxicity and biocompatibility of materials had shown there was considerable variation in tissue responses, depending on the site of implantation. It was also important to test the materials actually used in the manufacturing process, as the processes could differ from those used in other studies. In addition, materials were implanted in two species of animals to help establish that there were no significant species differences, so the results would be more applicable to humans. Not only was it important to carry out these biocompatibility tests to determine the toxicity of the materials per se, but they also formed the control for any assessments on the safety of electrical stimulation. Without these baseline data it was not possible to be certain whether the effects of electrical stimulation were due to toxicity or the electrical current. The materials finally chosen for the implantable receiver-stimulator were evaluated for cytopathic effects by placing the material in direct contact with a layer of human embryonic cells. The extracted materials were injected intravenously and intraperitoneally to see that there were no systemic effects. They were also injected intracutaneously to see there was no irritation. The results are outlined in more detail in the monograph by Clark, Blamey, et al. (1987).

Tissue Responses and the Effects of Trauma Following Implantation of the Electrode Array and Receiver-Stimulator

The effects of implantation of the electrode array on the cochlea of the experimental animal, other than biocompatibility, also needed to be assessed prior to intracochlear implantations in patients. The studies (Clark, 1973; Clark, 1977; Clark, Kranz, Minas, & Nather, 1975; Schindler, Merzenich, & White, 1977; Simmons, 1967) first examined whether implantation per se would lead to a loss of the peripheral processes of the auditory neurons. It was also important to determine the effects of insertion trauma on the cochlear structures, especially auditory neurons. The initial studies showed that the cochlea could be implanted with minimal effects on the peripheral processes and spiral ganglion cells, provided there was no tearing of the basilar membrane or fracture of the spiral lamina. Trauma also increased the amount of new bone formation. The introduction of infection, either at the time of surgery or subsequently, also led, in many cases, to marked pathological changes within the scala tympani, extending to the other scalae and throughout the cochlear turns in severe cases. Labyrinthitis resulted in a marked loss of neural elements and significant new bone formation.

A subsequent study (Shepherd, Clark, & Black 1983) examined the effects of intracochlear implantation in more detail. This study showed that, with the insertion of the smooth free-fitting banded electrode, hair cells as well as neural elements beyond the tip of the electrode were preserved, but hair cells adjacent to the electrode array were generally lost. The loss of hair cells was also associated with a loss of peripheral processes, but not spiral ganglion cells. Studies by Sutton and Miller (1983) and Leake-Jones and Rebscher (1983) also established these findings.

As the experimental studies in animals revealed that trauma could cause the loss of auditory neurons, it was considered important to see if the insertion of the smooth free-fitting banded array in the human would result in significant cochlear damage. In the first study by Shepherd, Clark, Pyman, and Webb (1985), the electrodes were inserted into nine temporal bones and then withdrawn, and the bones prepared for histological analysis. The study showed there was no significant damage of the spiral lamina and basilar membrane, provided force was not applied to the electrode after it first met resistance during its insertion. The results of this study were confirmed by Clifford and Gibson (1987) and Kennedy (1987), who removed the bone overlying the basal turns of the cochleas so the electrode could be seen both during and after insertion.

The atraumatic nature of the Nucleus flexible banded multiple-electrode array, which was graded in stiffness, was confirmed in a study by Patrick and MacFarlane (1987). The Nucleus array, which is fabricated from 22 platinum (90%)-iridium (10%) wires each with a diameter of 0.025 mm, was shown to be 10 times more flexible and applied 25 times less force than a single platinum electrode with a diameter of 0.21 mm and ball at the tip, as used with the 3M-House system.

The effects of inserting the Nucleus banded electrode array in the human have also been studied in temporal bones from implanted patients postmortem. The studies (Clark, Shepherd, Franz, Dowell, Tong, et al., 1988; Kawano, Seldon, & Clark, 1995; Kawano, Seldon, Clark, Ramsden, &

Raine, 1996; Linthicum, Fayad, Otto, Galey, & House, 1991; Marsh, Coker, & Jenkins, 1992; Zappia, Niparko, Kemink, Oviatt, & Altschuler, 1991) have confirmed the findings of the previous human temporal bone studies, that the array can be inserted with minimal trauma to the spiral lamina and no significant loss of neural elements.

Studies have also examined the effects of electrode shape and size on cochlear histopathology. In particular, Sutton, Miller, and Pfingst (1980) compared the effects of implanting a free-fitting smooth flexible electrical array with those for a moulded array. The moulded array was shown to cause significantly more trauma than the free-fitting array and hence, loss of neural elements. Studies have also shown that if the electrode array has discrete ball electrodes, which are either independently inserted or protrude beyond the surface of the array, they too will cause more trauma than the smooth free-fitting array (Shepherd, Matsushima, Martin, & Clark, 1994). When there has been a need to explant the ball arrays, the explantation can be extremely difficult because the protruding balls can be encircled with fibrous tissue and/or bone which holds the electrodes in place, and they can break when pulled out, or remain within the cochlea. This is considerably less of a problem with the smooth free-fitting banded array.

As new bone growth and excessive fibrous tissue have been seen in some experimental animals following electrode implantation, as well as in the cochleas of deceased patients who have previously had a cochlear implant, there is a need to determine their cause. This is especially necessary as they could effect the spread of current within the cochlea, and so lead to nonoptimal results. It was also thought bone growth itself might lead to the loss of neural elements. First, when comparing the degree of bone formation in the cochlea with psychophysical findings in patients (Clark et al., 1988, Kawano, Seldon, & Clark, 1995), we found that bone growth could affect the spread of current and hence dynamic range and place pitch resolution. Second, in the experimental studies by Ni, Shepherd, Seldon, Xu, Clark, and Millard (1992); Shepherd, Clark, and Black (1983); Shepherd et al. (1994); and Xu, Shepherd, Millard, and Clark (in press) we showed that bone growth was not induced by electrical stimulation and was not correlated with ganglion cell loss.

In research by Chow, Seldon, and Clark (1995) and Clark, Shute, Shepherd, and Carter (1995) electrode insertions were carried out in controlled studies where localized trauma was specifically applied to the endosteum of the basal turn, in combination with the installation of blood clot and/or bone paste. The results showed there was a significant increase in new bone formation if there was specific endosteal trauma when compared with the control, and it was aggravated by the installation of bone paste, but not blood clot. The findings from these investigations indicate that the production of excessive fibrous tissue and new bone formation should be kept to a minimum, and this can be achieved by minimizing the trauma to the endosteum, keeping drilling to a minimum, and ensuring that bone dust does not enter the cochlea.

Insertion Trauma and Tissue Responses with Peri-Modiolar Electrodes

There is physiological evidence in the cat that thresholds are lower when the electrodes are placed close to the spiral ganglion cells (Shepherd, Hatsushika, & Clark 1993), and this also suggests place coding might be improved. We therefore have been studying how best to place a smooth free-fitting electrode array close

to the modiolus where the ganglion cells are located.

One way of having the array close to the modiolus is to precurve it and mold it with a radius of curvature matching the basal turn of the cochlea, to hold it straight at insertion, and release it after insertion so it can be placed, or come to lie, close to the modiolus. One method of doing this is to hold the array straight prior to insertion in a special tool, and release it after it has been inserted a distance of 8–10 mm. The tool is then withdrawn and the electrode advanced by the usual means. Its tip will be hugging the modiolus and it will remain in this position as it is advanced (Treaba, Xu, Xu, & Clark 1995).

The placement of this precurved array within the scala tympani has been evaluated radiographically and histologically by Donnelly, Cohen, Xu, Xu, and Clark (1995). It was shown to lie significantly closer to the modiolus than the present straight array, and generally midway between the inner and outer walls. In sections of an undecalcified temporal bone where the electrode was left in situ, it was close to the modiolus proximally, but more distally it tended to lie laterally (Donnelly et al., 1995). A histological study has been carried out to examine human temporal bones after the precurved array has been inserted and withdrawn, and no significant trauma was seen. More work is needed to optimize the curvature and other specifications of this array.

An alternative method of holding a precurved array straight and have it come to lie close to the modiolus following insertion is to coat it in polyvinyl alcohol (PVA). When the electrode is inserted the PVA dissolves to release its curvature, so it can come to lie against the modiolus. As the array will be stiffened by the PVA it is desirable to also initially insert it 8–10 mm, and then wait until the PVA starts to dissolve before advancing it further. This electrode is being compared with other peri-modiolar electrodes to determine optimal placement and minimal trauma.

Another promising peri-modiolar electrode is bilaminar in design, with the outer layer of a material such as high molecular weight polyacrylic acid (PAA) as a filler in a Silastic matrix, which expands when it absorbs water. As the outer layer increases in length it causes the electrode to curl, and come to lie close to the modiolus (Seldon, Dahm, Clark, & Crowe 1995). The PAA-Silastic has been examined for biocompatibility by implantation subcutaneously and within the scala tympani of the cat cochlea. There was no significant inflammatory reaction, indicating the material to be biocompatible. Studies also showed that it did not stimulate macrophage activity, indicating that it was unlikely to induce excessive fibrous tissue or new bone formation. These perimodiolar electrodes are being compared in anatomical and histological studies to establish whether they can be placed close to the modiolus while evoking minimal trauma (Shepherd, Treaba, Pyman, & Clark, 1996).

Finally, an alternative method of placing an array close to the modiolus is to attach a strip of Teflon to its tip, and when it reaches the limit of its insertion, pressure on the strip will force the array against the modiolus (J. Kuzma, personal communication). The addition of the strip could make this array stiffer and lead to trauma unless care is taken with its orientation during insertion along the scala tympani.

Electrical Stimulus Parameters

An important feature of our safety studies has been to ensure that the electrical stimulus parameters do not lead to damage of the spiral ganglion cells. This may occur if either toxic or corrosive products are produced at the electrode-tissue interface, or stimulus parameters themselves have a direct effect on the ganglion cells.

Initially, we carried out in-vitro studies to see whether electrical stimulus parameters appropriate for stimulating nerves would lead to corrosion of platinum electrodes. If this occurred, platinum ions could combine with protein and lead to an adverse tissue reaction (Agnew, Yuen, Pudenz, & Bullara, 1977). Corrosion was measured by a spectrophotometric technique (Black & Hannaker, 1979). Results showed that the concentration of platinum in solution was greater for direct rather than biphasic current stimulation, and dissolution decreased markedly for biphasic stimulation using pulse durations of less than 500 µs, and reduced current densities. It was therefore important to develop a stimulus strategy where the current density was kept low and the pulse duration short. The banded electrode has an advantage in this regard, as it is circumferential and has a large area and therefore current density can be kept to a minimum. When this study was repeated in-vivo, the corrosion was much less. The reason for this is not clear, however, it may have been due to the presence of protein on the electrode surface (Roblee, McHardy, Marston, & Brummer, 1980). Furthermore, we found that, when stimulating in-vivo at a charge density of up to 32 $\mu C.cm^{-2}$ geom. per phase, there was no evidence of corrosion, as measured by scanning electron microscopy of the electrode surface (Shepherd & Clark, 1991; Shepherd, Murray, Houghton, & Clark, 1985). This indicated that corrosion at the charge densities to be used with the banded array would not be an issue for safe electrical stimulation of nerve fibers.

Research studies stimulating nonauditory neurons (Mortimer, Shealy, & Wheeler, 1970) showed that damage to neurons was minimized by using short duration charge-balanced biphasic current pulses. This was due to the fact that the electrochemical reactions at the electrode-tissue interface are reversible and this ensured that no toxic electrochemical products were formed. A maximum electrochemically safe stimulus regime of short duration 100–200 μs biphasic current pulses, having a maximum charge density of 300 μC.cm^{-2} geom. per phase was defined for platinum electrodes by Brummer, McHardy, and Turner (1977). Above this limit electrolysis of water occurs, resulting in the evolution of hydrogen and oxygen and the release of chlorine and organic molecules. These latter chemical products are likely to be harmful to biological tissue.

Stimulus parameters that would not lead to the corrosion of platinum, or produce harmful electrochemical products, could still cause neural damage through overstimulation and a direct metabolic effect. Studies by Walsh and Leake-Jones (1982) and Leake-Jones, Rebscher, and Aird (1985) demonstrated local neural degeneration adjacent to scala tympani electrodes following stimulation at charge densities up to 200 μC.cm^{-2} real per phase for stimulus periods up to 800 hours. The charge densities used for thresholds for the banded array in our first patient (Tong, Black, Clark, Forster, Millar, O'Loughlin, & Patrick, 1979) ranged from 2–20 μC.cm^{-2} geom. per phase for stimuli at rates of 200 pulses/s and 1,000 pulses/s. It was necessary to establish that a stimulus regime for parameters to be used by the Nucleus receiver-stimulator would not cause long-term neural damage. A study by Shepherd, Clark, and Black (1983) demonstrated that continuous stimulation for up to 2000 hours at 500 pulses/s, 200 μs/phase, charge densities from 18 to 32 μC.cm^{-2} geom. per phase, and charge asymmetries between phases of 0.01% to 0.1% showed there was no significant loss of ganglion cells. In this study DC current levels less than 0.1μA were achieved by electrode shorting between pulses. A stimulus rate of 500 pulses/s

was used, as the psychophysical studies on the first two patients had shown poor rate difference limens above about 250 pulses/s (Tong, Clark, Blamey, Busby, & Dowell, 1982).

In the mid 1980s we realized, however, that speech processing strategies could possibly benefit from higher stimulus rates (Clark, Blamey, et al., 1987). It was therefore necessary to determine the effects of higher stimulus rates on the auditory neural pathways. We initially carried out an acute study, comparing the effects of stimulation at 200 and 800 pulses/s with biphasic stimuli at 52 μC.cm^{-2} geom. per phase (Clark, Pyman, et al., 1987; Shepherd & Clark, 1986, 1987). The results showed there was a significant and prolonged decrement in the neural response as seen with the electrically evoked auditory brainstem response (EABR), and this indicated the need for more safety studies before speech processing strategies at rates higher than 500 pulses/s could be used with patients.

Further acute studies were undertaken by Tykocinski, Shepherd, and Clark (1995), which confirmed that at stimulus rates of 400 and 1000 pulses/s for charge densities of 75 μC.cm^2 geom. per phase, and high stimulus intensities (0.34–1.0 μC/phase) there were marked decrements in the EABR response. In assessing the effects of high rates of stimulation on neural tissue it is important to understand there is a complex interrelationship between rate, charge density, and current level, as well as stimulus mode and electrode geometry. These relationships have not been well defined, and for that reason it is very important that safety studies are conducted using a stimulator, stimulus mode (bipolar, common ground, monopolar), and charge recovery system that is intended for clinical application.

Not only may high stimulus rates and charge densities of biphasic pulses lead to neuronal damage, but so may DC currents. We have, for example, shown in a study by Shepherd, Matsushima, Millard, and Clark (1991) that a DC current of 2 μA could cause severe neuronal degeneration and marked pathological changes in the cochlea.

When stimulating at high rates there is a greater likelihood of a DC current occurring, due, for example, to a build-up of current if the two phases of the biphasic pulse are not completely symmetrical. This possibility has been avoided with the Nucleus receiver-stimulator by ensuring that the two phases of the pulses are symmetrical, and that any build-up of current is shorted between pulses. Alternatively, stimulating with the DC current may be avoided by using capacitors placed in series with the electrodes.

As discussed, if high rates of stimulation are to be used, then safety studies should be carried out using the rates, charge densities, stimulus mode, electrode configuration, and DC removal design in the device to be used clinically. Furthermore, long-term studies are mandatory, as long-term effects may not be seen in acute studies, or EABR reduction and histological changes in acute studies may not reflect long-term neuronal loss.

For these reasons a chronic study was undertaken by Xu, Shepherd, Clark, Tong, and Williams (in press) in which 13 normal hearing cats were stimulated continuously for periods up to 2100 hours, using receiver-stimulators of the same design as the Nucleus receiver-stimulators, and, in particular, their methods of charge recovery. For bipolar stimulation, two pairs of electrodes were used at rates of 2000 pulses/s, and for monopolar stimulation, three electrodes at rates of 1000 pulses/s. The study showed no statistically significant difference between the stimulated cochleas or between the stimulated cochleas and controls, indicating that chronic electrical stimulation

using these high rates, and operating at intensities within clinical limits, does not adversely affect the auditory nerve or cochlea.

Prevention of Infective Labyrinthitis Post-Implantation

Initial experimental studies on animals (Clark & Shepherd, 1984), where the scala tympani electrode arrays were implanted to determine tissue response, showed postoperative labyrinthitis could occur in approximately 10% of animals. This may have been due to lack of asepsis at surgery, or associated with preoperative or postoperative upper respiratory and middle ear infections. The infections often resulted in widespread loss of spiral ganglion cells. The findings made it essential to study how best to prevent labyrinthitis postoperatively to make sure that it would not be a problem in adults, and certainly not for children, where the incidence of otitis media is much higher.

The first undertaking was to develop an experimental model of otitis media, so the effect of implantation and round window sealing procedures could be studied. A successful model was developed by impregnating Gelfoam with the pathogenic organisms and placing it within the animals' bulla. By selecting an adequate concentration of organisms it was possible to produce an infection in a high proportion of animals (Brennan & Clark, 1985; Franz, Clark, & Bloom, 1987). Initially, the two organisms used in the model were Staphylococcus aureus and Streptococcus pyogenes, as it was easier to induce an infection with these species, even though they were not common infective agents in otitis media.

The first investigation examined whether autologous grafts of fibrous tissue and muscle, or heterologous grafts glued to the electrode, such as Teflon felt or Dacron mesh, prevented infection from Streptococcus pyogenes spreading from the middle to inner ear, in particular, causing labyrinthitis compared with not sealing the electrode entry point. The studies were undertaken by inserting the electrode through the round window membrane, and also via a cochleostomy (Clark & Shepherd, 1984; Cranswick, Franz, Clark, & Shepherd, 1987; Franz, Clark, & Bloom, 1984; Franz et al., 1987). The findings suggested that fascia gave a better seal than muscle, and that heterologous material, in particular Dacron, could in fact encourage the development of infection. The use of a fascial seal was marginally better than no seal. A key factor appeared to be the development of a substantial electrode sheath. Even if infection traveled between the sheath and electrode, a well developed fibrous tissue sheath was a significant barrier, and at worst, a localized infection developed.

SPECIFIC QUESTIONS FOR PEDIATRIC COCHLEAR IMPLANTATION

Effect on Skull Growth

In implanting infants and young children one of the concerns was whether drilling a package bed down to dura in the region of one or more cranial sutures would lead to premature closure of the suture (synostosis) and cranial deformity. The sutures are the site for bone growth, and the optimal placement of the electrode package was where the mastoid, parietal, and occipital bones joined at the asterion (Xu et al., 1993).

The experimental study was undertaken on four 6-month-old monkeys, because of their greater similarity to humans. Beds were made across sutures, down to dura, leaving an island of bone centrally to be depressed, and dummy implants were then positioned in the beds.

The animals were monitored radiographically for up to 3 years and there were no significant differences in cranial cavity dimensions to indicate asymmetric development. This was confirmed when the skulls were examined postmortem, using computed tomographic scans to calculate volume of the skull on each side. The region of the package bed was also examined histologically (Burton, Shepherd, Xu, Xu, Franz, & Clark, 1994) and no closure of sutures seen. A layer of new bone was present beneath the package in most animals, but in one there was only a layer of fibrous tissue. The findings suggest that long-term cochlear implantation in very young children will not cause any significant deformation of the skull.

Effect of Skull Growth on the Electrode and Lead Wire Assembly

In studying the effect of skull growth on the electrode and lead wire assembly, it was first necessary to know the degree of growth changes in the temporal bone from birth to adulthood. Previous studies by Nokubi (1969) and Dahm (1970) have examined postnatal growth of the temporal bone by direct anatomical measurement of its external features. The results showed that different parts varied in their growth patterns. The width of the facial recess, of importance when completing the posterior tympanotomy for cochlear implant surgery, has been studied by Su, Marion, Hinojosa, and Matz (1982) and Young and Nadol (1989) and found not to vary in size from newborns to adults. There have, however, only been three studies of the temporal bone growth, with reference to cochlear implantation. Sims and Neely (1989) examined the change in different surface landmarks, and demonstrated an increase in the distance between the external auditory canal and the mastoid tip and several points along the suture lines. A study by O'Donoghue,

Jackler, and Schindler (1986) used CT scans of temporal bones to examine dimensions relevant to cochlear implant surgery. They estimated the need for a 10–30 mm redundancy in the lead wire for a pediatric cochlear implant. A study by Eby and Nadol (1986) examined plain X-rays and histological sections of temporal bones. They concluded from this study that at least a 25 mm lead wire expansion should be allowed for. These studies have examined either external features of the temporal bone or used two-dimensional techniques to evaluate postnatal growth patterns relevant to cochlear implantation. However, to better understand the relative growth of different parts of the temporal bone of importance for

cochlear implantation, we dissected 60 bones of all ages, so we could make measurements in three dimensions (Dahm, Shepherd, & Clark, 1993). This meant we could obtain a more accurate assessment, not only of the lead wire redundancy needed, but where best to fix the lead wire, so there would be little growth change between the point of fixation and the round window. The study showed the best point to fix the electrode away from the round window was the floor of the mastoid antrum (fossa incudis). As shown in Figure 3–1, there was virtually no relative growth between these two points from birth to adulthood. The growth between the round window and the posterior superior point of Macewen's triangle, where

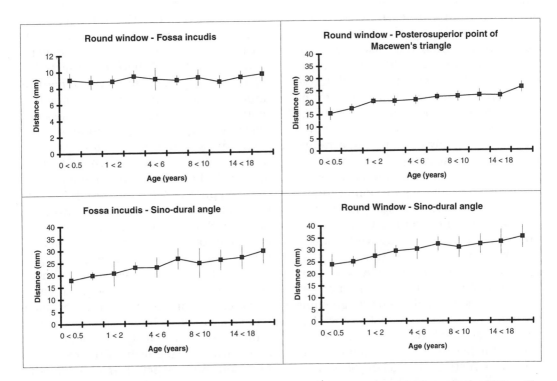

FIGURE 3–1. Graphs of the increased dimensions with age from birth to adult in the human temporal bone. *Top Left:* Round window—fossa incudis; *Top Right:* Round window—Posterosuperior point of Macewen's triangle; *Bottom Left:* Fossa incudis—Sino-dural angle; *Bottom Right:* Round window—Sino-dural angle. (From Dahm, M. C., Shepherd, R. K., & Clark, G. M. [1993]. The postnatal growth of the temporal bone and its implications for cochlear implantation in children. *Acta Otolaryngologica, 505,* 1–39. Reprinted with permission.)

the lead wire had been fixed in the adult (Webb, Pyman, Franz, & Clark, 1990 [Figure 9–13]) was, on average, 10 mm (Figure 3–1) indicating this was not an appropriate place to fix the lead wire in an infant or young child. Furthermore, the growth change between either the fossa incudis or the round window and the sino-dural angle (where the package bed would lie) was, on average, 12 mm. To allow for the variation between bones as shown by the standard deviation, a redundancy of 25 mm would be required.

The effect of skull growth on the ability of the lead wire assembly to lengthen was examined by Xu et al. (1993). First, a series of designs were implanted in the experimental animal for 3 months to 2 years, and then examined after removal, with the surrounding tissue intact. The ends of the lead wire assembly were connected to a strain gauge, and the force required to lengthen the assembly measured. Force versus lead wire expansion functions were determined for different lead wire assemblies, and it was found that it was very important that the redundancy be in the form of a U rather than a loop, and certainly not a helical arrangement. There appeared little difference between a U lying freely in the tissue or a U protected from tissue adhesions within a Teflon or Silastic bag. However, to ensure that the lead wire retains a U shape, it is preferable that it be enclosed within a bag, rather than lie free, so that lead wire lengthening can take place. A bag would also prevent the electrode being encircled in bone, which can also limit lengthening during head growth. The risk of the electrode being withdrawn from the cochlea can be further reduced by tying the lead wire to a structure, such as the floor of the antrum, as described by Webb et al. (1990). The point of fixation lies between the cochlea and the U-shaped redundancy.

In-vivo studies of lead wire lengthening were also carried out. The assemblies were attached to either the spines of the lumbar vertebrae or the spine of the scapula in young kittens, where rapid growth changes take place over a few months. The devices were X-rayed as growth took place, and it was found that the growth changes in vivo caused problems if the lead wire system did not lengthen, and could lead to a fracture of the wire or evulsion from the points of fixation. Again, the best design was one where there was a U shape in the assembly to allow for lengthening.

The Effect of Implantation on the Cochlea in the Young Animal (Kitten and Monkey)

Further studies were undertaken in the young animal (kitten and monkey) to ensure that there were no specific effects on the cochlear tissue at this young age. Results of the research (Burton, Shepherd, & Clark, 1996; Ni et al., 1992; Shepherd et al., 1994) showed there was a slight increase in the propensity of the immature animal cochlea to produce new bone formation, but otherwise no differences between young and adult animals were seen. Implantation in the young animal was examined not only in the cat (Ni et al., 1992), but also in the monkey (Burton, Shepherd, & Clark, 1996). The effects of implantation were examined both on the cochlea and the mastoid bone. The advantage of using the monkey as well as the cat was that as the monkey is a primate, its tissue responses would be more similar to humans. In addition, the monkey has mastoid air cells and a cochlea more closely resembling the human anatomy than in the cat. Consequently, the histopathological effects of the electrode insertion could be better assessed, as the electrode array could be inserted for a distance more comparable to that in humans. The study on the monkey (Figure 3–2) showed there were no significantly different adverse histopathological effects

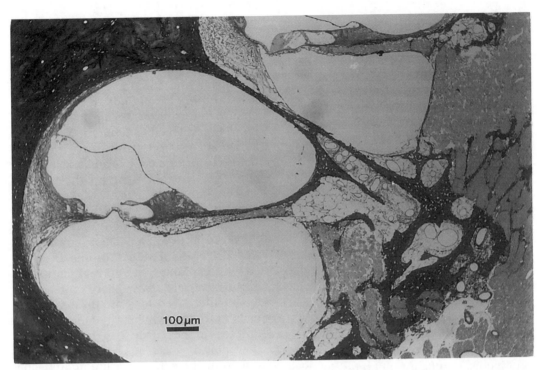

FIGURE 3–2. Photomicrograph of the upper basal and upper middle turns of a Macaca fascicularis cochlea. This cochlea was implanted for a period of 24 months with a Nucleus banded electrode array. The electrode array lay completely within the scala tympani and evoked a minimal tissue response, indicating its biocompatible nature. Although hair cells were absent adjacent to the array, presumably associated with a slight displacement of the basilar membrane, apicalward normal hair cell populations were observed (Bar = 100 μm) (From Shepherd, R. K., Clark, G. M., Xu S-A., & Pyman, B. C., [1995]. Cochlear pathology following reimplantation of a multichannel scala tympani electrode array in the macaque. *The American Journal of Otology, 16*, 186–199. Reprinted with permission.)

from those previously seen in the cat. In addition, in some monkey cochleas, the electrode was inserted along the scala media, and this too did not result in a significant loss of neural elements.

In the young monkey the surgery for the implant produced a strong inflammatory reaction in the extracochlear tissues, particularly where the bone over the mastoid had been drilled away (Burton et al., 1994). This new bone encircled the lead wire, and adhered to the platinum bands to an extent that could make its lengthening difficult with head growth. This emphasized the need to design the lead wire assembly for infants and very young chil-

dren, preferably with a U-shaped redundancy in a Teflon bag, so that lead wire lengthening could take place, even if there was considerable bone formation.

The Effect of Electrical Stimulation on the Cochlea in the Young Animal

To ensure that the electrical stimulus parameters found safe for adults were also safe for children, we undertook two further studies in young animals. The first (Ni et al., 1992) was on 8-week-old kittens with normal hearing, using bipolar stimulation. The stimuli were charge balanced biphasic current pulses at charge densities in the range 21-52 µC.cm^{-2} geom. per phase for periods of up to 1,500 hours. In the second study (Shepherd et al., 1994) bipolar and monopolar stimulation were used for kittens that had been deafened. They received stimulation for up to 1,730 hours at charge densities of 0.6-0.9 µC.cm^{-2}geom. per phase for monopolar, and 12-26 µC.cm^{-2}geom. per phase for bipolar stimulation.

Histological examination of the cochleas in the first study on kittens with residual hearing showed no evidence of stimulus-induced damage to cochlear structures when compared with implanted unstimulated controls. Hair cell loss, which was restricted to regions adjacent to the electrode array, was not influenced by the degree of electrical stimulation. In the second study the kittens were systematically deafened and implanted at 40–80 days after birth. The study also showed no significant difference in spiral ganglion cell numbers between either bipolar and monopolar stimulation, or between these and control cochleas. Interestingly, the cochleas with bipolar stimulation had increases in EABR response amplitudes during the course of stimulation and this was associated with more widespread fibrous tissue and new bone, which could have influenced the spread of current.

Insertion/Reinsertion

Another biological safety issue of importance when implanting young children is whether the electrode array can be explanted easily with minimal trauma to the cochlea, and another array inserted, also with minimal trauma. The ease with which the Nucleus banded smooth free-fitting, tapered electrode with graded stiffness could be explanted and another reimplanted was first reported by Clark, Blamey et al. (1987). This finding was the reason a connector has not been used with the receiver-stimulator for either the

present Nucleus-22 or new Nucleus-24 systems. Nevertheless, to be as sure as possible there were minimal effects on the cochlea or spiral ganglion cells, the array was implanted in a series of monkeys and left for periods of 5 months to ensure that a fibrous tissue sheath would be well developed (Shepherd, Xu, Clark, & Pyman, 1995). Both cochleas were implanted, one as a control and one as a test ear. The electrode array in the test ear was explanted without any difficulty and another one reinserted. After a further 5 months, the animals were sacrificed and the cochleas examined. This study showed that there was minimal trauma associated with explantation and reimplantation of the electrode array. There was, however, an increased loss of spiral ganglion cells in those cochleas where it was difficult to find the entrance to the round window after the electrode had been removed due to the presence of granulation tissue, and associated difficulty with reinsertion. In other words, if a series of abortive electrode insertions took place prior to the definitive replacement, because it was not quite clear where the previous channel was, then local trauma could occur. The above results were consistent with the findings of Jackler, Leade, and McKerrow (1989), who evaluated cochlear pathology in cats following explantation and reimplantation of an electrode array.

These studies indicate that care must be taken with the reimplantation to ensure that a good view is obtained of the passage before the insertion. The results do not necessarily apply to other electrode designs, as explained before, as electrodes that have protruding balls can cause trauma to the cochlea if an explantation is carried out.

Prevention of Labyrinthitis Post Implantation

Finally, further research was undertaken to help ensure that infection would not be a problem in young children (Dahm et al., 1995). In young children Streptococcus pneumoniae is a common cause of otitis media. We felt it necessary to carry out a further series of studies to ensure that this particular organism, which had different biological characteristics to the Streptococcus pyogenes and Staphylococcus aureus, could not spread into the implanted cochlea. Twenty-one kittens were used in the study and the ears were divided into those implanted with a fascial seal; implanted with Gelfoam seal; implanted with no seal; and unimplanted controls. Labyrinthitis was present in 44% of the unimplanted controls (Figure 3–3), 50% of the implanted ungrafted cochleas, and 6% of the implanted grafted (fascia and Gelfoam) cochleas. No statistically significant difference was seen between the unimplanted control and implanted cochleas. There was, however, a statistically significant difference between the implanted-ungrafted and implanted-grafted cochleas, but not between the use of fascia and Gelfoam. The data therefore indicate that cochlear implantation does not increase the risk of labyrinthitis following pneumococcal otitis media, but it is desirable to graft the round window. Al-

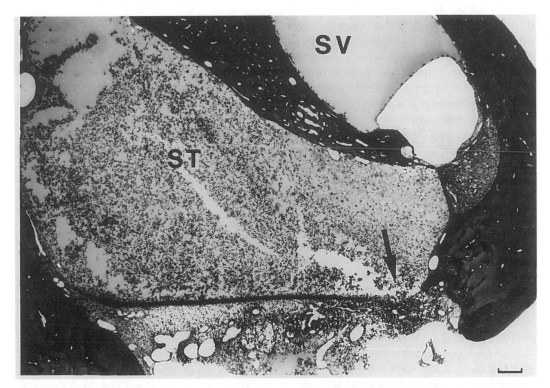

FIGURE 3–3. Photomicrograph of the lower basal turn of an unimplanted control cochlea that exhibited a suppurative labyrinthitis indicating an acute inflammatory response in the scala tympani and a proteinaceous exudate within the scala vestibuli. The bulla swab showed a high level growth of pneumococci. Note that the round window is incomplete in this example (*arrow*). ST = scala tympani; SV = scala vestibuli. Bar = 200 μm. (From Dahm, M. C., Shepherd, R. K., & Clark, G. M. [1993]. The postnatal growth of the temporal bone and its implications for cochlear implantation in children. *Acta Otolaryngologica, 505,* 1–39. Reprinted with permission.)

though there was no statistically significant difference between fascia and Gelfoam, it is recommended that fascia and not Gelfoam be used. Gelfoam was used in our animal models to produce otitis media as described previously. Therefore, if bacteria are introduced at surgery with Gelfoam around the electrode entry point it could act as a nidus for infection.

CONCLUSION

In summary, the studies examining the biocompatibility of cochlear implantation and electrical stimulation in the experimental animal have shown the procedure to be safe and not lead to adverse responses. The materials used cause minimal inflammatory responses and implantation per se does not lead to a loss of spiral ganglion cells unless there is a fracture of the spiral lamina, tear of the basilar membrane, or infection develops. Electrical stimulus parameters used with the Nucleus implant system have been shown to be safe at low as well as high stimulus rates. Moreover, electrical stimulus parameters shown to be safe in the adult are also safe in the young animal. In the young animal implantation does not lead to abnormal skull growth, and the lead wire assembly can be designed so that it is not affected by skull growth when optimal sites for lead wire fixation have been established. If at some stage there is a need to replace the electrode array, a similar type can be reinserted if care is taken to define the entry to the inner ear, and finally, the incidence of postoperative labyrinthitis following middle ear infection is no greater than in the unimplanted ear, and can be reduced in incidence by a fascial graft around the electrode entry point.

ACKNOWLEDGMENTS

We wish to acknowledge our colleagues who played an important role in the collection of data reviewed in this chapter: Dr. R. C. Black, Dr. M. J. Burton, Dr. J. K. K. Chow, Dr. N. E. Cranswick, Dr. M. C. Dahm, Dr. M. J. Donnelly, Dr. B. K. Franz, Dr. A. Kawano, Dr. J. Matsushima, Dr. D. Ni, Dr. H. L. Seldon, Dr. S. A. Shute, Mr. C. G. Treaba, Dr. M. Tykocinski, Dr. J. Xu, & Dr. S. A. Xu. In addition we would like to gratefully acknowledge Dr. F. T. Hambrecht, Head of the Neural Prosthesis Division of NINDS, for his constant support of our pediatric studies, Mr Frank Nielsen and Mr Trevor Carter for the figures, and Mrs. Sue Davine and Ms. Jacky Gray for secretarial help.

REFERENCES

Agnew, W. F., Yuen, T. G. H., Pudenz, R. H., & Bullara, L. A. (1977). Neuropathological effects of intracerebral platinum salt injections. *Journal of Neuropathology and Experimental Neurology, 36*, 533–546.

Black, R. C., & Hannaker, P. (1979). Dissolution of smooth platinum electrodes in biological fluids. *Applied Neurophysiology, 42*, 366–374.

Brennan, W. J., & Clark, G. M. (1985). An animal model of acute otitis media and the histopathological assessment of a cochlear implant in the cat. *Journal of Laryngology and Otology, 99*, 851–856.

Brummer, S. B., McHardy, J., & Turner, M. J. (1977). Electrical stimulation with Pt electrodes: Trace analysis for dissolved Platinum and other dissolved electrochemical products. *Brain Behaviour and Evolution, 14*, 10–22.

Burton, M. J., Shepherd, R. K., & Clark, G. M. (1996). Cochlear histopathologic characteristics following long-term imlantation: Safety studies in the young monkey. *Archives of Otolaryngology—Head and Neck Surgery, 122*, 1097–1104.

Burton, M. J., Shepherd, R. K., Xu, J., Xu, S., Franz, B. K.-G., & Clark, G. M. (1994). Cochlear implantation in young children: Histological studies on head growth, leadwire design and electrode fixation in the monkey model. *Laryngoscope, 104*, 167–175.

Chow, J. K. K., Seldon, H. L., & Clark, G. M. (1995). Experimental animal model of intra-cochlear ossification in relation to cochlear implantation. *Annals of Otology, Rhinology and Laryngology 104*(Suppl. 166), 42–45.

Clark, G. M. (1973). A hearing prosthesis for severe perceptive deafness—experimental studies. *Journal of Laryngology and Otology, 87,* 929–945.

Clark, G. M. (1977) An evaluation of per-scala cochlear electrode implantation techniques. An histopathological study in cats. *Journal of Laryngology and Otology, 9,* 185–199.

Clark, G. M., Blamey, P. J., Brown, A. M., Busby, P. A., Dowell, R. C., Franz, B. K.-H., Pyman, B. C., Shepherd, R. K., Tong, Y. C., & Webb, R. L. (1987). *The University of Melbourne–Nucleus Multi-Electrode Cochlear Implant. Advances in Oto-Rhino-Laryngology.* Switzerland: Karger.

Clark, G. M., Kranz, H. G., Minas, H., & Nather, J. M. (1975). Histopathological findings in cochlear implants in cats. *Journal of Laryngology and Otology, 8,* 495–504.

Clark, G. M., Pyman, B. C., Webb, R. L., Franz, B. K.-H. G. Redhead T. J., & Shepherd, R. K. (1987). Surgery for the safe insertion and reinsertion of the banded electrode array. *Annals of Otology, Rhinology and Laryngology, 96*(Suppl. 128), 10–12.

Clark, G. M., & Shepherd, R. K. (1984). Cochlear implant round window sealing procedudres in the cat. An investigation of autograft and heterograft materials. *Acta Otolaryngologica (Stockh),* (Suppl. 410), 5–15.

Clark, G. M., Shepherd, R. K., Franz, B. K.-H. G., Dowell, R. C., Tong, Y. C., Blamey, P. J., Webb, R. L., Pyman, B. C., McNaughtan, J., Bloom, D. M., Kakulas, B. A., & Siejka, S. (1988). The histopathology of the human temporal bone and auditory central nervous system following cochlear implantation in a patient. Correlation with psychophysics and speech perception results. *Acta Otolaryngologica (Stockh),* (Suppl. 448), 1–65.

Clark, G. M., Shute, S. A., Shepherd, R. K., & Carter, T. D. (1995). Cochlear implantation: Osteoneogenesis, electrode-tissue impedance and residual hearing. *Annals of Otology,* *Rhinology and Laryngology, 104*(Suppl. 166), 40–42.

Clifford, A., & Gibson, W. (1987). The anatomy of the round window with respect to cochlear implant insertion. Proceedings of the International Cochlear Implant Symposium and Workshop, Melbourne 1985. *Annals of Otology, Rhinology and Laryngology, 96*(Suppl. 128), 17–19.

Cranswick, N. E., Franz, B. K.-G., Clark, G. M., & Shepherd, R. K. (1987). Middle ear infection postimplantation: Response of the round window membrane to streptococcus pyogenes. *Annals of Otology, Rhinology and Laryngology, 96*(Suppl. 128), 53–54.

Dahm, P. (1970). *Über die postnatale Entwicklung der Form und Größe des menschlichen Os temporale.* Thesis, Würzburg.

Dahm, M.C., Clark, G.M., Franz, B.K., Shepherd, R.K., Burton, M.J., & Robins-Browne, R. (1995). Cochlear implants in children: The value of cochleostomy seals in the prevention of labyrinthitis following pneumococcal otitis media in unimplanted and implanted cat cochleas. *Acta Otolaryngologica, 114,* 620–625.

Dahm, M. C., Shepherd, R. K., & Clark, G. M. (1993). The postnatal growth of the temporal bone and its implications for cochlear implantation in children. *Acta Otolaryngologica, 505,* 1–39.

Donnelly, M. J., Cohen, L. T., Xu, J., Xu, S. A., & Clark, G.M. (1995). Investigations on a curved intracochlear array. *Annals of Otology, Rhinology and Laryngology, 104*(Suppl. 166), 409–412.

Eby, T. L., & Nadol, J. B. (1986). Postnatal growth of the human temporal bone. Implications for cochlear implants in children. *Annals of Otology, Rhinology and Laryngology, 95,* 356–364.

Franz, B. K.-H. G., Clark, G. M., & Bloom, D. M. (1984). Permeability of the implanted round window membrane in the cat—An investigation using horseradish peroxidase. *Acta Otolaryngologica,* (Suppl. 410), 17–23.

Franz, B. K.-H. G, Clark, G. M., & Bloom, D. M. (1987). Effect of experimentally induced otitis media on cochlear implants. *Annals of Otology, Rhinology and Laryngology, 96,* 174–177.

Jackler, R. K., Leade, R. A., & McKerrow, W. S. (1989). Cochlear implant revision: The effects of reimplantation on the cochlea. *Annals of Otology, Rhinology and Laryngology, 98*, 813–820.

Kawano, A., Seldon, H. L., & Clark, G. M. (1995). Intracochlear factors contributing to psychophysical percepts following cochlear implantation: Case studies.*Annals of Otology, Rhinology and Laryngology, 104*(Suppl. 166), 54–57.

Kawano, A., Seldon, H. L., Clark, G. M., Ramsden, R., & Raine, C. (1996). *Intracochlear factors contributing to psychophysical percepts following cochlear implantation.* Manuscript in preparation.

Kennedy, D. W. (1987). Multichannel intracochlear electrodes: Mechanism of insertion trauma. *Laryngoscope, 97*, 42–49.

Leake-Jones P. A., & Rebscher, S. J. (1983). Cochlear pathology with chronically implanted scala tympani electrodes. *Annals of New York Academy of Sciences, 405*, 203–223.

Leake-Jones, P. A., Rebscher, S. J., & Aird, D. W. (1985). Histopathology of cochlear implants: safety considerations. In M. M. Merzenich & R. A. Schindler (Eds.), *Cochlear implants* (pp. 55–64). New York: Raven Press.

Linthicum, F. H. Jr., Fayad, J., Otto, S. R., Galey, F. R., & House, W. F. (1991). Cochlear implant histopathology. *American Journal of Otology, 12*, 245–311.

Marsh, M. A., Coker, N. J., & Jenkins, H. A. (1992). Temporal bone histopathology of a patient with a Nucleus 22-channel cochlear implant. *American Journal of Otology, 13*, 241–248.

Mortimer, J. T., Shealy, C. N., & Wheeler, C. (1970). Experimental non destructive electrical stimulation of the brain and spinal cord. *Journal of Neurosurgery, 32*, 553–559.

Ni, D., Seldon, H. L., Shepherd, R. K., & Clark, G. M. (1993). Effect of chronic electrical stimulation on cochlear nucleus neuron size in normal hearing kittens. *Acta Otolaryngologica (Stockh), 113*, 489–497.

Ni, D., Shepherd, R. K., Seldon, H. L., Xu, S., Clark, G. M., & Millard, R. E. (1992). Cochlear pathology following chronic electrical stimulation of the auditory nerve. I: Normal hearing kittens. *Hearing Research, 62*, 63–81.

Nokubi, K. (1969). Post-natal growth of the Japanese temoral bone. *Journal Tokyo Medical College, 27*, 217–228.

O'Donoghue, G. M., Jackler, R. K., & Schindler, R. A. (1986). Observations on an experimental expansile electrode for use in cochlear implantation. *Acta Otolaryngologica (Stockh), 102*, 1–6.

Patrick, J. F., & MacFarlane, J. C. (1987). Comparative mechanical properties of single and multi-channel electrodes. *Annals of Otology, Rhinology and Laryngology, 96*(Suppl. 128), 46–48.

Roblee, L. S., McHardy, J., Marston, J. M., & Brummer, S. B. (1980) Electrical stimulation with Pt electrodes. V. The effect of protein on Pt dissolution. *Biomaterials, 1*, 135–139.

Schindler, R. A., Merzenich, M. M., & White, M. W. (1977). Multielectrode intracochlear implants—nerve survival and stimulation patterns. *Archives of Otolaryngology, 103*, 691–699.

Seldon, H. L., Dahm, M. C., Clark, G. M., & Crowe, S. (1995). Silastic with polyacrylic acid filler: Swelling properties, biocompatibilty and potential use in cochlear implants. *Biomaterials, 15*, 1161–1169.

Shepherd, R. K., & Clark, G. M. (1986). Electrical stimulation of the auditory nerve: Effects of high stimulus rates. *Proceedings of the Australian Physiological and Pharmacological Society, 18*, 14P.

Shepherd, R. K., & Clark, G. M. (1987). Effect of high electrical stimulus intensities on the auditory nerve using brainstem response and audiometry. *Annals of Otology, Rhinology and Laryngology, 96*(Suppl. 128), 50–52.

Shepherd, R. K., & Clark, G. M. (1991). Scanning electron microscopy of platinum scala tympani electrodes following chronic stimulation in patients. *Biomaterials, 12*, 417–425.

Shepherd, R. K., Clark, G. M., & Black, R. C. (1983). Chronic electrical stimulation of the auditory nerve in cats. Physiological and histopathological results. *Acta Otolaryngologica (Stockh.).* (Suppl. 399), 19–31.

Shepherd, R. K., Clark, G. M., Pyman, B. C., & Webb, R. L. (1985). Banded intracochlear electrode array: Evaluation of insertion trauma in human temporal bones. *Annals of Otology, Rhinology and Laryngology, 94*, 55–59.

Shepherd, R. K., Clark, G. M., Xu S-A., & Pyman, B.C. (1995). Cochlear pathology following reimplantation of a multichannel scala tympani electrode array in the macaque. *The American Journal of Otology, 16*, 186–199.

Shepherd, R. K., Franz, B. K.-H. G., & Clark, G. M. (1990). The biocompatibility and safety of cochlear prostheses. In G. M. Clark, Y. C. Tong, & J. F. Patrick (Eds.), *Cochlear prostheses* (pp. 69–98). Edinburgh: Churchill Livingstone.

Shepherd, R. K., Hatsushika, S., & Clark, G. M. (1993). Electrical stimulation of the auditory nerve. The effect of electrode position on neural excitation. *Hearing Research, 66,* 108-120.

Shepherd, R. K., Matsushima, J., Martin, R. L., & Clark, G. M. (1994). Cochlear pathology following chronic electrical stimulation of the auditory nerve. 2 Deafened kittens. *Hearing Research, 81,* 150–166.

Shepherd, R. K., Matsushima, J., Millard, R. E., & Clark, G. M. (1991). Cochlear pathology following chronic electrical stimulation using non charge balanced stimuli. *Acta Otolaryngologica (Stockh), 111,* 848–860.

Shepherd, R. K., Murray, M. T., Houghton, M. E., & Clark, G. M. (1985). Scanning electron microscopy of chronically stimulated platinum intracochlear electrodes. *Biomaterials, 6,* 237–242.

Shepherd, R. K., Treaba, C. G., Pyman, B. C., & Clark, G. M. (1996) *Peri-modiolar electrode arrays: A comparison of insertion trauma and electrode position in the human temporal bone.* World Congress submission in preparation.

Simmons, F. B. (1967). Permanent intracochlear electrodes in cats. Tissue tolerance and cochlear microphonics. *Laryngoscope, 77,* 171–186.

Simms, D. L., & Nealy, J. G. (1989). Growth of the lateral surface of the temporal bone in children. *Laryngoscope, 99,* 795–799.

Su, W.-Y., Marion, M. S., Hinojosa, R., & Matz, G. J. (1982). Anatomical measurements of the cochlear aqueduct, round window niche and facial recess. *Laryngoscope, 92,* 483–486.

Sutton, D., & Miller, J. M. (1983). Cochlear implant effects on the spiral ganglion. *Annals of Otology, Rhinology and Laryngology, 92,* 53–58.

Sutton, D., Miller, J. M., & Pfingst, B. E. (1980). Comparison of cochlear histopathology following two implant designs for use in scala tympani. *Annals of Otology, Rhinology and Laryngology, 89,* 11–14.

Treaba, C. G., Xu, J., Xu, S.-A., & Clark, G. M. (1995). Precurved electrode array and insertion tool. *Annals of Otology, Rhinology and Laryngology, 104*(Suppl. 166), 438–441.

Tong, Y. C., Black, R. C., Clark, G. M., Forster, I. C., Millar, J. B., O'Loughlin, B. J., & Patrick, J. F. (1979). A preliminary report on a multiple-channel cochlear implant operation. *Journal of Laryngology and Otology, 93,* 679–695.

Tong, Y. C., Clark, G. M., Blamey, P. J., Busby, P. A., & Dowell, R. C. (1982). Psychophysical studies for two multiple-channel cochlear implant patients. *Journal of the Acoustical Society of America, 71,* 153–160.

Tykocinski, M., Shepherd, R. K., & Clark, G. M. (1995). Reduction in excitability of the auditory nerve following electrical stimulation at high stimulus rates. *Hearing Research, 88,* 124–142.

The United States Pharmacopeia (20th revision). (1980). (pp. 950–953). Rockville, MD: United States Pharmacopeial Convention, Inc.

Walsh, S. M., & Leake-Jones, P. A. (1982). Chronic electrical stimulation of the auditory nerve in cat: Physiological and histological results. *Hearing Research, 7,* 281–304.

Webb, R. L., Pyman, B. C., Franz, B. K.-G, & Clark, G. M. (1990). The surgery of cochlear implantation. In G. M. Clark, Y. C. Tong, & J. F. Patrick. (Eds.), *Cochlear prostheses* (pp. 153–180). Edinburgh: Churchill Livingstone.

Xu, S. A., Shepherd, R. K., Clark, G. M., Tong, Y. C., & Williams, J. F. (1993). Evaluation of expandable leadwires for pediatric cochlear implants. *American Journal of Otology, 14,* 151–160.

Xu, J., Shepherd, R. K., Millard, R. E., & Clark, G. M. (in press). Chronic electrical stimulation of the auditory nerve at high stimulus rates: A physiological and histopathological study. *Hearing Research.*

Xu, J., Shepherd, R. K., Xu, S. A., Seldon, H. L., & Clark, G. M. (1993). Pediatric cochlear implantation: Radiological observations of skull growth. *Archives of Otolaryngology—Head and Neck Surgery, 119,* 525–534.

Young, Y.-S., & Nadol, J. B. (1989). Dimensions of the extended facial recess. *Annals of Otology, Rhinology and Laryngology, 98,* 336–338.

Zappia, J. J., Niparko, J. K., Kemink, J. L., Oviatt, D. L., & Altschuler, R. A. (1991). Evaluation of the temporal bones of a multichannel cochlear implant patient. *Annals of Otology, Rhinology and Laryngology, 100,* 914–921.

4

The Melbourne Cochlear Implant Clinic Program

ROBERT S. C. COWAN
GRAEME M. CLARK

The Melbourne Cochlear Implant Clinic program involves a multidisciplinary clinical team, collaborating with those engaged in more fundamental research, and with the biomedical company Cochlear Limited. This chapter reflects the contributions of many professionals to managing children with cochlear implants.

AIMS OF THE CLINIC PROGRAM

The multiple-channel cochlear implant provides the severely to profoundly deaf child with access to the spectral and temporal components of speech. The implanted child must (re)learn to "listen" and to effectively use the information provided through the implant. The degree to which each implanted child develops auditory skills will be influenced by diverse factors such as the cause of deafness, age at onset of hearing loss, length of profound deafness prior to implantation, age at implantation, degree of residual hearing present preoperatively, presence of other handicaps or diseases affecting the central audi-

tory pathways and cognition, number of active electrodes in the cochlea, experience in implant use, communication mode, educational setting, and the consistency of habilitation and support from family, peers, and professionals. Innate characteristics such as auditory memory, neural plasticity of the auditory pathways, auditory and cognitive attention, as well as the child's own motivation and personality, may influence this learning process in the same way as they influence the learning of a child with normal hearing.

The Clinic's first aim is to assess the child in terms of these factors and make a realistic recommendation to the parents and child on candidature and the potential for benefits to speech perception, speech production, and language development.

A second aim is to ensure that the implantation can be carried out safely and effectively, and that there are no long-standing or intermittent diseases that can affect the success of the implant.

The Clinic's third aim is to maximize the potential for the implanted child to improve speech perception and articulation,

47

to acquire language, and to develop communication skills through effective coordination of the efforts of the child, parents, Clinic team, teachers, and consultants.

Although the degree to which each implanted child will develop auditory skills varies, given improved auditory skills, there is also the potential, particularly for younger children, to develop articulation patterns that more closely approximate those of normally hearing peers. Auditory skills, developed through cochlear implant use, may impact on the child's acquisition of oral receptive and expressive vocabulary and his or her ability to acquire the knowledge of syntax and grammatical constructs necessary for effective use of language. The development of language is a critical step in broadening educational options and resultant life options for hearing-impaired children.

The Melbourne Cochlear Implant Clinic program for children was established in 1985 as an extension of the Clinic's work with deaf adults. From its inception, there has been a strong emphasis on a multidisciplinary approach, involving medical, audiological, speech and language, and educational expertise. The Clinic's management aim is to show children how to gain the most benefit from their cochlear implants in all aspects of their lives (Dowell et al., 1991).

The program's emphasis for each child is determined in part by the extent to which auditory skills may have already developed. In the case of postlinguistically deafened children, children with progressive deafness, or children with severe-to-profound hearing impairment, some auditory skills may have already been acquired through normal hearing prior to the onset of profound deafness, or through hearing aid use prior to implantation. For these children, the program emphasizes helping them to adjust to the new auditory signal presented through the cochlear implant, and relies on their pre-existing auditory skills or knowledge of language to assist teaching the child to make use of the information provided through the implant. In contrast, congenitally deaf children may have had no opportunity to develop auditory skills or knowledge of language, and the program emphasizes encouraging them to learn to "listen" as a first step. Then, through intensive habilitation, the child is helped to develop the auditory skills necessary for improved speech perception, speech production, and language acquisition.

The Cochlear Implant Clinic assumes a responsibility for the long-term management of each child receiving a cochlear implant, including otological and audiological review and habilitation (Clark et al., 1991). To effectively provide this management, the Clinic also receives technical support from the manufacturer Cochlear Limited. Cochlear Limited has demonstrated a strong commitment to patient support through its corporate philosophy, and arrangements regarding upgrades to new speech processors, and in assuming responsibility for device support of 3M and Ineraid patients following the purchase of those companies by Cochlear Limited.

The activities of the Cochlear Implant Clinic are not limited to coordinating the selection of pediatric candidates and the long-term postoperative management of implanted children. It also has important roles in pediatric cochlear implant research and in disseminating information to parents of deaf children considering the cochlear implant procedure, teachers of the deaf, other professionals, and members of the public involved in the management of children with cochlear implants.

HISTORY RELEVANT TO THE MELBOURNE CLINIC PROGRAM

The development of the 22-channel cochlear implant has been reviewed in Chapter 2 and in other publications (Clark, 1995; Clark et al., 1992; Webb et al., 1988). Prior to discussing the current Clinic program, it is relevant to review the experiences of The University of Melbourne Cochlear Implant team, which led to establishing cochlear implants as a management option for deaf children and to the evolution of the present Melbourne Clinic program.

In 1978, the first adult patient was implanted with the Melbourne multiple-channel cochlear implant. Initial studies using a formant-based speech processing strategy developed by The University of Melbourne showed that these patients could understand running speech when using the implant in combination with lipreading, or through electrical stimulation alone. As a result, the Australian biomedical company Nucleus Limited collaborated with The University of Melbourne to develop the 22-channel cochlear implant (Patrick & Clark, 1991). On the basis of success in improving the speech perception of six deaf adults who received the Nucleus device in Melbourne during 1982, The University of Melbourne and The Royal Victorian Eye and Ear Hospital established the first public hospital Cochlear Implant Program in Australia in 1983.

Before proceeding with cochlear implantation in children, a number of criteria were met:

■ Benefits to speech perception, including supplementation of lipreading and understanding of words and sentences using electrical stimulation alone were achieved with postlinguistically deaf adults.
■ Experience with two prelinguistically deaf young adults, using the multiple-channel cochlear implant, was gained which suggested that speech perception benefits might be greater for patients with a shorter period of profound deafness and auditory/oral experience prior to implantation.
■ Subsequently, experience with a 14-year-old boy, deafened at 16 months by meningitis, and a 22-year-old woman,

who had experienced a progressive hearing loss, was gained. Both of these patients achieved good supplementation to lipreading, but no open-set speech recognition with electrical stimulation alone. These results suggested that benefits from use of the cochlear implant might be greater for younger children who had a shorter period of profound deafness and auditory deprivation.
■ Issues relevant to surgery for children were investigated and the implant procedure was adapted for them (Clark, Cohen, & Shepherd, 1991).
■ A redesigned implant (the CI-22M) was produced which incorporated a smaller and flatter receiver-stimulator (for thinner skull dimensions) and a rare earth magnet to affix and align the transmitter coil without headbands (Clark et al., 1987).
■ A smaller and lighter Mini Speech Processor (MSP) was developed.
■ A multidisciplinary team comprising otologists, pediatric audiologists, speech pathologists, and educators of the deaf was established.
■ An intensive program of long-term habilitation and assessment suitable for young children was developed (Nienhuys et al., 1987).

The first implant was undertaken in September 1985 on a 10-year-old who went deaf at the age of 3 years 6 months following meningitis. This was followed by an operation in April 1986 on a 5-year-old boy who had been deafened at age 3 following meningitis. Experiences with these and subsequent children helped to evolve and establish our management and habilitation procedures. In particular, they emphasized that care was necessary in setting threshold and comfortable listening levels and that a positive approach by the habilitationist was an important factor. In addition, traditional methods of speech therapy were found to be insufficient to achieve good voice quality. Postoperative results obtained following 1 year of intensive habilitation with the initial group of implanted children showed significant benefits in speech perception when the implant was used in combination with lipreading and, in addition, some open-set speech recognition with electrical stimulation alone (Clark, Dawson, et al., 1991). These results were encouraging and the Clinic Program was formally extended to include young children, including those who were congenitally deaf. Implant use by young children was facilitated through developing an improved speech processing strategy (Multipeak), which was approved by the U.S. Food and Drug Administration (FDA) for use in children from 2 years of age in 1990 (Clark et al., 1992; Dowell, Seligman, Blamey, & Clark, 1987).

Over 6,000 children have now received the Nucleus 22-channel device worldwide. Studies in Melbourne and elsewhere have reported that children using the implant can gain significant benefits to speech perception, speech production, and language development (Blamey et al., 1992; Dawson et al., 1992, 1995; Dowell et al., 1991; Dowell, Blamey, & Clark, 1995; Geers & Moog, 1994; Staller et al., 1991; Tobey & Hasenstab, 1991). In addition, longer term experience in the management of implanted children has provided a growing understanding of the factors that may potentially influence outcomes. On the basis of reported benefits and accumulated experience, the original selection criteria for candidacy used in the Melbourne Clinic have been revised to include children with severe-to-profound hearing impairment (Dowell et al., 1995; Pyman et al., 1991).

RESEARCH INPUT TO THE MELBOURNE CLINIC PROGRAM

The Melbourne Cochlear Implant Clinic program has evolved through a strong underpinning and interaction with cochlear implant research. Developments in research have often arisen from the needs of clinical practice.

For example, a significant direction in clinical practice has been the need to provide implants to children under the age of 2 years, who are at a critical period of development for communication and language and who have greater neuronal plasticity in the auditory system. This has meant undertaking a series of biological safety studies prior to implanting this age group (Burton et al., 1994; Clark, 1995; Shepherd, Hatsushika, & Clark, 1993). These studies, discussed in more detail in the Chapter 3, established that (a) implanting over cranial suture lines would not affect skull growth; (b) fixation techniques and lead wire redundancy were required to allow for head growth and the fixation of the electrode array; (c) implantation or electrical stimulation of the young cochlea would not adversely affect the spiral ganglion population; and (d) middle ear infection in an implanted ear would not lead to any greater chance of labyrinthitis postimplantation.

Plans for implanting young children under 2 years of age also identified clinical needs in selection, mapping, and habilitation. The use of steady state evoked potentials to provide accurate and objective assessment of hearing thresholds in infants and young children was developed from research at The University of Melbourne (Rickards & Clark, 1984). Studies in normal neonates and hearing-impaired children showed behavioral thresholds and steady state evoked potential thresholds to be within 10 dB across a range of carrier frequencies from 250–4000 Hz (Rance et al., 1995). The steady state procedure is now routinely used in the clinical program as an objective measure of hearing thresholds.

New techniques were also required for evaluating device function and speech discrimination in children who had not yet developed spoken language and for whom formal pediatric speech perception tests were linguistically or cognitively inappropriate. The Vowel Imitation task, developed at The University of Melbourne, relies on the natural tendency of young children to imitate speech sounds (Dawson, 1990). Results obtained for the Vowel Imitation task with implanted children were highly correlated with scores on PBK monosyllabic words and the closed-set Picture Vocabulary test (Dettman et al., 1995). The Vowel Imitation task is routinely used in the Clinic for the early assessment of speech perception, to alert the clinician to the need to modify the speech processor mapping to ensure effective discrimination of individual speech sounds, or to provide input to the habilitation program.

Research has also resulted in clinical application of the Computer-Aided Speech and Language Analysis (CASALA) software in the assessment of phonetic inventories of implanted children before and after implantation. Initial results have shown that postimplantation, the acquisition of sounds became closer to that of normal-hearing children, and that, as a group, children with a cochlear implant improved on segmental features of speech production in everyday conversation over time (Grogan, Barker, Dettman, & Blamey, 1995; Serry, Blamey, & Grogan, 1996). The CASALA software is used in the Clinical Program for analysis of videotaped speech samples.

More recently, research has shown that implanted children who were experienced users of the Multipeak strategy were able to successfully change over to the Speak speech processing strategy (Cowan et al., 1995). Repeated evaluations over an 18-month period have shown that children using the Speak strategy were able to obtain significantly improved speech perception compared to Multipeak, particularly in background noise. Children changing from Multipeak to Speak required only a short period of adjustment, which was an important finding for the counseling of

parents who were considering changing their child to Speak. All children in the Melbourne Clinic are now fitted with the Spectra-22 speech processor and programmed with the Speak strategy.

These studies highlight the interaction between research and clinical practice which has been instrumental in the development of the Melbourne Clinic program. It is also important to note that the research and clinical interaction has benefited from close collaboration with Cochlear Limited, who has maintained a research and development unit within the Cochlear Implant Clinic and University of Melbourne since the inception of the program.

THE CLINIC TEAM

The Melbourne Clinic stresses the acquisition and improvement of skills in speech perception and speech production, and the use of these skills in developing language and enhancing general communication (Clark et al., 1992; Nienhuys et al., 1987). The need for close, long-term cooperation between the Clinic team, the child, the parents, extended family, and teachers involved with the child in both preimplant and postimplant stages is also stressed. The Clinic also has a vital role in providing information and counseling support, with particular emphasis on the need for the family to accept and understand the capabilities and limitations of the cochlear implant (Clark et al., 1991; Mecklenburg et al., 1990).

The child, along with the parents and family, must be considered as an integral part of the Cochlear Implant team. The child must be motivated to use his or her device and to learn to listen. The child needs to be a willing participant in habilitation and accept the necessities of long-term review. Most important, the child will be required to accept responsibility for the management of his or her own device as early as practicable. In the earliest stages, this may involve simply telling the parent when the implant is not working. In later years, the child should be encouraged to assume responsibility for maintaining batteries and changing spare parts. The parent's involvement will have greater impact on the child's potential outcomes than that of professionals in the Clinic team. It is sometimes the case that the caring professional may unintentionally "take over" in an effort to maximize the benefits of an implant for a child. It is important for the Clinic team professional to remember that involvement with any implanted child may be transitory, in contrast to the lifelong commitment of the parent.

The Melbourne Clinic has developed a multidisciplinary team approach, involving primarily the surgeon/otologist, audiologist, and speech pathologist working together with each child. The individual roles of team members have been outlined previously in greater detail for the Melbourne Clinic (Clark, Dawson, et al., 1991), and for other clinical programs in the United States and Europe (Archbold, 1994; Bertram, 1996; Fraser 1991; Sillon et al., 1996; Tye-Murray, 1993). Each of these programs is multidisciplinary, involving close collaboration between medical and nonmedical professionals. The current staffing profile is shown in Figure 4–1.

As the otologist is ultimately responsible for making the decision to undertake a cochlear implant operation on the child, he or she must assume the responsibility of being head of the Clinic. This is also in accord with the principles of the Helsinki Declaration of the World Medical Association (1993), which states that biomedical research involving human subjects should be conducted only by scientifically qualified persons under the supervision of a clinically competent medical person. To adequately fulfill the role as head of a Cochlear Implant Clinic, it is important that the otologist obtains knowledge and experience in the participating disciplines

of pediatric audiology and speech and language science. Without this knowledge, it may prove difficult to adequately evaluate the opinions of members of the Clinic team concerning the management of a particular child.

Although cochlear implantation in children has evolved from primarily research to accepted clinical practice, it is in the interest of the child that the high standards required for monitoring biomedical research be maintained in the Clinic program. The active involvement of the otologist in all facets of patient management is essential. For example, fluctuations in thresholds may occur in the mapping phase due to middle ear effusion. In addition, pain or other discomfort in the ear or head can result from many etiologies requiring medical investigation. Most important, in the case of implanted children who fail to make satisfactory progress, the otologist, audiologist, speech pathologist, and educator must work as a team to investigate the medical factors (e.g., mental retardation, neurological disorders) and audiological or development factors that might be responsible. Furthermore, as progress in medicine depends heavily on research, there should be continuing review of research proposals and studies conducted in association with the Clinic.

Although acknowledging the otologist's ultimate responsibility for the management of each child, in practice and for logistic reasons, in the Melbourne Clinic program either the audiologist or speech pathologist assumes the role of case manager. The case manager is responsible for coordinating the program for the child, making necessary arrangements for medical and audiological assessments, reporting on progress of preoperative and postoperative phases during Clinic meetings, managing the child during postoperative mapping, and providing any one-to-one habilitation. The case manager collaborates with the audiologist or speech pathologist as a consultant, providing specialist

Head and Director
(Otologist)

Assistant Director
(Policy Implementation & Training)

Deputy Director
(Medical Selection & Surgery)

Hearing, Speech, and Language Specialists

Clinic Coordinator

Social Worker

Education Consultants

Research Consultants
(Department of Otolaryngology)
(CRC for Cochlear Implant, Speech Hearing Research)

Senior Secretary

Deputy Director
(Audiological Selection & Habilitation)

Surgeons

Consultants
(Pediatric Medicine, Psychology, etc)

Consultants
(Cochlear Limited)

Financial Officer

FIGURE 4–1. Cochlear Implant Clinic Program Staff Profile.

input to the assessment, habilitation, or management. Each team member is trained to cross disciplines to allow them to fulfill all of the necessary activities of the case manager and to function effectively as a "hearing communication specialist" for cochlear implantation.

Efforts are made to maintain the same case manager and consultant throughout the preoperative assessments and in the postoperative period up to 12 months. The continuity of case manager provides a single contact for the parents and child involved in the implant procedure and a single source of reference about the child for other members of the implant team, which facilitates the transition through the preoperative assessment, surgery, programming, and postoperative habilitation.

In addition to the otologist, audiologist, and speech pathologist, the team involves educators of the deaf, social workers, administration, and technical support staff. The Clinic team may also consult with pediatricians and psychologists regarding opinions on management of specific children, in particular, those with multiple handicaps.

Educators of the deaf provide specialist knowledge of early intervention techniques relevant to developing auditory, language, and communication skills in the implanted child. Their input is useful in advising parents on communication mode and educational setting, and in helping them to develop more effective strategies to encourage early language development postoperatively. In addition, educators of the deaf assist the Clinic in reviewing the child's progress in acquiring language and communication skills, investigating factors contributing to language delays, and planning a strategy for intervention.

The Clinic team includes an experienced pediatric social worker who can assist in a number of areas. For example, parents may have significant difficulties in adjusting to the special needs of their hearing-impaired child. In particular, a period of "grieving" is often experienced, and is viewed as a necessary stage in the parent's acceptance of their child's disability. Although the otologist, audiologist, speech pathologist, and educator are cross-trained in the counseling of parents regarding the social impact of hearing loss, the pediatric social worker can often advise the Clinic team on the parents' progress in acceptance of the hearing loss, and whether they are realistically assessing the information provided on the benefits and potential risks of cochlear implants for their child. In addition, there is a significant trend toward single parents and other styles of families. The social worker will be the person best placed to advise a parent or guardian of their responsibilities.

Pediatricians may be called on to provide specialized medical advice regarding the selection, management, or (re)habilitation of the child. This is particularly important for the Melbourne Clinic, which has a significant proportion of children with other disabilities in addition to their deafness. Pediatricians may also assist the team in counseling parents regarding genetic factors in their child's deafness, and on expectations for their child's development.

Children with hearing impairment may have acquired inappropriate behavioral patterns, which must be addressed before completing the assessment or undertaking habilitation. Child psychologists or psychiatrists may be required in this situation to provide specialized behavior modification programs to help the parent in managing the child, or advise on development issues relevant to the child's management.

The input from the consulting specialists is very important in reviewing patients. This occurs on a regular basis, and is particularly needed for those who fail to show acceptable progress. In the latter case, the Clinic benefits from the close association with Cochlear Limited staff in

Melbourne, who can assist with advice on implant function and programming issues. Worldwide, similar support is provided to other clinics by Cochlear Limited staff.

To function smoothly, administration and technical support staff are necessary to help ensure the smooth transition of children through the various phases of the Clinic program. In Melbourne, the role of Clinic Coordinator has evolved for managing day-to-day operations of the Clinic and coordinating activities of the Clinic staff, who are drawn from a number of diverse organizations, including university, hospital, private clinic, and research. The Coordinator is also responsible for liaison between the Clinic and outreach programs located at various schools for hearing-impaired children throughout Melbourne.

COMPONENTS OF THE CLINIC PROGRAM

The preoperative and postoperative components of the Melbourne Clinic program have been described previously (Clark, Dawson, et al., 1991; Osberger et al., 1991). Dettman et al. (1996) presented a detailed framework for the Melbourne Clinic program, and a revised version of this framework is shown diagrammatically in Figures 4–2 and 4–3. The following discussion is intended to illustrate the integration between phases of the preoperative, surgery, and postoperative management. Individual phases are discussed in detail in respective chapters.

The Initial Interview and Referral

Children may be referred to the Cochlear Implant Clinic from a variety of sources, including Australian Hearing Services (a Commonwealth Government hearing health statutory authority), early intervention centers, individual otologists, medical practitioners, and audiologists both in private

practice and in hospital audiology units. Occasionally, initial inquiries come from teachers at schools where other implanted children are in attendance, or directly from concerned parents. Regardless of the initial referral source, a referral letter from the child's medical practitioner to the Clinic Director is required.

Referral at an early stage is desirable, as recent research and clinical practice have suggested that children receiving cochlear implants at an early age may potentially show rapid acquisition of listening skills (Gibson, 1996; Waltzman et al., 1996). Early detection is an essential precursor to early implantation. In Victoria, severe and profound deafness is detected in "at risk" children at a very early age, due to the implementation of an ABR and hearing screening program (F.C. Jarman, S.A. Aldridge, & Z. Poulakis, personal communication, 1996). Over the first 24 months of its operation, the median age of detection declined significantly ($p < 0.05$) from 22.5 months to 17.5 months. In particular, there was a significant increase in the proportion of deaf children detected between the ages of 6 and 12 months. This is an important development, as the preoperative phase of assessments, counseling, and candidature in general require from 3–6 months to complete. Early detection allows time for a number of steps to be completed while the child is still quite young. The parents have time to accept their child's deafness, and to plan strategies to deal with the consequences. The Clinic team has time to complete the preoperative assessments, and to make a recommendation to the parents on benefits. Most important, the parents have time to make a considered and informed decision regarding implantation on behalf of their child while the child is still at a critical stage of development for learning auditory skills and language development.

Once phone contact is established with the family, they are invited to visit the Coch-

Initial Interview Referral
- Clinical History and Examination
- Initial Counselling
- Discussion on Cochlear Implant Program (Melbourne)

Establishing Cochlear Implant Candidacy
- Unaided Threshold Testing
- Aided Threshold Testing
- Impedance Testing
- Objective Audiometry (SSEP) for all children < 5 yrs
- Complete Otological Examination
- CT Scan
- Other assessments as required

Hearing-Aid Trial/Auditory Habilitation
- Speech Perception Assessment
- Auditory Habilitation
- Play and Communication
- Counselling
- Video Recordings
- Formal Team Review and Recommendation
- Liaison with other professionals, schools

Preparation for the Cochlear Implant Procedure
- Preoperative Review and Examination
- Ward Visit
- Meeting other parents/children

Surgery and Hospital Stay
- 5–6 days in hospital
- One parent may stay with child

FIGURE 4–2. Preoperative Program.

Medical Monitoring and Postoperative Management
- Otological review 2–3 days after discharge
    - weekly for 1 month
    - monthly for 6 months
    - at least every 6 months
- Postoperative X-rays
- Impedance Testing if required

Speech Processor Mapping
- Measuring threshold and comfort levels.
    - weekly for 1 month
    - monthly for 6 months
    - at least every 6 months
- Order and fit Radio Frequency device if required

Postoperative Habilitation
- Resume individual program
- One-to-one work
- Guide parents to optimize listening
- Facilitate learning language through listening
      detection, discrimination, identification, & comprehension
- Develop speech sounds and self-monitoring
- Consultation with other professionals, schools, etc.

Evaluation of Benefit
- Sound Detection/Sound Imitation (daily)
- Video Analysis of parent/child interaction (monthly)
- Speech Perception Testing (every 6–12 months)
- Speech and Language Sample Analysis (every 6–12 months)

Technical Support
- Guide parents to check listening daily
- Guide parents to check/maintain speech processor & headset
- Complete minor repairs and provide spare parts

Professional Education, Support, & Public Awareness
- Liaison with school regarding implanted children.
- Education of professionals and public

FIGURE 4–3. Postoperative Program.

lear Implant Clinic for a meeting with members of the team. At the initial discussion, the Clinic team (otologist, audiologist, and speech pathologist, in the case of younger children) will provide information on medical, surgical, audiological, and developmental issues relevant to the implant procedure and to their individual child. The primary focus of the initial discussion is on providing information. Table 4–1 provides examples of the diverse range of topics that might be addressed in the initial discussion.

The otologist will also obtain relevant medical and audiological case history details regarding the child and his or her hearing at this interview. This may include details of the mother's pregnancy, the child's birth and physical progress since birth, medical history, educational programs, communication skills, and details of the hearing loss and hearing aid use.

The parents are encouraged to bring any other support persons or members of the child's extended family to the initial discussion and to subsequent appointments. Occasionally, an audiologist or teacher who is already working with the child may attend appointments with the parents. In the case of parents of younger hearing impaired children, it may be nec-

essary to arrange a first visit without the child, so that they may concentrate on the information being provided and have the time to formulate and ask questions. Older hearing-impaired children and adolescents will need to have a very responsible part in deciding whether to proceed with the cochlear implant investigations and ultimately, the operation.

At the end of the initial discussion, the parents and child, if of an appropriate age, should have a clear understanding of the implant procedure and program. If they wish to proceed, further appointments are made, but no pressure is placed to make a decision. It is stressed that a recommendation on candidature cannot be made until the preoperative assessments are completed. They are also counseled that their decision to proceed with the next phases of the assessment does not commit the child to proceeding with an implant.

Establishing Cochlear Implant Candidacy

For those deciding to proceed, a number of assessments are completed over the next weeks. These assessments, shown in Table 4–2, are discussed in subsequent chapters

Table 4–1. Examples of topics addressed in the initial discussion.

- How much hearing will my child have?
- Will my child be able to learn to speak normally?
- Is it too late to gain help with my child's hearing problems?
- What do unaided or aided audiograms mean?
- How does the hearing system function, and why can't a hearing aid provide enough help?
- How does the cochlear implant work, and what equipment is involved?
- What is involved in the Clinic program and how long is each component?
- What does the device cost and what are the costs for the procedure?
- What funding options through public health care or private insurance are available?
- What other options are available to improve hearing?
- Is signing possible with an implant?
- What alternatives for communication are possible?

Table 4–2. Summary of assessments for candidacy.

- **Otological examination**
  (to examine the child, review the medical history, and assess the child's fitness/need for general anesthetic for a CT scan, and middle ear function including impedance testing)

- **CT scan**
  (performed 2 to 4 weeks later, to provide the surgeon with evidence on whether the cochleas are implantable)
  - CT scans for young children are completed under a general anesthetic in order to ensure that the child will remain still during the procedure.
  - CT scans for older children who are able to keep still during the 15–20 minute procedure do not require a general anesthetic.

- **Steady state evoked potential testing**
  (for younger children, to objectively measure hearing thresholds performed while the child is under general anesthetic immediately following the CT scan)

- **Unaided and aided hearing threshold assessment**

- **Speech perception and language assessments**
  - if child has sufficient auditory skills to cooperate with formal testing.
  - for children under 5 years of age the Vowel Imitation task is used.
  - videotaped samples of play are recorded and later analyzed.

---

detailing the Preoperative Medical Evaluation and the Preoperative Audiological, Speech, and Language Evaluation. These assessments detail the child's hearing and communication status and medical suitability for the implant procedure. The constellation of results is considered by the multidisciplinary team to ensure that due consideration is given to medical, audiological, developmental, and educational issues. The team considers the results of the assessments and establishes whether the child is a candidate for the cochlear implant procedure. For some children, additional assessments may be required, for example, to provide information on potential medical contraindications or complications inherent in genetic syndromes, or to seek advice on developmental issues in the case of multiply handicapped children.

Candidature requires that the child is medically fit for surgery, has an implantable cochlea, and has no other medical contraindications. Given this, the team will establish whether the results confirm that the child is also a candidate on audiological criteria. Given the child is a suitable candidate, a recommendation is made that they proceed with the next phase of the preoperative program, which involves a period of habilitation using hearing aids.

Hearing Aid Trial and Auditory Habilitation

The preoperative habilitation period includes three specific tasks: hearing aid trial and auditory habilitation; the development of play and communication; and intensive counseling of the child and parents.

Auditory Habilitation and Hearing Aid Trial

The first step in the hearing aid trial is to ensure that the child's hearing aid fitting is optimal. The child's current skills in using the hearing aid(s) and any associated radio-frequency devices, and any improvements made during habilitation are then assessed. The hearing aid trial will in general be a minimum of 10 weeks of intensive one-to-one therapy. The length of the hearing aid trial and the likelihood that the child will make significant progress with conventional amplification will depend on the degree of hearing impairment of the individual child, previous history of hearing aid use, and whether adjustments were required to optimize the hearing aid fitting.

In each case, the primary question is whether the child shows evidence of using residual hearing to develop communication. This can be difficult to assess, particularly for profoundly deaf children for whom it may be unreasonable to expect significant progress in a 10-week hearing aid trial. It is also well-known that variation exists in the ability of individual hearing-impaired children to gain benefit from their residual hearing. However, children with a profound or total hearing loss would be unlikely to have access to the full spectrum of speech sounds, even when optimally fitted with conventional hearing aids. For this reason, it is necessary to assess speech and language acquisition in relation to previous hearing aid use, and the child's hearing thresholds. If the child demonstrates significant progress using hearing aids, the audiologist may recommend continuing the hearing aid habilitation and monitoring progress before a decision is made to proceed with an implant. If speech and language acquisition are not progressing satisfactorily, the cochlear implant is the preferred option.

The decision to proceed with the implant is often more difficult for parents of infants and very young children, particularly those who have significant residual hearing. However, experience in the Melbourne Clinic has shown that severely to profoundly deaf children, who preoperatively have good lower frequency residual hearing, may not make good progress with a hearing aid but show significant benefits from the cochlear implant, including understanding of open-set words using electrical stimulation alone (Cowan et al., 1996; Dowell et al., 1995).

The hearing aid trial also provides the opportunity to teach the child to cooperate with play audiometry or conditioned reinforcement techniques. These techniques will be used in postoperative mapping of the speech processor. In some cases, the decision to proceed with the implant may need to be delayed until a reliable stimulus-response paradigm has been established for mapping the child.

Development of Play and Communication

In young children, an important focus of the preoperative habilitation is to establish the parent as the facilitator of the child's auditory learning (Dettman et al., 1996). It also provides opportunities for the parent to develop behavior management strategies and techniques to enhance the development of play and communication skills. Nienhuys, Cross, and Horsborough (1984) reported that mothers of hearing impaired children displayed a different pattern of interaction in communication as contrasted with mothers of normally hearing children. As a group, they were more likely to act as "teachers" of their hearing impaired child, focusing on the production of words, rather than as "facilitators" who encouraged developmental dialogue without requests for labels. Plapinger and Kretschmer (1991) emphasized the role of the hearing rehabilitationist as an observer, analyzer, and modifier of the parent-child interaction, stressing that parents be helped to learn to use a variety of interaction styles that encourage the development of communication with their hearing impaired child. In the case of the child with acquired hearing loss, the parents' successful strategies should be encouraged and they should be shown techniques that maintain auditory skills already developed.

Counseling

Counseling is an important focus of the preoperative habilitation period. The Clinic stresses two-way counseling, providing ample opportunity for parents to air concerns. This is vital in ensuring that the parents feel in control of the decisions regarding their child. To facilitate clear understanding of the potential benefits and risks, the Clinic encourages the parents and the child considering the implant to become involved with the Cochlear Implant Parents Support Group. The Clinic also arranges for the family to meet with families of implanted children who are of a similar age and have similar etiologies and hearing history. Luterman (1984) stressed the importance of shared experiences and support among parents of hearing-impaired children. As discussed previously, counseling parents regarding sudden deafness involves a sensitive approach and understanding of the parent's need to progress through stages of guilt, questioning, and acceptance. This emphasizes the need for early referral so that the Clinic team can manage the child and parents, and have the time to call on specialized consultants if required.

Counseling will also address the issues involved in deciding on or maintaining progress in the educational and communication setting for the hearing-impaired child. In the course of the preimplant period, parents may have received conflicting advice from professionals and friends. They may already have formed strong opinions as to the communication mode of choice for their child. The Clinic respects the rights of the parents to make their own decision regarding communication mode and education setting. Within the Melbourne program, implanted children are enrolled in both Oral and Total Communication settings. However, as noted in greater detail in Chapter 12, analysis of pediatric performance has shown that children enrolled in oral settings may progress at a more rapid rate. On the basis of these findings, it is generally recommended that young children with cochlear implants who do not have special needs related to additional handicaps should be in an oral communication setting emphasizing the development and use of auditory skills.

Team Review and Recommendation to Parents

At the end of the preoperative habilitation period, the progress of the child in developing auditory, speech, and language skills through his or her aided residual hearing is reviewed by the interdisciplinary team. After careful consideration of all available information, the team will make a recommendation to the parents regarding the potential for their individual child to benefit from the implant. The otologist and case manager provide a comprehensive summary of the factors that may influence the performance of children with cochlear implants and discuss with the parents (and child) how these factors might apply to outcomes. The risks associated with the procedure and the demands that will be placed on the parents' time are also clearly identified and discussed. The surgeon will also discuss the hospital's Patient Consent form and plain language statement of the risks and benefits with the parents. The team must ensure that the parents understand their ongoing commitments regarding programming, habilitation, and medical/clinical review. During the counseling process, the parents and the child should also be informed about the opinions of the Deaf community and its advocates regarding cochlear implants.

Once parents and the child have been counseled regarding realistic expectations of the implant and its limitations, they can make an informed decision regarding proceeding with a cochlear implant. Parents who decide not to proceed are provided with information about alternative support services.

A preferred ear for the implant procedure will have been identified by the otologist. In general, the approach has been to implant the ear with the least residual hearing, given no other contraindicating factor. Considerable emphasis however is given to ensuring that the child will in fact benefit from electrical stimulation. In cases of symmetrical bilateral hearing loss, and where no other surgical or audiological factors suggest a preferred ear for implantation, consideration should include the "handedness" of the child, and the ease with which he or she will be able to manipulate the device. These issues are explored in more detail in Chapters 6 and 7.

As discussed, the Clinic philosophy stresses the annual review of all patients, including those who do not make significant progress, and those who do not progress to implantation. For children not proceeding with an implant, the review process will detect any children who have experienced progressive hearing loss, for example, retinitis pigmentosa (Usher's syndrome). In addition, continuing developments in cochlear implant speech processing may result in revised selection criteria. Regular review of the status of hearing-impaired children allows for reevaluation of the progress of the child in developing auditory and language skills using conventional hearing aids and their future possible implant candidature.

Preparation for the Cochlear Implant Operation

If the parents and child elect to proceed, a surgery date is planned, and the child and family enter the next phase of preparing for the surgical procedure and hospital stay. Any necessary otological procedures, such as repair of perforations, correction of middle ear effusion, or treatment of otitis media, will also require completion prior to proceeding with surgery. A suffi-ciently long period needs to elapse to show that the otitis media is resolved. In the event of a significant delay, the child would continue to use hearing aids if possible, or use The University of Melbourne's electro-tactile Tickle Talker™ (Cowan et al., 1990) to ensure that auditory skills or articulation did not deteriorate from an absence of auditory or sensory feedback.

The preparatory phase will vary with the needs of the individual family and child, but may include the use of books, stories, photos, and role toys to help the young child to understand the entry to hospital. Familiarization visits to the hospital ward may also be included. In the case of older children and adolescents, it is important to ensure their understanding and consent for the cochlear implant procedure, as the child's motivation to use the implant is a vital factor contributing to a successful outcome.

Surgery and Hospital Stay

The child's preoperative medical examination is completed approximately 2 weeks prior to the selected date of surgery. This will include review by an anesthetist to exclude any specific problems associated with syndromes or general health. Careful monitoring of the middle ear status continues up to admission. Any indication of the presence of a middle ear effusion or incipient infection will result in a postponement of the procedure.

The child is hospitalized for a period of 5–6 days, during which time one parent may remain in the hospital with the child. The operation occurs on the day following admission and in general takes 3 hours. Other issues relevant to the surgery are discussed in detail in Chapter 7. At the conclusion of the operation, intraoperative EABR testing of the electrode array is used to ensure proper function of the receiver-stimulator and electrode array. A postoperative X-ray of the position of the array within the cochlea is also taken. This serves both as a record of the position of the electrode and to assist in making decisions regarding programming (i.e., identifying electrodes that are outside of the cochlea and likely to produce nonhearing sensations). It is good for the nonmedical team members to visit the theater on occasions and support the parents during surgery. In addition, the case manager will be present when the surgeon reports the operation outcomes to the parents.

Medical Monitoring and Postoperative Management

The child will be reviewed by the visiting otologist or hospital medical staff. Approximately 2 or 3 days following discharge, the otologist will again review the child and a schedule for initial fitting of the speech processor will be decided. In general, "start-up" occurs no sooner than 2 weeks following surgery, although this will depend on the individual child's recovery from the procedure. Continuing otological review is an important component of patient management, and reviews are conducted at weekly intervals for the first month, then monthly for the next 6 months, and subsequently at 12-month intervals.

Speech Processor Mapping

Speech processor mapping, discussed in more detail in Chapter 9, requires establishing which electrodes produce useful hearing sensations and measuring a threshold and comfortable level of electrical stimulus for each of these electrodes. The speech processor must be mapped for each child, and this progresses over several weeks at a pace geared to the child. Continued monitoring is required to check that the map remains suitable. Experience has shown that levels may vary initially as swelling over the receiver-stimulator reduces. In addition, the ability of the child to subjectively report minimum thresholds will gradually improve with age. Mapping

also ensures that the loudness of individual electrodes is balanced across the electrode array, which is important in ensuring an optimum dynamic range. The comments and observations of parents, family, and teachers concerning the child's responses to everyday sounds and speech can provide valuable input regarding the suitability of the child's map, particularly for young preverbal children. At this stage, the parents will also be familiarized with using a seven-sound detection task on a daily basis as a quick check that the full spectrum of speech sounds are being detected by the child through the implant.

Postoperative Habilitation

The habilitation of children of different age ranges and at different stages of development is discussed in detail in subsequent chapters. In brief, habilitation aims to ensure that the child acquires skill in discriminating auditory input through the cochlear implant. In addition, habilitation is focused on maximizing the potential for improved auditory comprehension, improved speech production, and the development of language and communication skills.

The need for intensive habilitation must be balanced with that for mapping sessions during the immediate postoperative period. In general, mapping will become less frequent during the first 2 to 6 months (depending on the age and progress of the individual child). Once the map has become stable, mapping reviews are scheduled at 6-month intervals. In the immediate period following implantation, the case manager (audiologist or speech pathologist) will be involved in one-to-one habilitation sessions with the child. Although emphasis is placed on an auditory-oral approach to habilitation, parents and children who have used total communication in the preoperative period may continue to use these skills to assist in habilitation postoperatively. However, examples of specific communication interactions that do not include manual supplements would be modeled for the parent. As the child gains confidence and improved skills in listening, the need for manual supplements may be naturally reduced.

In younger children, habilitation emphasizes developing the child's listening skills and enhancing the parent's abilities as a facilitator of speech and language development. As the child progresses, habilitation may shift from the clinic to the home or school. In the case where a number of children are enrolled at one school, the Clinic has established outreach programs, in which clinic staff visit on a regular basis to deal with particular mapping, habilitation, or management issues for implanted children and to provide ongoing in-service training and support for teachers. In the longer term, the Clinic role evolves from providing one-to-one habilitation to providing long-term support for parents and teachers in the child's educational facility.

In the case of children and families living some distance from the clinic, the Clinic may utilize the help of local teachers, audiologists, or speech pathologists in the provision of weekly intervention at an earlier stage. In such cases, the role of the clinician will be primarily in providing liaison and support for the implanted child and these local professionals, and in providing contact between the Clinic and the parent for reviews.

The issues involved in the educational management of children with cochlear implants are complex, and beyond the scope of this chapter (Barnes, Franz, & Bruce, 1994). However, the Melbourne Clinic has established and maintained close interaction with teachers responsible for the educational management of implanted children. In the case of younger children, the pediatric educational consultants provide expertise in the development of language in normally hearing and hearing-impaired children, including children with cochlear implants.

Evaluation of Benefit

Evaluation (a) allows the long-term progress of individual children with their implants to be monitored; (b) identifies specific targets in speech perception, speech production, language development, or communication skills requiring remediation or training; (c) investigates possible factors for children who do not make acceptable progress with their implant; and (d) examines specific research issues and questions through well-designed and controlled studies.

A range of formal assessment tests and informal techniques are necessary to cover differing developmental stages, attentive abilities, and language sophistication of preverbal versus school-aged children. In addition, there is an overlap between testing to provide input to the postoperative management of the individual child, and testing to provide data to answer specific research questions. It is important that evaluation materials used routinely in the Clinic are carefully selected, and that protocols and test procedures are consistently adhered to, if the information collected for clinical management is to be of use in answering important research questions regarding candidature and outcomes. Differing considerations may also apply to the analysis of data and procedures used in prospective versus retrospective studies. These issues are discussed in more detail in Chapter 12.

Technical Support

Instruction and practice in proper device function, troubleshooting, and replacement of spare parts and batteries is an important component of long-term management. Initially, the parent assumes primary responsibility for the speech processor. As noted earlier, it is important that the child be involved in troubleshooting at the earliest possible age. For example, the child should be encouraged to report when the speech processor is "off the air." The assumption of responsibility by the child for device management is an important factor in maintaining motivation for continuing and effective use of the implant.

The Parents' Support Group, established by families of implanted children, assists the Clinic in disseminating technical support and information to parents and implanted children, through their newsletter, informal parents' nights with Clinic staff, and information days organized in cooperation with CICADA, the Cochlear Implant Support Group.

Professional Education, Support, and Public Awareness

Although the numbers of implanted children have continued to increase, additional funding for team members has not kept pace. This places an added imperative on ensuring that the parent gains skills as a facilitator of the child's auditory skills and language development and in actively pursuing the involvement and collaboration of educators and other professionals in providing habilitation and support for implanted children in early intervention and school settings.

The Clinic has a responsibility to ensure that professionals involved in working with implanted children are well informed regarding the device and its proper function, as well as revisions to selection procedures and candidature based on reported outcomes. Clinic staff provide significant in-service and school-based professional education and support activity. This has included production of a professional information video summarizing key issues and components of the Cochlear Implant Program, which is made freely available to parents, teachers, and interested professionals. The Melbourne Clinic, in collaboration with the Bionic Ear Institute and with support from Cochlear Limited, has also established an International Workshop program for surgeons and habilitationists, providing hands-on experience and training in cochlear implantation in children.

APPROACHES TO CLINIC MANAGEMENT

Although we have focused on the development and procedures adopted by the Melbourne Cochlear Implant Clinic, it is important to recognize that a range of programs managing cochlear implants in children are in use worldwide. It is also important to recognize that programs are continually under review as the body of world experience with pediatric cochlear implants expands.

For example, The Melbourne Clinic, primarily because of its role in initiating research in the clinical application of the Nucleus multiple channel cochlear implant to different patient groups, has evolved a selection procedure that assesses each child individually, without restricting candidature to particular groups of hearing-impaired children. As a result, the Melbourne Clinic has implanted children with a range of age, length of deafness, etiology, preoperative residual hearing, and communication mode, as well as a number of children with additional disabilities and congenitally deaf adolescents.

In contrast, other clinics may restrict candidacy to particular groups. For example, at the present time, the Nottingham program (Archbold, 1996) has focused on children younger than 5 years. Similarly, some clinics may be reluctant to include congenitally deaf adolescents or children enrolled in signing programs. Although these decisions regarding candidacy are based on individual experience and published reports of pediatric implant users, results such as those reported by Sarant et al. (1994) stress the need to assess the potential benefits for each child individually. In that study, two of three congenitally deaf adolescents showed significant open-set scores on monosyllabic word tests using electrical stimulation alone. Additional factors such as the costs of the device, device supply by public health authorities or private insurance, the staff and resources required to manage multiply handicapped children, or the educational options available locally may also influence the decisions on candidacy. The assessment of benefits versus economic costs is an important issue that is addressed in more detail in Chapter 13.

Habilitation is also provided to implanted children through a variety of programs (Allum, 1996). In some, an emphasis is placed on an intensive postoperative program provided in a specially built residential setting at the clinic (Bertram, 1996). Alternatively, habilitation may be provided in a clinic-based intensive rehabilitation program operated on an outpatient basis (Sillon et al., 1996) or through a habilitation program based in a school facility (Barnes et al., 1994). Although the approach varies, in each case the need for intensive habilitation involving the parent as a facilitator has been recognized.

Pediatric programs all involve multidisciplinary cooperation of professionals from diverse backgrounds who possess specialized knowledge relevant to the surgical and medical management of children, the assessment of auditory function in young children, the development and facilitation of auditory learning, the educational management of hearing impaired children, and in the counselling of hearing impaired children and their parents. It has been suggested that the management of cochlear implants in children is best accomplished through establishing a separate pediatric team and clinic facility which is tightly focused and has specific expertise in pediatric assessment and management (Lutman et al., 1996). In contrast,

other programs have stressed that initial experience in the implantation of deaf adults can be a useful prerequisite to implantation of deaf children (Tye-Murray, 1993). Although the need for specialized pediatric knowledge is not disputed, there are a number of advantages inherent in the latter approach. Pediatric team members can acquire experience and skill with the function of the hardware, programming software, and the procedures of the cochlear implant program through experience with adult patients prior to commencing work with children. Although the congenitally deaf child's perceptions may differ substantially from that perceived and reported by a postlinguistically deaf adult using an implant, reports of implanted adults can provide useful knowledge for dealing with mapping problems in the young child.

There can also be social benefits for the young implanted child and parents in coming into contact with adult implant users, raising awareness of the long-term nature of the commitment to implant use and management in children. In addition, it is recognized that the management of young hearing-impaired children and their families can be physically and mentally demanding. The opportunity of varying the caseload with both pediatric and adult candidates can be an advantage in the process of broadening the expertise of clinic staff, through cross discipline training of clinicians. From an administrative standpoint, the ability to share staff, facilities, equipment, technical, nursing, and secretarial support across a combined clinical program allows a "critical mass" of expertise to be achieved in one facility and can yield significant cost savings through avoidance of duplication.

SUMMARY

The selection, habilitation, and management of children with cochlear implants requires a multidisciplinary team of professionals with specialized knowledge in the medical and nonmedical issues relating to hearing impairment. The Clinic coordinates the assessment, selection, habilitation, medical and surgical management and review, and counseling of severely to profoundly hearing-impaired children and their parents who are considering or who have proceeded with cochlear implantation. Through coordination of the activities of the child, parents, Clinic team members, and other professionals, the program aims to facilitate the child's use of the cochlear implant to acquire auditory skills, and to maximize the potential for these auditory skills to enhance speech production, use of language, and general communication behavior.

The concepts of benefit, candidacy, and habilitation approach are fluid and undergoing review in clinics world-wide, as experience and research with cochlear implants in children continues to expand. In particular, the candidacy of children with severe hearing impairment will require careful review of results from severely hearing-impaired adult implant patients, and research to evaluate the comparative benefits of cochlear implants and hearing aids for these children. The use of cochlear implants in babies and infants under the age of 2 years is a further issue that will require intensive research and investigation of the issues of neural plasticity and the potential for the cochlear implant to make a significant impact on language development for children implanted at this early age.

ACKNOWLEDGMENTS

We would like to acknowledge our colleagues Julia Sarant, Shani Dettman, and Karyn Galvin for their comments and assistance in producing this chapter. Many researchers, otologists, audiologists, speech pathologists, educators, speech scientists, engineers, administrative, and technical support staff have contributed to the development and evolution of the Melbourne Cochlear Implant Clinic over the past 15 years. This chapter is written on behalf of, and with special thanks to, all these dedicated professionals both past and present.

REFERENCES

Allum, D. J. (Ed). (1996). *Cochlear implant rehabilitation in children and adults.* San Diego: Singular Publishing Group.

Archbold, S. (1994). Implementing a paediatric cochlear implant programme: Theory and practice. In B. McCormick, S. Archbold, & S. Sheppard (Eds), *Cochlear implants for young children* (pp. 86–102). London: Whurr.

Barnes, J. M., Franz, D., & Bruce, W. (1994). *Pediatric cochlear implants: An overview of alternatives in education and rehabilitation.* Washington, DC: Alexander Graham Bell Association for the Deaf.

Bertram, B. (1996). An integrated rehabilitation concept for cochlear implant children. In D. J. Allum (Ed.), *Cochlear implant rehabilitation in children and adults* (pp. 52–65). London: Whurr.

Blamey, P. J., Dawson, S. J., Dettman, S. J., Rowland, L. C., Brown, A. M., Busby, P. A., Dowell, R. C., Rickards, F. W., & Clark, G. M. (1992). Speech perception, production and language results in a group of children using the 22-electrode cochlear implant. *Australian Journal of Otolaryngology, 1,* 105–109.

Burton, M. J., Shepherd, R. K., Xu, S. A., Xu, J., Franz, B. K-H., & Clark, G. M. (1994). Cochlear implantation in young children: Histological studies on head growth, leadwire design, and electrode fixation in the monkey model. *Laryngoscope, 104,* 167–175.

Clark, G. M. (1995). Historical perspectives. In G. Plant & K-E. Spens (Eds), *Profound deafness and speech communication* (pp. 165–218). London: Whurr.

Clark, G. M., Blamey, P. J., Busby, P. A., Dowell, R. C., Franz, B. K-H., Musgrave, G. N., Nienhuys, T. G., Pyman, B. C., Roberts, S. A., Tong, Y. C., Webb, R. L., Kuzma, J. A., Money, D. K., Patrick, J. F., & Seligman, P. M. (1987). A multiple-electrode intracochlear implant for children. *Archives of Otolaryngology—Head and Neck Surgery, 113,* 825–828.

Clark, G. M., Busby, P. A., Dowell, R. C., Dawson, P. W., Pyman B. C., & Webb, R. L. (1992). The development of the Melbourne/Cochlear multiple-channel cochlear implant for profoundly deaf children. *Australian Journal of Otolaryngology, 1*, 3–8.

Clark, G. M., Cohen, N. L., & Shepherd, R. K. (1991). Surgical and safety considerations of multichannel cochlear implants in children. *Ear and Hearing, 12*(Suppl.), 15S–24S.

Clark, G. M., Dawson, P. M., Blamey, P. J., Dettman, S. J., Rowland, L. C., Brown, A. M., Dowell, R. C., Pyman, B. C., & Webb, R. L. (1991). Multiple-channel cochlear implants for children: The Melbourne program. *Journal of Otolaryngological Society of Australia, 6*, 348–353.

Cowan, R. S. C., Blamey, P. J., Sarant, J. Z., Galvin, K. L., & Clark, G. M. (1990). Perception of sentences, words and speech features by profoundly hearing-impaired children using a multichannel electrotactile speech processor. *Journal of the Acoustical Society of America, 87*, 1374–1384.

Cowan, R. S. C., Brown, C., Whitford, L. A., Galvin, K. L., Sarant, J. Z., Barker, E. J., Shaw, S., King, A., Skok, M., Seligman, P. M., Dowell, R. C., Everingham, C., Gibson, W. P. R., & Clark, G.M. (1995). Speech perception in children using the advanced Speak speech-processing strategy. In G. M. Clark & R. S. C. Cowan (Eds), *International Cochlear Implant, Speech and Hearing Symposium 1994. Annals of Otology, Rhinology and Laryngology*, (Suppl. 166), 318–321.

Cowan, R. S. C., Deldot, J., Barker, E. J., Sarant, J. Z., Dettman, S. J., Pegg, P., Galvin, K. L., Rance, G., Larratt, M., Hollow, R., Herridge, S., Skok, M., Dowell, R. C., Pyman, B., Gibson, W. P. R., & Clark, G. M. (1996, June 6–8). *Speech perception for children with different levels of preoperative residual hearing.* Paper presented at the Third European Symposium on Paediatric Cochlear Implantation, Hannover, Germany.

Dawson, P. W. (1990). Development of a vowel imitation speech perception test for very young children. *Human Communication Research Centre Annual Report* (p. 13).

Dawson, P. W., Blamey, P. J., Rowland, L. C., Dettman, S. J., Clark, G. M., Busby, P. A., Brown, A. M., Dowell, R. C., & Rickards, F. W. (1992). Cochlear implants in children, adolescents, and prelinguistically deafened adults: speech perception. *Journal of Speech and Hearing Research, 35*, 401–417.

Dawson, P. W., Blamey, P. J., Dettman, S. J., Barker, E. J., & Clark, G. M. (1995). A clinical report on receptive vocabulary skills in cochlear implant users. *Ear and Hearing, 16*, 287–294.

Declaration of Helsinki. (1983). *Recommendations guiding physicians in biomedical research involving human subjects.* 18th World Medical Assembly, Helsinki, Finland, June 1964, amended 35th World Medical Assembly, Venice, Italy.

Dettman, S. J., Barker, E. J., Dowell, R. C., Dawson, P. W., Blamey, P. J., & Clark, G. M. (1995). Vowel imitation task: Results over time for 28 cochlear implant children under the age of eight years. In G. M. Clark & R. S. C. Cowan (Eds), *International Cochlear Implant, Speech and Hearing Symposium 1994. Annals of Otology, Rhinology and Laryngology, 104*(Suppl. 166), 321–324.

Dettman, S., Barker, E., Rance, G., Dowell, R., Galvin, K., Sarant, J., Cowan, R., Skok, M., Hollow, R., Larratt, M., & Clark, G. (1996). Components of a rehabilitation program for young children using the multichannel cochlear implant. In D. J. Allum (Ed), *Cochlear implant rehabilitation in children and adults* (pp. 144–166). London: Whurr.

Dowell, R. C., Seligman, P. M., Blamey P. J., & Clark, G. M. (1987). Speech perception using a two-formant 22-electrode cochlear prosthesis in quiet and in noise. *Acta Otolaryngologica (Stockh.), 104*, 439–446.

Dowell, R. C., Dawson, P. W., Dettman, S. J., Shepherd, R. K., Whitford, L. A., Seligman, P. M., & Clark, G. M. (1991). Multichannel cochlear implantation in children: A summary of current work at The University of Melbourne. *American Journal of Otology, 12*(Suppl.), 137–143.

Dowell, R. C., Blamey, P. J., & Clark, G. M. (1995). Potential and limitations of cochlear implants in children. In G. M. Clark & R. S. C. Cowan (Eds), *International Cochlear Implant, Speech and Hearing Symposium 1994. Annals of Otology, Rhinology and Laryngology, 104*(Suppl. 166), 324–327.

Fraser, G. (1991). The cochlear implant team. In H. Cooper (Ed), *Cochlear implants, A practical guide* (pp. 84–92), London: Whurr.

Geers, A. E., & Moog, J. S. (Eds). (1994). Effectiveness of cochlear implants and tactile aids for deaf children. *The Volta Review, 96,* 1–231.

Gibson, W. P. R. (1996, April). *The importance of age in the selection of congenitally deaf children for cochlear implant surgery.* Paper presented at The First Asia Pacific Symposium on Cochlear Implant and Related Sciences, Kyoto, Japan.

Grogan, M. L., Barker, E. J., Dettman, S. J., & Blamey, P. J. (1995). Phonetic and phonologic changes in the connected speech of children using a cochlear implant. In G. M. Clark & R. S. C. Cowan (Eds), *International Cochlear Implant, Speech and Hearing Symposium 1994. Annals of Otology, Rhinology and Laryngology, 104*(Suppl. 166), 390–393.

Luterman, D. (1984). *Counselling the communicatively disordered and their friends.* Boston: Little, Brown.

Lutman, M. E., Archbold, S., Gibbon, K. P., McCormick, B., & O'Donaghue, G. M. (1996). Monitoring progress in young children with cochlear implants. In D. J. Allum (Ed), *Cochlear implant rehabilitation in children and adults* (pp. 31–51). London: Whurr.

Mecklenburg, D. J., Blamey, P. J., Busby, P. A., Dowell, R. C., Roberts, S., & Rickards, F. W. (1990). Auditory (re)habilitation for implanted deaf children and adults. In G. M. Clark, Y. C. Tong, & J. F. Patrick (Eds), *Cochlear prostheses* (pp. 207–222). Edinburgh: Churchill Livingstone.

Nienhuys, T., Cross, T., & Horsborough, K. (1984). Child variables influencing maternal speech style: Deaf and hearing children. *Journal of Communication Disorders, 17,* 187–207.

Nienhuys, T. G., Musgrave, G. N., Busby, P. A., Blamey, P. J., Nott, P., Tong, Y. C., Dowell, R. C., Brown, L. F., & Clark, G. M. (1987). Educational assessment and management of children with multichannel cochlear implants. *Annals of Otology, Rhinology & Laryngology, 96*(Suppl. 128), 80–82.

Osberger, M. J., Dettman, S. J., Daniel, K., Moog, J. S., Siebert, R., Stone, P., & Jorgensen, S. (1991). Rehabilitation and education issues with implanted children: Perspectives from a panel of clinicians and educators. *American Journal of Otology, 12*(Suppl.), 204–211.

Patrick, J. F., & Clark, G. M. (1991). The Nucleus 22-channel cochlear implant system. *Ear and Hearing, 12*(Suppl.), 3S–9S.

Plapinger, D., & Kretschmer, R. (1991). Effect of context on interaction between normally-hearing mother and her hearing-impaired child. *Volta Review,* 75–87.

Pyman, B. C., Dowell, R. C., Brown, A. M., Clark, G. M., Webb, R. C., Franz, B. K-H., Dettman, S. J., Rowland, L. C., & Blamey, P. J. (1991). Revised selection criteria for the multiple-channel cochlear implant. *Journal of Otolaryngological Society of Australia, 6,* 467–471.

Rance, G., Rickards, F. W., Cohen, L., De Vidi, S., & Clark, G. M. (1995). Automated patterns of hearing thresholds in sleeping subjects using auditory steady state evoked potentials. *Ear and Hearing, 16,* 499–507.

Rickards, F. W., & Clark, G. M. (1984). Steady-state evoked potentials to amplitude modulated tones. *Evoked Potentials, 2,* 163–168.

Sarant, J. Z., Cowan, R. S. C., Blamey, P. J., Galvin, K. L., & Clark, G. M. (1994). Cochlear implants for congenitally deaf adolescents: Is open-set speech perception a realistic option? *Ear and Hearing, 15,* 163–168.

Serry, T., Blamey, P. J., & Grogan, M. (1996, June). *Phoneme acquisition in the first four years of implant use.* Paper presented at The Third European Symposium on Paediatric Cochlear Implantation, Hannover, Germany.

Shepherd, R. K., Hatsushika, S., & Clark, G. M. (1993). Electrical stimulation of the auditory nerve: The effect of electrode position on neural excitation. *Hearing Research, 66,* 108–120.

Sillon, M., Vieu, A., Piron, J-P., Rougier, R., Broche, M., Artieres-Reuillard, F., Mondain, M., & Uziel, A. (1996). The management of cochlear implant children. In D. J. Allum (Ed), *Cochlear implant rehabilitation in children and adults* (pp. 83–102). London: Whurr.

Staller, S. J., Beiter, A. L., Brimacombe, J. A., Mecklenburg, D. J., & Arndt, P. (1991). Pediatric performance with the Nucleus 22-channel cochlear implant system. *American Journal of Otology, 12*(Suppl.), 126–136.

Tobey, E. A., & Hasenstab, M. S. (1991). Effects of a Nucleus multichannel cochlear implant upon speech production in children. *Ear and Hearing, 12*(Suppl.), 48S–54S.

Tye-Murray, N. (1993). Aural rehabilitation and patient management. In R. S. Tyler (Ed), *Cochlear implants—audiological foundations* (pp. 87–144). San Diego: Singular Publishing Group.

Waltzman, S., Cohen, N., Gomolin, R., Shapiro, W., & Green, J. (1996, June). *Auditory perception and speech production results in congenitally deaf young children using a multichannel cochlear prosthesis.* Paper presented at The Third European Symposium on Paediatric Cochlear Implantation, Hannover, Germany.

Webb, R. L., Clark, G. M., Shepherd, R. K., Franz, B. K-H., & Pyman, B. C. (1988). The biological safety of the Cochlear Corporation multiple-electrode intracochlear implant. *American Journal of Otology, 9,* 8–13.

5

PREOPERATIVE MEDICAL EVALUATION

GRAEME M. CLARK
BRIAN C. PYMAN

The aim of the medical assessment of infants and children is to determine the cause, severity, and duration of any hearing loss, as well as the presence of any medical conditions that may influence their management with a cochlear implant. There should also be an initial assessment of the child's communication skills and the parental expectations for his or her education.

A thorough clinical history and examination should be carried out at the initial and/or subsequent visits. In deciding whether infants or children are suitable candidates for a cochlear implant they should also receive thorough assessments by a pediatric audiologist and a speech pathologist, and their teacher of the deaf should be consulted.

If the child has no medical contraindications and a severe or profound communication handicap that is not remedied with hearing aids, further assessments will be needed to decide whether a cochlear implant would be helpful. Important medical contraindications are uncontrolled otitis media, autism, severe intellectual disability, and possibly, central nervous system disorders likely to affect the auditory pathways and compromise speech perception.

Special medical investigations would be serological tests to help determine the causes of deafness, X-rays, and possibly, electrocochleography and electrical stimulation of the promontory. In addition, a more detailed assessment of the child's auditory thresholds, speech perception, speech production, and expressive and receptive language will be required. The decision to proceed with a cochlear implant can only be made after a thorough review of all the investigations and assessments, and a consultation to determine whether the parents have realistic expectations for their child.

ETIOLOGY

Genetic

At the Cochlear Implant Clinic at the Royal Victorian Eye and Ear Hospital the causes of severe-to-profound hearing loss in people ranging in age from 17 months to 18 years who have had a cochlear implant have been analyzed.

Many of the children presenting for a cochlear implant at our clinic have deafness of unknown origin (O'Sullivan et al.,

1997) and no family history. However, a significant number may be of genetic origin and autosomal recessive (Gorlin, Toxielo, & Cohen, 1995), and a small proportion X-linked recessive or autosomal dominant.

Dominant inheritance is suspected if one of the parents was deaf. Similarly, if neither parent had a hearing loss, then it is likely to be recessive. With a recessive loss there may, however, occasionally be siblings of the patient with a hearing loss or consanguinity of the parents. In evaluating the pedigree it is important to remember that deaf people often marry deaf people so that two parents with a recessive loss may have deaf children in whom the inheritance will appear to be dominant, but in reality is pseudo-dominant. It has been shown in epidemiological studies that there are two broad categories of non-syndromic recessive loss. They are, first, a loss that is early in onset and rapidly progressive, and second, a moderately slowly progressive loss. Deafness that is dominant may also appear *de novo* when it is due to a mutation. Furthermore, in the case of incomplete penetrance, dominance may not be apparent in the history, as parents and other relatives can be unaware they have a hearing loss if it is unilateral or mild to moderate in degree. For this reason audiograms should be obtained from all members of the family. Deafness may also be X-linked, in which case it is present in the male offspring. Rarely deafness can be due to mitochondrial DNA mutations.

The syndromes associated with a hearing loss are usually hereditary and in most cases the genetic defect affects the development of both the ear and related systems. The degree of expression of the phenotype can vary so that all the features of the syndrome are not necessarily expressed in the child. Some syndromes are, however, sporadic and have therefore not been inherited. Syndromes may also present as two or more types. For example, in Usher syndrome, three types are described

(Gorlin et al., 1995). Type I, divided into A, B, and C groups, has congenital severe-to-profound hearing loss, absent vestibular function, and reduced visual fields early in life. Type II, divided into A and B groups, has congenital moderate-to-severe hearing loss, normal vestibular function, and the onset of visual symptoms in the teens to twenties. Type III has a progressive hearing loss with a variable onset in visual loss.

The cochlear lesion associated with these genetic causes of deafness can vary. The lesion of the inner ear can be a bony malformation in the case of the Michel aplasia where there is a complete agenesis of the temporal bone. The Mondini dysplasia with failure to form interscalar septa has, on the other hand, a decreased number of cochlear turns (Figure 5–1). Deafness may be associated with vestibular abnormalities which can be visualized radiographically. In particular, the commonest anomaly is a widely patent vestibular aqueduct and enlarged vestibule (Figure 5–2). This inherited disorder typically presents with stepwise loss of hearing and sometimes vertigo at the same time as the sudden threshold shifts. The cochlea and vestibule may also be represented as a single cavity as shown in Figure 5-3. In addition, in a number of children with a hearing loss only the membranous structures are affected. For instance, in the Bing-Siebenmann dysplasia both the cochlear and vestibular components are malformed, whereas with the Scheibe dysplasia only the membraneous structures of the cochlea are affected.

The cochlear lesions responsible for a hearing loss may be inherited as autosomal dominants or recessives, and occur both with and without associated syndromes. The Michel aplasia is an autosomal dominant, and can be associated with the Klippel-Feil syndrome. The Mondini dysplasia is usually an autosomal dominant without associated syndromes, but may also be present with the Pendred, Waardenburg, Treacher Collins, Klippel-Feil, and Trisomy

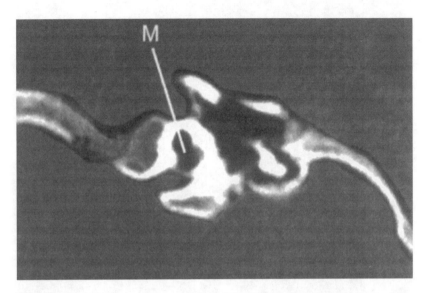

FIGURE 5-1. CT scan of the cochlea showing the Mondini dysplasia (M).

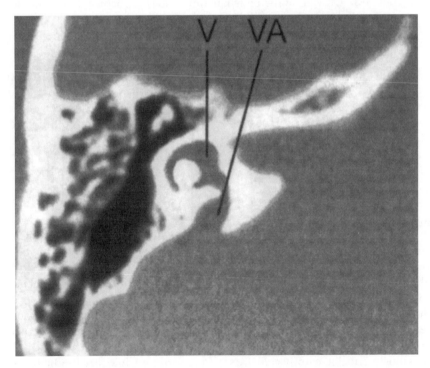

FIGURE 5-2. CT scan of the bony labyrinth with enlarged vestibule (V) and vestibular aqueduct (VA).

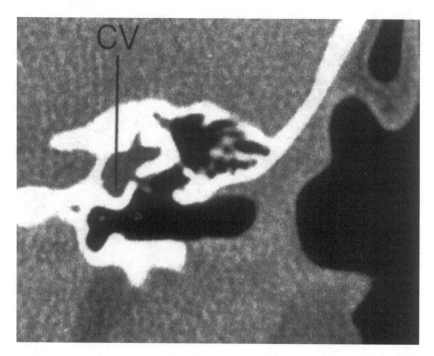

FIGURE 5–3. CT scan of the bony labyrinth with the cochlea and vestibule represented as a single cavity (CV).

13 and 18 syndromes. The Bing-Siebenmann and Scheibe dysplasia are inherited as autosomal recessives, and they too may be present with deafness alone or in association with a syndrome. The syndromes associated are retinitis pigmentosa, Jervell and Lange-Nielsen, Refsum, Usher, Waardenburg, and Trisomy 18.

Acquired

Approximately half the causes of a sensorineural hearing loss are acquired. This may be the result of an infection or conditions occurring during pregnancy. It may also be due to difficulties at birth or conditions after birth. The most common infections during pregnancy causing deafness are toxoplasmosis, rubella, cytomegalovirus (CMV), and herpes simplex (TORCH). In our own study CMV and rubella were identified as the commonest infections causing a hearing loss (O'Sullivan et al., 1997).

Toxoplasmosis results from the ingestion of cysts of the protozoan, *Toxoplasma gondii,* excreted in the feces of the primary host, the cat. The symptoms are nonspecific and flu-like with lymphadenopathy in 20%. There is a 50% probability of transplacental transmission in the first and second trimesters. Up to 10% of infected children have severe involvement at birth, and others have gradual development of retinal and central nervous system (CNS) symptoms and signs. The resulting chorioretinitis can lead to loss of sight, and the CNS involvement to cerebral calcification. Hearing loss occurs in up to 25% of children born with untreated toxoplasmosis. It may be diagnosed by the detection of antibodies in the serum and other body fluids, the presence of IgM antibodies appearing 1 week after the infection, and IgG antibodies 6–8 weeks after the infection.

Congenital rubella is very likely to lead to a severe hearing loss (30% of babies born to mothers with subclinical but laboratory confirmed infection become deaf, and in 25% the hearing loss is progressive). It has also been shown that nearly half the viral infections are subclinical and the effects are most profound if the infection occurs in the first trimester, but second trimester infection can also lead to deafness, microcephaly, cataracts, and mental or motor retardation. Widespread use of the vaccine should eliminate the disease.

Cytomegalovirus (CMV) as a cause of deafness should be determined, as it has been shown that the hearing loss is often severe to profound and can progress, and impaired vision or cerebral palsy, epilepsy, and intellectual disability may be associated. CMV infections are very prevalent and can be detected in 0.5 to 2.4% of all live births (Pass et al., 1980; Spreen et al., 1984); Rasmussen (1990) estimated that 10% of infected newborns are at risk for hearing loss, impaired vision, or neuromuscular abnormalities. Although 90% of cases are without symptoms, there may be swollen lymph nodes and enlargement of the liver and spleen. In children presenting with a severe-to-profound hearing loss, it is considered important to undertake serological tests on both the mother and child as well as viral cultures from the saliva and urine of the child up to the age of approximately 4 years (Lochernini, personal communication). This will help in deciding whether the child has had a CMV infection, and whether it was of congenital origin when the effects are more severe.

Herpes simplex encephalitis is a viral infection usually from genital herpes. It may present neonatally as a localized mucocutaneous or disseminated infection. When it is disseminated there is a 30% risk of meningoencephalitis which is likely to occur in the second or third week of life. Herpes simplex infections leading to sensorineural hearing loss may also involve the central auditory pathways.

The most important infection occurring postnatally that can lead to a severe to profound hearing loss is meningitis. With meningitis there is a high incidence of hearing loss due primarily to labyrinthitis. The incidence, which varies from 5%–30%, depends on the causal organism. The hearing loss is likely to be severe to profound, and may have been exacerbated by the use of ototoxic antibiotics. In addition, the meningitis may have caused specific learning disorders, intellectual disability, loss of vision, motor weakness, and balance problems which will influence the management of the child.

It is also necessary to know whether there has been a history of recurrent middle ear infections as these can result in a severe sensorineural hearing loss or affect the assessment of the hearing thresholds and subsequent treatment. Middle ear effusions would also influence the scheduling of a cochlear implant operation. It is certainly not appropriate to operate if there is any active infection in the middle ear or mastoid, as a labyrinthitis is likely to ensue as has been demonstrated in our animal experiments (Clark & Shepherd, 1984). A low grade infection may also be present with an asymptomatic middle ear effusion, and this should be corrected before surgery.

CLINICAL HISTORY

At the first visit it is important to learn about the parents' expectations for a cochlear implant, and what educational options they have explored. It is necessary to determine when the parents first became aware of their child's hearing loss. A mother having her first baby will be less aware than a multiparous woman that her child has a difficulty. Most parents realize that a child with a severe-to-profound hearing loss has a disability by 6 months of age. At an early age children should respond to their mother's voice, and to other familiar sounds, as well as startle to loud noises.

Next, determine if there are factors in the clinical history that could have precipitated or predisposed to a sensorineural hearing loss. Enquire specifically whether a hearing loss occurred after an illness, which would be the case with meningitis or the childhood exanthemata. Note too whether the mother has been a child care worker, as they have an increased risk of exposure to CMV. Ask if there are other symptoms related to the ear such as discharge or problems with the gait in children starting to walk. It is also important to know whether the baby or infant has any general medical problems such as neural, motor, renal, or cardiac. These may be associated with a hearing loss, and influence the management of the child.

Enquire about events during pregnancy and delivery to determine if there are any factors predisposing to a hearing loss. Ask specifically for evidence of prenatal factors, in particular, toxoplasmosis, rubella, cytomegalovirus (CMV), herpes simplex, and syphilis infections, as well as maternal illnesses such as toxemia. Also determine if there were difficulties with labor, and the condition of the baby after birth, especially the Apgar score. Enquire too if there was jaundice after birth. Jaundice is a symptom of kernicterus, a neurological syndrome due to the deposition of bilirubin in brain cells. The raised level of bilirubin manifests as jaundice, and it is due to the hemolysis of red cells when the antigens of the Rh blood group in particular cross the placenta and produce antibodies in the mother.

A hearing loss will be present in the family history if it is inherited as a dominant gene. More than half the cases of genetic deafness are, however, recessive, and are therefore not usually evident. Enquire also for evidence of X-linked deafness. If deafness has been present in members of the family determine if it has been associated with any other condition such as abnormalities in facial appearance (e.g., Treacher-Collins syndrome), eye disorders (e.g., Usher syndrome), musculoskeletal

disorders (e.g., severe autosomal recessive osteoporosis, or Albers-Schönberg disease), renal disorders (e.g., Alport syndrome), nervous system disorders (e.g., Cockayne syndrome), endocrine and metabolic disorders (e.g., Pendred syndrome), integumentary disorders, (e.g., Waardenburg syndrome), and miscellaneous disorders (e.g., Jervell and Lange-Nielsen syndrome). A detailed description of hereditary hearing loss and its syndromes can be obtained from texts such as Gorlin et al. (1995). Furthermore, not all syndromes are associated with a severe-to-profound hearing loss.

Enquire also whether the infant or young child has reached normal developmental milestones. This is best done through one of the established questionnaires for development assessment. The Denver Developmental Screening Test (DDST), for example, provides pass-fail ratings in personal, social, fine and gross motor, and language development for children from birth to 6 years. It has been reissued as the DDST-II with a greatly expanded language section. This is important because of the relation between language and hearing and cognitive development.

CLINICAL EXAMINATION

The physical examination of the child should commence with general observation of communication skills, demeanor and gait, and by establishing how the child relates to the parent(s). Notice too how the parents relate to each other. This will help provide essential information on how much mutual support they would give if the child was implanted. Observe also any developmental anomalies, particularly in the head and neck, including a cleft palate, that would indicate a syndrome associated with deafness.

In examining the ears it is necessary to obtain a good view of the tympanic membrane. This may not be possible at the initial consultation, but should be completed later after the removal of any wax or debris. This should be accomplished before a complete audiological assessment is carried out. Attention should also be paid to the nose and throat for evidence of upper respiratory tract infection or developmental anomalies.

A general medical examination should also be completed to assess developmental milestones and evaluate neurological deficits. The child's height, weight, blood pressure, and head circumference must always be measured and recorded. The general appearance of the skull can suggest the presence of macroencephaly, microencephaly, or craniostenosis. Examine the head and neck region for any dysmorphic features. In particular, look for evidence of cerebral palsy, congenital syphilis, microphthalmia, cataract, and cranial nerve palsies, as well as cutaneous lesions. Note the condition of the teeth which may indicate antenatal defects or kernicterus. Note too the location of the hair whorl, and the appearance of the palmar creases. The whorl pattern can indicate the presence of cerebral malformations.

A neurological examination in older children can be carried out in much the same way as with an adult. In a younger child, however, information can be gained during play, especially handedness, motor ability, and cerebellar function. After the consultation, if there appear to be any abnormalities, specialist advice should be sought from a pediatrician.

SPECIAL EXAMINATIONS

If the child has a severe-to-profound hearing loss when examined by a pediatric audiologist, then further assessing the child's suitability for a cochlear implant requires objective assessment of hearing, plain X-rays of the skull and temporal bone, and a CT scan of the temporal bone, focusing on the cochlea. An objective assessment of hearing is needed when the child is under 5 years of age, when an anesthetic will be required. An anesthetic will also be necessary for the X-rays. It is best if the X-rays and auditory assessment are carried out under one anesthetic. This will be easier to do if the objective auditory assessment uses a steady state evoked potential (SSEP), or auditory brainstem evoked potential (ABR) procedure rather than electrocochleography.

The SSEP is a noninvasive procedure allowing accurate thresholds to be obtained over the speech frequency range. As originally described by Rickards and Clark (1984), a Fourier analysis is carried out on the averaged EEG activity to amplitude modulated tones. Thresholds are obtained automatically by an on-line statistical analysis of the phase of the response. The thresholds have been shown to correlate well with the behavioral thresholds in children with normal hearing and adults with severe-to-profound hearing loss (Rance et al., 1995).

To obtain thresholds at low as well as high frequencies using the ABR technique it is necessary to average the responses to tone pips and not clicks. Masking noise is required to ensure that the acoustic "splatter" caused by the rapid onset of the tone does not stimulate regions of the cochlea other than that corresponding to the frequency of the tone. With these provisos the ABR also gives a good prediction of behavioral thresholds (Stappels, Gavel, & Martin, 1995).

Alternatively, under some circumstances it may be desirable to carry out electrocochleography. This procedure is invasive and cannot be as readily performed under the same anesthesia as the CT scan. It provides a good signal for the high and even middle frequencies, but an accurate threshold for the low frequencies cannot be obtained because the current from this area of the cochlea is attenuated at an electrode near the round window. Electrocochleography is useful in children where there is a need to explore the middle ear, for example, if a mixed severe-to-profound hearing loss is suspected, and where a Type I afferent dysfunction is suspected (Berlin et al., 1993: Starr et al., 1996).

It is a good practice to also routinely test for otoacoustic emissions. This test is not as useful as the former procedures in assessing the hearing threshold in the low frequencies, but can help exclude the child who has normal cochlear hair cell function, but a retrocochlear lesion including Type I afferent neuron dysfunction.

Plain X-rays of the skull may be needed, but CT scans of the temporal bone are essential. It is recommended that coronal and axial views (horizontal plane) be taken, and they should cover the whole inner ear. The axial views demonstrate the overall relationship of the inner ear to related structures, and the coronal projections are useful for confirming the extent of new bone formation in the cochlea. The features to be checked are the state of development of the cochlea and labyrinth, evidence of a communication between the basal turn and internal meatus if there is dysplasia, the presence of bone in the cochlear turns, the degree of the mastoid pneumatization, the presence of fluid in the middle ear, and aeration of the middle ear. Three-dimension CT scans (Figure 5–4) are also useful for better visualization of cochlear and temporal bone anatomy especially in guiding the surgery. The CT scans used should allow good definition and this requires 1 mm cuts. Finally, if there is any concern that the basal turn is filled with fibrous tissue following labyrinthitis, then it is necessary to carry out an MRI examination.

MANAGEMENT

In deciding whether to undertake a cochlear implant operation it is important not only to be sure the child has a communication handicap that cannot be relieved adequately with hearing aids, but also that the parents will provide a satisfactory home environment for auditory habilitation. In addition, the child's management can often depend on underlying medical problems. The three most common that present at our Cochlear Implant Clinic are multiple handicaps, labyrinthitis due to meningitis, and chronic suppurative otitis media.

Multiple Handicaps

Multiple handicaps present special problems in the management of implanted children. If the child has impaired vision that can be remedied, for example, congenital cataracts, this should be corrected before implantation so that maximum help can be obtained with lipreading. On the other hand, with Usher syndrome and progressive visual loss the operation should be carried out as soon as convenient to provide good lipreading assistance for habilitation before the vision deteriorates.

Diseases of the musculoskeletal system can have implications for the management of implanted children. With the Klippel-Feil anomaly the degree of fusion of the cervical vertebrae is a concern as it will restrict the ability to take coronal X-rays, and make intubation of the trachea for anesthesia a risk. If the child has Jervell and Lange-Nielsen syndrome there will usually be a history of syncopal attacks or fits. The condition, which is manifest as a prolonged QT interval on the ECG, leads to ventricular arrythmias that can result in death, which is a high risk under anesthesia. Therefore, it should be corrected prior to cochlear implant surgery.

When mental retardation is present and of mild degree this will not seriously affect the habilitation program. When the retardation is severe the child will not be able to adequately understand or attend to the commands required for training, and at this stage should not be implanted. In

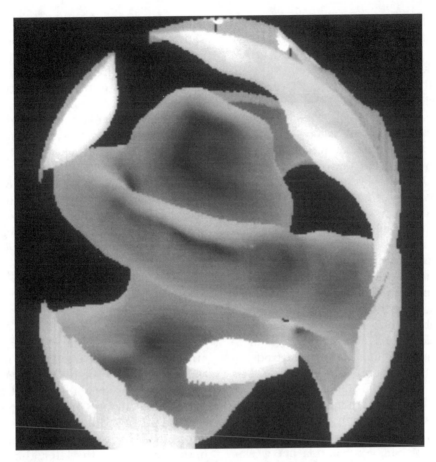

FIGURE 5–4. Three-dimensional CT scan of the cochlea.

assessing the level of retardation an opinion from a clinical psychologist or neuropsychologist will be very helpful. This will be particularly necessary if there are other disabilities such as cerebral palsy.

Labyrinthitis Due to Meningitis

In considering when to undertake cochlear implantation on a child with labyrinthitis following meningitis a number of factors need to be considered. First, it has been shown by Brookhouser and Auslander (1989) that 3 out of 25 children with post-meningitic hearing loss and limited or no auditory responses had an increase in aided thresholds 16–66 months post-illness.

It has been argued that if useful hearing could return then it would be appropriate to wait before carrying out a cochlear implant, especially as the implant could damage hearing. On the other hand, it does not seem reasonable to wait up to 66 months when the child's speech perception, speech production, and language development is going to suffer. Furthermore, cochlear implant speech processing results have improved considerably since Brookhouser and Auslander (1989) cautioned about the need to wait many months before carrying out a cochlear implant.

In postlinguistically deaf adults cochlear implants now provide speech perception scores that are better than some severely profoundly deaf people get with a hearing aid (Flynn, Dowell, & Clark, 1966). Our studies in children (Cowan et al., 1996) have also demonstrated that children with a limited amount of hearing do better with an implant. For these reasons it is not appropriate to wait for many months before implanting a child following meningitis providing the audiological findings show a severe-to-profound hearing loss, and aided word in sentence speech perception scores are less than 30–40%.

The decision when to operate needs to be made on medical grounds. This decision must also take into consideration the need to counsel the family so they can adjust to the hearing loss. There must be sufficient time for the period of "grieving" over the loss. From the medical point of view it is desirable to operate when the scala tympani does not have sufficient bone or fibrous tissue to impede a good electrode insertion. Experimental studies on animals (Dahm et al., 1995) have shown that fibrous tissue starts to form 2 weeks after the infection, and can be quite mature at 6 weeks. New bone likewise develops at 2 to 3 weeks and can be substantial at 6 weeks. The studies also indicate that acute infection can continue for some weeks.

It is important that surgery not be undertaken until the infection has resolved, especially as antibodies will not easily reach the organisms in the scala tympani when there is an accumulation of round cells and development of fibrous tissue. Consequently, although it is an advantage to operate as early as possible so loose fibrous tissue and soft bone can be removed, this should not be at the risk of exacerbating infection. This is a risk if a foreign body in the form of an electrode array is introduced into the infected area. For this reason it is recommended that implantation not occur for at least 6 months. During that time the extent of fibrous tissue and bone production can be monitored with MRI and CT scans. Surgery

could be considered earlier if the CT scan shows significant new bone formation.

Furthermore, there are new improved surgical procedures for managing the new bone and fibrous tissue formation, and these include drilling along the scala tympani, drilling a double barrelled canal along the scala vestibuli and scala tympani and joining the two cavities (Gibson, 1995); inserting an array along the scala vestibuli when patent (Balkany, Gantz, & Nadol, 1988); inserting a split array along each scala; and drilling the bone overlying the scala tympani to exteriorize the cavity for an onlay placement of the electrode array.

Otitis Media and Middle Ear Effusion

If there has been a history of recurrent suppurative otitis media then it is essential the condition be resolved before any implant surgery is conducted. It may remain quiescent for 6 months or longer. We have found in adults after conventional tympanomastoid surgery with a well-healed middle ear 6 months later, that if a cochlear implant is then performed a recurrence of the suppurative otitis could occur 12 months after implant surgery with adverse results (Donnelly, Pyman, & Clark, 1995). It is therefore necessary in some children to be quite aggressive in the management of tympanomastoid infections. Irving and Grey (1994) described an obliterative technique involving creating a radical mastoid cavity, obliterating the Eustachian tube, obliterating the mastoid cavity with abdominal fat, and closing the external auditory canal.

In the case of a middle ear effusion this will need correction before implant surgery. In some children it will resolve with a course of antibiotics, but if not, myringotomy and insertion of grommets will be required. These should be removed a few weeks before implant surgery, and should leave the tympanic membrane healed and the middle ear free of fluid.

In summary, the young child will be considered for surgery only if a thorough otological, audiological, communication, and educational assessment has been made by the implant team. This team management will continue through the child's postoperative habilitation, and continue as long as they have their implant.

ACKNOWLEDGMENTS

We would like to thank Dr. L. Sheffield, Dr. I. Hopkins, Departments of Genetics and Pediatric Neurology, the Royal Children's Hospital, Melbourne, Associate Professor H. McLean, Department of Ophthalmology, The University of Melbourne; and Dr. M. Scott, Department of Radiology, Royal Victorian Eye and Ear Hospital, for their helpful comments; Mrs Sue Davine and Ms Jacky Gray for secretarial help; and Mr Frank Nielsen and Mr Trevor Carter for technical support.

REFERENCES

Balkany, T., Gantz, B., & Nadol, J. B. (1988). Multichannel cochlear implants in partially ossified cochleas. *Annals of Otology, Rhinology and Laryngology, 97*, 3–7.

Berlin, C. I., Hood, L. J., Cecola, R. P., Jackson, D. F., & Szabo P. (1993). Does Type I afferent neuron dysfunction reveal itself through lack of efferent suppression? *Hearing Research, 65*, 40–50.

Brookhouser P. E., & Auslander, M. C. (1989). Aided auditory thresholds in children with postmeningitic deafness. *Laryngoscope, 99*, 800–808.

Clark, G. M., & Shepherd, R. K. (1984). Cochlear implant round window sealing procedures in the cat. *Acta Otolaryngologia (Stockh.),* (Suppl. 410), 5–15

Cowan, R. S. C., Del Dot, J., Barker, E. J., Sarant, J. Z., Dettman, S., Pegg, P., Galvin, K. L.,

Rance, G., Larratt, M., Hollow, R., Herridge, S., Skok, M. C., Dowell, R. C., Pyman, B. C., Gibson. W. P. R., & Clark, G. M. (1996, June). *Speech perception results for implanted children with different levels of preoperative residual hearing.* The Third European Symposium on Paediatric Cochlear Implantation, Hannover, Germany.

Dahm, M. C., Clark, G. M., Franz, B. K-H., Shepherd, R. K., Burton, M. L., & Robins-Browne, R. (1995). Cochlear implantation in children labyrinthitis following pneumococcal otitis media in unimplanted and implanted cat cochleas. *Acta Otolaryngologica, 114,* 620–625.

Donnelly, M. J., Pyman, B. C., & Clark, G. M. (1995). Chronic middle ear disease and cochlear implantation. *Annals of Otology, Rhinology and Laryngology, 104*(Suppl, 166), 406–408.

Flynn, M. C., Dowell, R. C., & Clark, G. M. (1996, December). *Speech perception for hearing aid users versus cochlear implantees.* Abstract for presentation at the 111rd Joint Meeting of the Acoustical Society of America and the Acoustical Society of Japan, Honolulu, Hawaii.

Gibson, W. P. R. (1995). Surgical technique for inserting the cochlear multielectrode array into ears with total neo-ossification. *Annals of Otology, Rhinology and Laryngology, 104* (Suppl. 166), 414–416.

Gorlin, R. J., Toxiello, H. V., & Cohen, M. M. (1995). *Hereditary hearing loss and its syndromes.* Oxford: Oxford University Press.

Irving, R. M., & Grey, R. F. (1994). Cochlear implants in chronic suppurative otitis media: Preparing the septic ear for a sterile device. In J. J. Hochmair-Desoyer & E. S. Hochmair (Eds), *Advances in cochlear implants* (pp. 223–227). Vienna, Austria: Manz.

O'Sullivan, P. G., Ellul, S. M., Pyman, B. C., & Clark, G. M. (1997, March). *The relationship between aetiology of hearing loss and outcome following cochlear implantation in a paediatric population.* Proceedings of the XVI World Congress of Otorhinolaryngology Head and Neck Surgery, Sydney, Australia 1997. Manuscript in preparation.

Pass, R. F., Stagno, S., Myers, G. J., & Alford, C. A. (1980). Outcome of symptomatic congenital cytomegalovirus infection: Results of long-term congenital follow-up. *Pediatrics, 66,* 758–762.

Rance, G., Rickards, F. W., Cohen, T., De Vidi, S., & Clark, G. M. (1995). The automated prediction of hearing thresholds in sleeping subjects using auditory steady-state evoked potentials. *Eye and Ear Hearing, 16,* 499–507

Rasmussen, L. (1990). Immune responses to human cytomegalovirus infection. In J. K. McDougall (Ed.), *Cytomegalovirus* (pp. 221–254). Berlin: Springer-Verlag.

Rickards, F. W., & Clark, G. M. (1984). Steady state evoked potentials to amplitude-modulated tones. *Evoked Potentials II, 163–168.*

Spreen, O., Tupper, D., Risser, A., Tuokke, H., & Edgell, D. (1984). *Human developmental neurophysiology.* Oxford: Oxford University Press.

Stappels, R. D., Gravel, J. S., & Martin, B. A. (1995). Thresholds for auditory brain stem responses to tones in notched noise from infants and young children with normal hearing or sensorineural hearing loss. *Eye and Ear Hearing, 16,* 361–371

Starr, A., Pictor, T. W., Sininger, Y., Hood, L. J., & Berlin, C. I. (1996). Auditory neuropathy. *Brain, 119,* 791–753.

6

PREOPERATIVE AUDIOLOGICAL, SPEECH, AND LANGUAGE EVALUATION

RICHARD C. DOWELL

This chapter covers the main audiological issues that arise in the preoperative selection of children for a cochlear implant. The structure of the preoperative program is outlined, the important issues are highlighted, and practical case examples are used to illustrate the process.

GOAL OF THE SELECTION PROCESS

In order to discuss the preoperative selection of children for cochlear implantation adequately, it is necessary to establish some basic principles about the purpose of the selection process. From an audiological perspective, this can be summed up as follows: Children recommended for cochlear implantation should have a good chance of improved hearing using the implant and a minimal chance of a reduction in auditory ability. This relatively straightforward statement presents a number of major difficulties for clini-

cians. What is improved hearing? Is this equivalent to improving the detection of sounds? To some extent this is so, as a child has little chance of understanding speech through audition if unable to detect the components of speech. On the other hand, detection is a necessary but not sufficient condition for discrimination and recognition of speech sounds. So we cannot equate improved detection with improved auditory ability. We must look further to discrimination, recognition, and comprehension of speech to evaluate the benefit of a cochlear implant. Even the recognition of speech sounds may not provide the desired outcome for children with implants unless this improved auditory ability is incorporated into an auditory language system.

On the other hand, cochlear implant devices are designed to provide improved peripheral auditory ability, and this must be the initial focus in young children in whom speech and language are yet to develop. Thus, it is reasonable to consid-

83

er the sound detection ability of a child preoperatively, using appropriate hearing aids, in comparison to that available with a cochlear implant as part of the selection process. If a cochlear implant is able to provide better access to speech sounds, a child has the potential to benefit from the procedure. A multiplicity of factors will then determine if improved access to acoustic signals leads to speech recognition, speech production, and auditory language development, and where possible, these must also be considered in the selection process.

PARTICULAR PROBLEMS IN ASSESSING YOUNG CHILDREN AND INFANTS

For hearing to be useful, auditory information must reach the central auditory pathways in an appropriate form and the central auditory system must be capable of processing this information in a variety of ways. Despite improved input at the periphery of the auditory system, limitations of the central processing system may prevent the development or improvement of speech perception. This problem is one reason for the motivation in many clinics to implant children as young as possible. The ability of the central auditory system to process speech sounds does not develop adequately in the absence of input. It has been demonstrated that early childhood is when maximum development of speech perception, speech production, and communication skills occurs (Ling & Nienhuys, 1983). Thus, in children with congenital or profound deafness the restoration of peripheral auditory input with a cochlear implant will not necessarily provide the desired improvements in these skills.

The earlier the auditory input is provided or restored, the better the child can learn to use this information. It is widely assumed that the ability for the central auditory system to develop and change reduces with age, an assumption now supported by speech perception results in implanted children (Dowell, Blamey, & Clark, 1995). These are powerful arguments for implanting children as young as possible and this is the clear trend in the clinical application of implants today. Unfortunately, due to the difficulty of obtaining any meaningful measures of speech perception ability in young children with profound hearing impairment, clinicians must make decisions about the potential of a certain level of residual hearing using conventional hearing aids compared with the potential of a cochlear implant. Some approaches to dealing with this problem are addressed later in this chapter.

MAIN CONSIDERATIONS IN THE SELECTION PROCESS

From an audiological perspective there are, perhaps, three main questions to consider in the selection of children for cochlear implantation. Can we provide more auditory information to the peripheral auditory system with a cochlear implant than by using a hearing aid? If so, will the child learn to discriminate and recognize speech sounds with this input? Finally, if they can, is the cochlear implant likely to allow adequate communication and educational development using audition without alternative communication strategies? These questions can be difficult to answer, particularly the third one, but they should be considered in the selection process so that the best possible advice can be provided to parents and other professionals. It is not the goal here to make absolute rules about the selection process but rather to highlight the important issues so that each individual case can be considered in a careful and flexible way.

STRUCTURE OF THE PREOPERATIVE PROGRAM FOR CHILDREN

This section will outline the fundamentals of the preoperative audiological, speech, and language evaluation program with an emphasis on the problems encountered in young children and infants.

Initial Referral

To provide the best possible chance for profoundly deaf children to benefit from cochlear implants, it is important for medical practitioners and health care professionals to be aware of implant surgery as a clinically proven procedure. Dissemination of information about cochlear implants is therefore an important activity for implant clinicians. A problem often encountered in the initial stages of referral for cochlear implant is the amount of inaccurate information about implants in the community. This arises from a number of different sources, including groups who are opposed to implants in children (Balkany, 1993), media information that is exaggerated or incomplete, opinions based on no objective information, or professionals with a little knowledge of the implant field who may consider themselves "experts." For these reasons, it is important to encourage families of hearing-impaired children to come to a specialist implant center to discuss the potential of cochlear implantation for their own child.

As mentioned before, children with profound congenital hearing impairment are likely to develop better speech perception and language skills if implanted as young as possible. Thus, the importance of early referral to an implant clinic cannot be underestimated. Although some professionals involved with hearing-impaired children are concerned that a referral to an implant center will automatically mean surgery, this should not be the case. An early referral allows time to plan the preoperative program, to ensure that preoperative testing is carried out rigorously, and to address all the difficult counseling issues that may affect parents' decisions. The earlier this can be completed, the earlier the child is ready for implantation if they do proceed to surgery. If they are not implanted, it is important that a consistent alternative approach (e.g., total communication or sign language) be initiated at as young an age as possible.

Another task at the time of referral is to obtain and collate existing medical and audiological records for the child. Audiological, psychological, and medical assessments of children are subject to variable interpretation. Due to the effect of hearing loss on other developmental indicators, the assessment of cognitive deficits in these children can be particularly difficult. The aim should be to build up a consistent picture of the child's hearing and medical history.

AUDIOMETRIC EVALUATION

Behavioral Techniques

The assessment of audiometric thresholds becomes more difficult, the younger the age of the child, but fortunately, standard techniques to obtain accurate results are well established for all but the youngest children. The audiogram is of such importance in the preoperative selection of candidates for implantation that it deserves a rigorous approach. The most accurate threshold information for children above the age of 6 to 9 months is obtained using behavioral audiometric techniques (visual reinforcement audiometry, play audiometry), providing the child is well conditioned and in a good response state. In children with severe, profound, or total hearing losses, conditioning may first need to be established using a vibrotactile stimulus before a "no response" can be accepted as no hearing. It is important that behavioral audiograms show a consistent profile. If genuine fluctuations in hearing can be ruled out, thresholds should be within ±5 dB from different test centers or on different occasions. Any inconsistencies should be investigated carefully until a reliable profile is obtained.

Effect of Middle Ear Pathology

An additional practical problem in determining accurate hearing thresholds in young implant candidates is the prevalence of middle ear pathology. Up to 30% of young children may have some degree of middle ear pathology at a particular time (McCormick, 1993; Northern & Downs, 1991). In potential cochlear implant candidates, it is difficult to measure the conductive component of the hearing loss as bone conduction testing is not generally useful in severe-to-profound losses due to the levels required. The effect of middle ear pathology must be deduced from fluctuations in hearing thresholds. This requires repeated testing over time and continuous monitoring of the middle ear status with tympanometry. It is helpful for the audiologist and otologist to work closely together in determining the persistence and effect on hearing of middle ear pathology. In many cases the insertion of ventilation tubes or more radical surgery may be required to clear middle ear effusion or infection and allow accurate threshold measurement. This may be crucial to decisions regarding implantation and will allow children with useful residual hearing to make use of their auditory ability.

Evoked Potential Testing

In recent years, evoked potential testing has become increasingly popular in the assessment of hearing in young children. In particular, click and tone burst ABRs are used extensively in hearing screening programs for newborn and young infants. Although click-evoked ABR testing can provide confirmation of behavioral results, and testing with tone bursts can also provide some frequency specific information, there are limitations in applying these techniques in evaluation of children for cochlear implantation. In profound or severe hearing impairment, ABR responses are often absent at maximum levels despite useful residual hearing in the high frequencies. Brookhauser, Gorga, and Kelly (1990) have shown that up to 40% of children with no response to click-evoked ABR testing at 100 dBnHL have useful aided hearing at 2kHz or above. In particular, there are limitations on the prediction of low frequency hearing from ABR assessments.

Steady-state evoked potential (SSEP) testing (Rance et al., 1995) provides a means of assessing hearing thresholds objectively up to high sound pressure levels (120 dB HL) with frequency-specific responses across the audiometric range. Rance (personal communication) has shown that use of the SSEP technique significantly reduces the chance of a child with useful hearing being diagnosed as totally deaf. Instances of children with useful residual hearing at 2 or 4 kHz with no response to an SSEP assessment are rare (less than 5%). Even with the SSEP technique, it is important that behavioral test results are obtained to support the objective findings. In approximately 2% of children with known risk factors for hearing loss (Rance, personal communication), children with no response to evoked potential testing have been shown to have only a mild hearing loss or even normal hearing. In such cases, mild neural pathology is thought to affect the evoked potential findings but may have only a limited effect on auditory ability.

Additionally, otoacoustic emissions, which are objective, noninvasive, and quick to administer, should be conducted on each child prior to implantation. If the hearing loss is of cochlear origin, no emissions should be recorded for either transient or distortion product stimuli.

In summary, behavioral and objective threshold testing in young hearing-impaired children requires experienced, well trained clinicians. This is becoming particularly important as otologists begin considering the implantation of children under 12 months of age. Separate behavioral assessments should show a consistent profile and be supported by objective measures. Middle ear pathology and other possible causes of fluctuation in hearing must be assessed carefully before threshold results are used in the selection process for cochlear implantation.

Optimization of Hearing Aids

It is important to establish that children being considered for cochlear implantation are adequately aided before proceeding with other tests of their auditory ability. In many cases, the decision to implant young children is based largely on the aided audiograms. The validity of using the aided audiogram in this way relies on the accuracy of the unaided audiogram, the quality of hearing aid fitting and optimization, and the correct functioning and setting of the hearing aids. Careful attention to detail in these areas is important, including the maintenance and calibration of audiometric and hearing aid test equipment.

Real-ear measurement of gain and saturation response of hearing aids can be difficult in children but provides important additional information to combine with the aided thresholds (Rickards et al., 1990). Prescription methods for the setting of gain and maximum power output (MPO) such as the NAL procedure

(Byrne & Dillon, 1986) provide a starting point for fitting hearing aids in young children but some flexibility may be needed to obtain the optimal response in individual cases. For instance, prescription methods can lead to gain settings that are inadequate for accessing acoustic features of speech in individual cases. The main prescription methods now incorporate adjustments for severe and profound losses that reduce this problem (Byrne, Parkinson, & Newall, 1990). The actual everyday acoustic environment of the child should also be considered. The main caregiver may have a particularly soft or loud voice, or background noise levels may be unacceptably high. These problems may be helped by hearing aid adjustments or modifying the acoustic environment. Tolerance problems also must be considered and appropriate adjustments made to the MPO or output limiting. Careful attention to ear molds is often required in young children to prevent feedback in high gain aids. Growing ears may require new ear impressions and special ear mold materials every few months to allow consistent use of the aids. To summarize, the optimization of hearing aids for young children with severe and profound hearing impairment is a difficult process, often requiring compromises due to practical constraints. It is, however, of fundamental importance to address this area thoroughly, particularly as children with more residual hearing are now being considered as possible cochlear implant candidates.

Speech Perception Assessment

Ideally, decisions about implant candidacy in young children should be based on speech perception ability, as is the case for adults and older children. The reader is referred to Busby et al. (1990), Tyler (1993), and Plant and Spens (1995) for summaries of the large number of tests that have been developed to assess speech perception in children. Unfortunately, it is rarely possible to apply standard speech perception tests below the age of 4 or 5 years in severely and profoundly hearing impaired children with associated speech and language delays. Perhaps 80–90% of children being considered for implantation are under the age of 4 years, and therefore, pursuit of formal test results is impractical.

New Techniques for Assessing Young Children

However, there are some new techniques that are beginning to provide some useful information about the auditory potential of these young hearing-impaired children. These involve elicited imitation of syllables to assess the discrimination of syllabic patterns or vowel information (Dettman et al., 1995), and the careful observation of behaviors within the child's play that can be related to auditory input (Tait, 1993). These techniques have been shown to have significant correlations with performance on more formal measures of speech perception in older children but more work is needed before these techniques can provide a complete picture of a child's auditory potential.

Use of Speech Perception Results in Selection

In children who are old enough and have adequate language abilities to perform formal speech perception tests, there is a need to formulate some guidelines to help in the selection process. Many of the tests available for assessing children use closed-set formats and measure specific acoustic phonetic discriminations. The basic auditory skills assessed by such tests are important, but it is the higher level skills involving the recognition of connected speech in an open-set context that are more relevant for assessing ben-

efit from a hearing aid or cochlear implant. Sentence tests are more reliant on language ability than isolated word or phoneme discrimination tasks so the language ability of the individual child must be adequate for sentence recognition for results to be valid. Provided these issues are considered carefully, it is possible to use preoperative speech perception data to compare with results on implanted children to assist with the selection process.

Results in Melbourne show mean open-set BKB (Bench & Bamford, 1979) sentence scores of 32% ($N = 38$, $SD = 29\%$) for children and adolescents aged between 5 and 19 years using the Nucleus implant system. This mean score is conservative as it includes scores for many congenitally deaf adolescents and reflects performance with the MSP-Multipeak speech processor rather than the latest processing scheme. If we consider a subgroup of children implanted before the age of 5 years, the mean BKB sentence score is 49% ($N = 11$, $SD = 25\%$). As the language ability of the younger children is often not adequate for sentence testing, open-set word tests are more appropriate. For the PBK open-set word test (Haskins, 1949), mean scores for 21 children implanted under 5 years of age were 43% (phoneme score) and 15% (word score). Thus, for young children with scores above approximately 40% on either phonemes in monosyllables or sentences preoperatively, the likelihood of improvement with a cochlear implant must be considered carefully in light of other factors. Particularly important is the possible loss of residual hearing in the implanted ear. These considerations will be highlighted again in the case discussions. In reference to our main goals in the selection process, it is reasonable to conclude that young children whose open-set scores do not exceed 20% for sentences or phonemes in monosyllabic words in their optimally aided condition have a good chance of speech perception benefit from use of a multiple-channel cochlear implant.

In most young children with profound hearing impairment, however, speech perception test scores will be poor due to (a) lack of perceptual ability, (b) lack of understanding or the necessary cognitive ability to do the test, or (c) lack of the necessary attention or cooperation to complete the test. Due to these factors, test scores for young children must always be interpreted carefully.

Dilemma of "Good" Speech Perception Performance in Cochlear Implant Candidates

Variation in perceptual ability is well known in adults with severe or profound hearing losses. It is reasonable to assume that this is also the case for children. If a profoundly hearing-impaired child performs relatively well on perceptual tasks, how should this affect the decision to proceed with cochlear implantation? Does it mean that this child is likely to do well with an implant as he or she is showing effective use of limited auditory information, or should the child continue to use his or her residual hearing without cochlear implantation? The information now available on postoperative performance of children with implants suggests that children with better preoperative auditory abilities also perform better with a cochlear implant. In general, it appears that good use of limited auditory input is a positive prognostic factor for cochlear implantation. As long as preoperative results are not significantly better than those obtained for implanted children, implantation should remain an option in these cases. Each child should be considered on an individual basis and the audiometric results viewed in conjunction with other results from the preoperative evaluation including radiological studies of temporal bones, speech and language evaluation, and educational placement.

Otological Evaluation

The otological review should occur early in the preoperative program as there may be medical conditions that affect candidacy for implant surgery in any profoundly hearing-impaired patient. For children in particular, the most common problem of this type is middle ear pathology, which must be treated prior to implantation to reduce the risk of postoperative infection and to enable accurate audiometric information to be obtained. It is also important to perform the radiological investigations of the temporal bone early in the preoperative program, as in rare cases this may change the candidacy of a child who is otherwise suitable. This is particularly important in cases of meningitis where new bone formation within the cochlea is relatively common.

There is often a need for referral to other medical specialists for implant candidates. This occurs when there are other medical conditions present that may be relevant to the success of the surgery, when an opinion is needed for multiply handicapped children, and when serious behavior problems are present or psychiatric illness is suspected. More details on the medical and otological considerations in the preoperative evaluation are given in Chapter 5.

Preoperative Speech and Language Program

Assessment of Speech and Language Ability

Many assessment tools are available to evaluate the speech production and language abilities of hearing-impaired children. These include formal tests of phonetic repertoire, articulation, speech intelligibility, receptive and expressive language, vocabulary, and other speech and language skills (Busby et al., 1990). Although such assessments have been useful within certain research contexts, their clinical use has declined as the number of children being implanted has increased and average age of implant candidates has decreased. Tests that require large amounts of time and provide limited useful information for the clinical management of the children have tended to be discarded. To provide more relevant information, naturalistic sampling of interactive play in young children and conversational samples in older children have begun to replace many of the formal tests. The emphasis is on how the child is using auditory information in his or her normal communication rather than what can be elicited within a formal test. Video-recorded samples can be structured to provide maximum opportunities for meaningful interaction and the child can interact with a parent or clinician depending on the desired information. Analysis of such conversational samples can provide direct information about problems in a communicative context that can be used within habilitation programs. More detailed analysis can provide much of the information more commonly obtained from formal tests, including phonetic repertoire, mean length of utterance, syntactic analysis, pragmatic analysis, and intelligibility (see Chapter 12 on evaluation of benefit). The sampling methods lack the direct control of formal tests but show what the child is actually doing in a communication situation. This information, preoperatively, can be integrated with audiometric results to provide a clearer picture of the child's use of audition. The speech and language assessments may not influence selection for cochlear implantation in all cases but are important in establishing the goals of habilitation programs both pre- and postoperatively.

Preoperative Habilitation Program

There are a number of reasons why the habilitation program should be well established prior to implant surgery. It is important for a therapist to develop rapport with the child and family well before the problems of surgery and programming of the implant are addressed. In young children, where speech perception testing is not possible, preoperative speech and language habilitation can provide information about the child's functional use of audition, and this can be correlated with audiometric information. Such information may be useful in the decision to proceed with implantation. The child's ability to cope cognitively with various tasks also provides useful information about the way to approach programming of the device after implantation. This type of information can only be gained after rapport has been established over a number of clinical sessions.

The preoperative habilitation program aims to facilitate the parent/child interaction during regular one-to-one sessions. In addition to fostering the child's use of the hearing-aid, the clinician aims to improve turn-taking skills and extend the range of early communication intentions. The parent and child should share attention to objects, people, and events as this will form the basis of future communication. The parent's skills in observing, engaging, and reinforcing the child are evaluated. The clinician may intervene if the play interactions are not mutually reinforcing for parent and child or are insufficient for developing communicative competence. Intervention generally involves discussion, modeling appropriate interactions, positively reinforcing successful interaction attempts between the parent and child, and occasionally reviewing videotapes.

Young children with an acquired or progressive course of hearing loss may require habilitation to reduce the effects of the sudden auditory deprivation. For example, the clinician may aim to maintain the child's existing lexicon, voice quality, and phonetic elements during the preoperative program.

This preoperative time also provides an opportunity for the family to become familiar with some of the major issues relating to cochlear implants in children. The parents of the preoperative child are encouraged to meet with other parents of children who have already received a cochlear implant. Where possible, the families are matched for child age and cause of hearing loss. This is also an important time for establishing liaison with schools and educators involved with the particular case. Closer to surgery, the preoperative visits can focus on preparing the child for the stay in the hospital so that he or she has some knowledge of what is about to happen. This can be useful in reducing the family's anxiety regarding the surgical procedure.

In terms of future research and clinical outcomes, it is also important to measure speech and language development as a baseline for postoperative investigations. As it would be expected that developing children will improve over time in many skills despite being profoundly hearing-impaired, two preoperative evaluations are useful to provide a comparison with the rate of progress postoperatively.

KEY ISSUES IN SELECTION FOR COCHLEAR IMPLANT SURGERY

Residual Hearing

It is somewhat difficult to define what the audiological profile for an implant candidate should be, particularly in infants, but it is certainly important to have some way of reaching a decision in children with useful residual hearing. There are two distinct approaches to this problem. One is to set guidelines based on the unaided and optimal aided thresholds and the other is to rely solely on speech perception results.

The approach with adult patients has been to consider preoperative speech per-ception results and compare them with those for implanted patients. By taking into account additional predictive factors for individual patients, an educated estimate of the patient's chances for improved speech perception can be made. As discussed before, there is usually not enough reliable speech perception information for young children to meaningfully compare with postoperative performance of implanted subjects. Even where scores are available, it is difficult to allow for the possible effect of cognitive development and delayed speech and language development on the results.

There is also evidence that children who perform well on speech perception tests despite a profound hearing loss may have relatively greater potential for benefit with a cochlear implant. If preoperative speech perception results are compared only to average postoperative scores without considering the individual child in detail, many children may be ruled out who could benefit significantly from an implant.

An approach based on the unaided and aided audiograms allows a decision to be made based on the detection of the auditory components of speech, irrespective of how well this information is used. By comparing optimal aided thresholds with the long term average speech spectrum, one can at least be certain that a child will have increased access to auditory information with the implant. This conclusion is justified as cochlear implants have been shown to provide detection of most components of speech across the main audiometric frequencies for virtually all subjects (see Chapter 9 on speech processor programming). Following this approach, a child can be considered suitable for cochlear implantation if appropriately fitted hearing aids cannot provide access to the majority of speech sounds under normal conditions. In particular, due to the configuration of most severe and profound hearing losses in children, aided thresholds at 2 and 4 kHz often do not provide detection of speech information. These children have the potential to benefit from a multiple-channel cochlear implant. How the auditory information provided by a cochlear implant is used by the child then depends on a number complex factors, many of which cannot be measured accurately in young children at the present time.

Multiple Handicaps

The main causes of hearing loss in children often produce other medical problems. Meningitis can cause various cognitive deficits. Maternal rubella is often associated with heart abnormalities and visual deficits. Cytomegalovirus (CMV) can be associated with cerebral palsy and developmental delay, along with hearing loss. Many of the genetic syndromes that cause deafness also produce additional deficits such as visual deterioration. Often, the children with these additional handicaps have very profound or total hearing losses, and thus may be the most in need of help via a cochlear implant.

It remains difficult, however, to provide clear recommendations to parents about some of these children regarding cochlear implantation. The long term results do not yet give a clear enough picture of how additional handicaps affect progress with an implant.

A significant cognitive deficit is likely to have some effect on how well a child can learn to use information from the implant. It is unknown how much of a deficit would render implantation useless. It is also difficult to assess such problems in young deaf children. At a practical level, there are certain skills required from a child to enable programming of the speech processor (see Chapter 9). If a developmental or cognitive delay precludes this initial step then the implant procedure would appear to be ill-advised.

Implantation in children or adolescents with visual deterioration also raises some difficult issues. For instance, children with Usher syndrome may become almost totally blind later in life. In this case an implant may help communication while they have partial vision but unless the implant provides enough information for communication using auditory input alone, it may not be as useful when their vision deteriorates. On the other hand, a number of teenagers with this condition have been implanted and are full-time users of their implants despite obtaining very little in terms of speech perception. It would appear to be better to identify and implant children with Usher syndrome as early as possible to provide the greatest chance of obtaining good speech perception through audition.

Psychosocial Issues

For many years, the stability of home life for a hearing-impaired child has been identified as a crucial factor in their progress along with the actual input from parents during their early intervention and habilitation program. At a basic level, if a child's speech processor is not working regularly (e.g., dead batteries, broken cables), there is little chance that the child will receive any useful information from the implant. If they do not receive any useful information, there is no chance of learning from auditory experience. Results for children and adults indicate that a good deal of experience is required before the full potential is reached, underscoring the need for consistent monitoring of the function and programming of the device.

On the other hand, it would be unfair to deny children the chance to improve their hearing, speech, and language through use of an implant merely because of the home situation. There are examples of good results despite a difficult family situation. Assessing these factors is an important part of the preoperative program. Input from social workers and other professionals may be needed to gain a clear idea of whether adequate support will be available to an implanted child. It should be remembered that it would never be considered ethical to deny a child hearing aids due to problems in the home situation.

RELEVANCE OF POSTOPERATIVE RESULTS TO SELECTION

In addition to the results of preoperative evaluations, the long-term results of implants in children can be used in the selection process. Multiple-channel cochlear implants have been in use with children and adolescents for over 10 years. The speech perception, speech production, and language of many of these children have been investigated in some detail (Fryauf-Bertschy et al., 1993; Osberger et al., 1994; Staller et al., 1991; Tobey & Hasenstab, 1991). There is now a body of speech perception results for children using cochlear implants and it is possible to determine some of the factors that have a significant effect on performance.

Comparison of Cochlear Implants with Hearing Aid Users

Boothroyd (1991) showed that children using multiple channel cochlear implants developed speech perception abilities in a range equivalent to children using hearing aids with average hearing losses of 80 to 100 dB HL. The pure tone average hearing losses for most implanted subjects in this study exceeded 110 dB HL. This type of data can be used in the selection process for young children as the unaided hearing thresholds can usually be obtained accurately from 6 months onward with appropriate pediatric audiology, whereas reliable speech perception in-formation may not be obtained until a child is 5 or 6 years old. Osberger et al. (1994) showed that children using multiple channel cochlear implants developed speech perception and production skills that, on average, were significantly better than hearing aid users, with pure tone average thresholds exceeding 100 dB HL after 3 years of experience with the cochlear implant. These results support Boothroyd's data and suggest that a reasonable audiometric criterion for implant candidacy is a pure tone average exceeding 100 to 110 dB HL. These studies, however, show a large range of performance for both hearing aid users with severe or profound hearing losses and cochlear implant users. This range of performance tends to be hidden when only the average results are considered. It may be more useful to investigate some of the factors that are affecting the performance of these children. By knowing more about why results are variable, it is possible to make a more informed decision about implant candidacy than simple reliance on the unaided audiogram. In addition, the implant devices, and in particular speech processing strategies, are improving rapidly. If we rely on data that apply to implant systems from 5 or 10 years ago this will perhaps underestimate the potential benefit of a cochlear implant for a particular child.

Predictive Factors for Speech Perception Results

A review of the speech perception results for 100 children implanted with the Nucleus 22 channel cochlear prosthesis (Dowell et al., 1995) in Australia has been completed. Statistical analysis of speech perception results showed that the duration of profound hearing loss had a significant ($p < 0.001$) negative association with speech perception performance. Postlinguistic hearing losses were associated with better perceptual performance ($p < 0.01$), as was useful preimplant residual hearing ($p < 0.001$). Experience with the implant also showed a significant ($p < 0.001$) positive association with perceptual performance, and an oral/aural educational placement had a weaker association with better performance ($p < 0.05$). There was no significant difference between the results for children with congenital hearing losses and those with acquired losses. Various other parameters relating to differences in the electrical stimulation parameters were not significant. The five significant variables, when included in a linear multiple regression analysis, accounted for 37% of the variance in the speech perception results. This shows that a large amount of unexplained variability remains in the data. Clinical experience suggests that factors such as the child's home environment and additional handicaps contribute to this variability.

Additional studies based on open-set sentence perception results in 38 school-aged children implanted in Melbourne were consistent with the previous findings (see Chapter 12 on evaluation). This study also found that a shorter duration of profound hearing loss, oral/aural educational placement, and hearing experience prior to implantation were associated with better performance to a significant extent. In particular, this study, which considered results of open-set sentence testing, showed a stronger effect of educational placement than previous studies. The ability to understand connected speech within a sentence test relies more on auditory language skills (use of syntactic and semantic redundancy) than other tests which assess discrimination of phonemes or recognition of single words. In this sense these results provide important information relevant to the optimal management of young children using cochlear implants. They highlight the need for an environment where audi-

tion is meaningful if the auditory abilities provided by cochlear implants are to be translated into improved language and communication skills.

The Use of Predictive Factors in the Selection Process

These results provide additional information helpful to the selection process. The hearing history of each candidate should be established as carefully as possible. The effective use of any residual hearing or a progressive nature to the hearing loss provide positive prognostic indicators for use of a cochlear implant. Similarly, a short duration of profound hearing loss is a positive indicator. In most cases, particularly for cases of congenital profound deafness, this means that the earlier the implant is performed, the better the expected outcome. The use of an oral/aural communication mode rather than a totally visual system would also be considered as favorable. Indeed, the use of a manual communication mode would appear to be incompatible with the goals of the cochlear implant in terms of developing auditory language. The dilemma is that many young implant candidates have so little hearing that manual communication provides the only realistic strategy.

Informed Decision-Making Process

These attempts at prediction of outcomes should be treated carefully at the present time and form only part of the preoperative assessment. Individual information about each child particularly regarding multiple handicaps or cochlea malformation may have a much larger impact on outcomes than some of the predictive factors mentioned before. However, it is important to provide the best possible information to parents, which should include predictive information derived from results in other children.

PRACTICAL CASE EXAMPLES

The following case studies bring some of the issues involved in the selection of cochlear implant candidates into perspective. Each case is based on a real example with names and some details altered to highlight particular issues. These cases are not particularly unusual or rare in cochlear implant work and they highlight the need for an individual approach to each case. It is also clear from these cases and others that it is difficult to rule out a particular child as a candidate unless there are compelling reasons that would prevent benefit from the procedure. This means that, in most cases, it is the parent(s) and child who should ultimately make an informed decision about proceeding with an implant. No consideration of the financial problems of funding cochlear implants for children has been given in these discussions. These considerations will vary from clinic to clinic and will obviously have some impact on selection issues. However, it is not possible to treat funding issues in a general sense because of this variation. Thus, it is assumed in what follows that implant devices are generally available.

CASE 1: SUSAN
(AGE: 2 YEARS 6 MONTHS)

History

Susan was diagnosed with a profound bilateral hearing loss at 14 months of age. The etiology was unknown and the loss was thought to be congenital. She was fitted with bilateral hearing aids at 15 months. Susan's mother decided to take an auditory-verbal approach to Susan's management and has worked intensively with this method. Susan has made good progress, given the extent of her hearing loss, and at the age of 2 years, when first reviewed in the cochlear implant clinic, had developed a small vocabulary of intelligible words. She also responded well to some environmental sounds and appeared to recognize familiar sounds around the home. Her parents have heard that a cochlear implant may provide better hearing for Susan and are enthusiastic for Susan to have an implant if she is a suitable candidate.

Main Issues to Be Resolved

There are a number of positive aspects to Susan's case. Her apparently good use of her residual hearing would suggest that she is well placed to make use of information from a cochlear implant. Her mother's focus on auditory communication also provides a good starting point for progress with an implant. However, it does appear that Susan's residual hearing is very useful and it is most important to assess this accurately and make some educated assessment of her auditory potential if she did not have a cochlear implant. This is problematic in a 2 year old as it is difficult to obtain comprehensive speech perception information in order to compare with results for implanted children. The fact that Susan has residual hearing means that she has something to lose as a result of implant surgery, so it is important to have clear audiometric information about each ear in deciding which ear should be implanted.

Investigations

Audiometry showed a profound bilateral hearing loss (see Figure 6–1). Objective audiometry was consistent with the behavioral testing. Evaluation of hearing aids showed useful aided hearing up to 1500 Hz, bilaterally. Both ears had aided thresholds within the speech spectrum but the right ear had slightly better results for the higher frequencies. The hear-

UNAIDED AUDIOGRAM

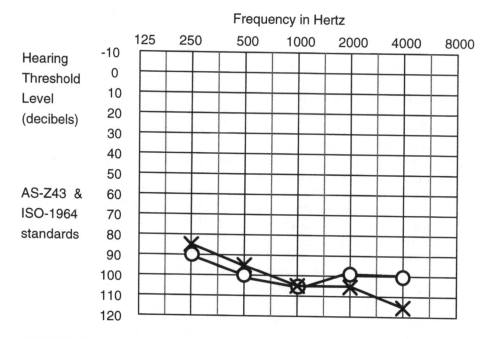

AIDED THRESHOLDS

FIGURE 6–1. Unaided and optimal aided audiometric thresholds for Case 1. Crosses denote left ear results, and circles denote right ear results. The shaded area of the aided audiogram chart represents the long-term average 70 dB SPL speech spectrum.

ing aids were functioning well and were appropriately fitted. Evaluation of video-taped interactive play sessions showed evidence of good pragmatic skills and early use of auditory information. Formal speech perception testing was not possible. CT scans showed normal cochleae on both sides. There was no history or evidence of middle ear problems and medical evaluation showed no contraindications to implant surgery. Susan lived approximately 30 km from the implant clinic and was receiving intensive support from an auditory verbal early intervention center.

Discussion

In this case, it is difficult to claim that a cochlear implant would definitely improve Susan's auditory capabilities and potential. Her aided hearing in the right ear is comparatively good for an implant candidate and she has shown clear progress in the development of speech and language through audition. It is possible that she will develop reasonable open-set speech perception using her hearing which would exceed the performance of at least some implanted children. On the other hand, there are many positive aspects in this case that tend to predict a good result if Susan is implanted. She is young and has some useful residual hearing which she is using effectively. In addition, her communication method and likely educational management are firmly in the oral/aural direction. All of these factors have been shown to correlate with good performance postoperatively. In terms of detection of speech sounds, it is possible to say that an implant would provide better aided thresholds in the high frequency region than Susan's current hearing aids. Given that there are no medical considerations regarding the implantation of either ear, the left (worse hearing) ear would be preferred for implantation.

Outcomes

Susan's parents were advised that there was no guarantee that she would hear better with an implant than with her hearing aids, but that some improvement with the implant was possible. They were also advised that Susan would lose the residual hearing in the left ear if it was implanted. With this information, they decided they would like to go ahead. Susan has progressed extremely well in using the cochlear implant and has developed good speech perception, speech production, and language skills since her implant. She scores 90% for open-set sentence material using the implant without lipreading. She attends a normal school with minimal additional support. She has continued to wear a hearing aid in the right ear and scores 10% for open-set sentences using the hearing aid alone.

CASE 2: CAROLINE (AGE: 14 YEARS 5 MONTHS)

History

Caroline was diagnosed with a profound bilateral hearing loss at 9 months of age. This loss was later found to be due to Usher syndrome, which in most cases causes profound congenital hearing loss and deteriorating vision. In particular, people with this syndrome develop night blindness and tunnel vision which can lead to total blindness by age 50. Caroline was fitted with hearing aids at 12 months of age and had been a consistent aid user. She had attended schools with a predominantly oral educational approach using cued speech, but had also spent 2 years in a total communication setting. Caroline had largely unintelligible speech but had a reasonably complete phonetic repertoire. She had an outgoing personality and was well motivated to improve her hearing with a cochlear implant despite the need for an operation. Her parents were very hopeful that a cochlear implant would improve Caroline's speech.

Main Issues to Be Resolved

As a teenager with a congenital profound hearing loss, Caroline has reduced potential for developing open-set speech perception with a cochlear implant. In general, these patients have struggled to develop good auditory skills, presumably due to the duration of sensory deprivation and consequent effects on central auditory processing. In this case there is the additional problem of deteriorating vision to consider. Even if an implant can provide only environmental sound awareness and assistance with lipreading, this may be of substantial benefit to a person with visual impairment. Looking at this case from another perspective, we know that Caroline will eventually lose most of her vision and unless the cochlear implant can provide an auditory communication channel, then perhaps she would need to learn deaf-blind sign language as a fall-back situation. Clinical experience has indicated that congenitally profoundly deaf patients implanted after the age of 12 years do not show substantial changes in speech production ability, even with long-term therapy. It is most important that Caroline understands the possible benefits of implantation and is well motivated to proceed. It may also be relevant to discuss the views of some deaf adults who are opposed to cochlear implantation, particularly if Caroline has many deaf friends.

Investigations

Audiometry showed a total bilateral hearing loss (see Figure 6–2). Hearing aid evaluation with the most powerful hearing aids available showed no useful aided hearing thresholds within the speech spectrum. CT scans of the temporal bones showed no abnormalities of the cochlea on either side. Promontory stimulation gave a positive result on both sides although Caroline was not sure that the sensation was hearing until halfway through the test. This test increased her motivation to have an implant as she found the "hearing" sensations quite pleasant. Aided speech perception assessment was not possible due to the very poor aided thresholds. Equivalent language age as determined from vocabulary testing was 5 years. Medical evaluation showed no evidence of middle ear disease and no contraindications to implant surgery. During the evaluation it became clear that Caroline did not know that her vision, which was already poor, was likely to deteriorate further.

Outcomes

After a good deal of discussion and counseling with Caroline and her parents, they decided to proceed with the implant. Caroline was advised that the implant may provide some improvement in conjunction with lipreading and for environmental awareness but would not provide auditory alone communication. It was also explained that changes in speech intelligibility were unlikely. Caroline, in contrast to many implanted adolescents, has maintained consistent use of the implant system for over 7 years. As predicted, speech perception is limited to closed-set vowel and consonant discrimination and some assistance to lipreading. Caroline reports that the implant keeps her in touch with her environment and she would not be without it. In this case, the success of the procedure was probably related to the strong motivation of the patient and the visual problems, which created a situation where any additional input was welcome.

UNAIDED AUDIOGRAM

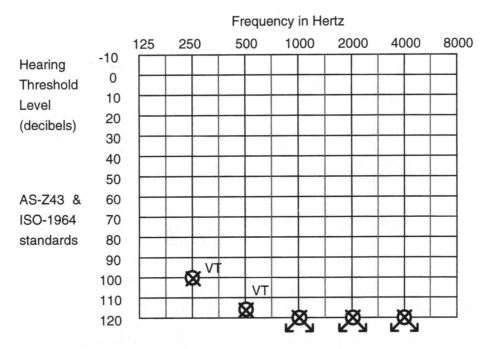

AIDED THRESHOLDS

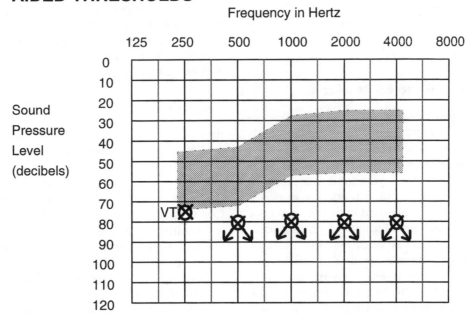

FIGURE 6-2. Unaided and optimal aided audiometric thresholds for Case 2. Crosses denote left ear results, and circles denote right ear results. The shaded area of the aided audiogram chart represents the long-term average 70 dB SPL speech spectrum.

CASE 3: ANGELA
(AGE: 5 YEARS 6 MONTHS)

History

Angela was born with multiple medical problems and was not expected to survive. She was subsequently diagnosed with cytomegalovirus (CMV). Following lengthy hospitalization, her main medical problems were resolved. However, CT scans provided direct evidence of brain damage. Severe motor problems and/or cognitive delay were anticipated. Total bilateral hearing loss was confirmed at 12 months of age. Angela made better developmental progress than expected, although motor development was delayed and restricted due to spastic muscle tone on the right side. Cognitive development had been difficult to assess due to the hearing loss. Although Angela was fitted with powerful hearing aids she had shown no evidence of effective use of audition and was fitted with a vibrotactile aid. Her mother had provided very intensive help for Angela and was generally positive about her potential.

Main Issues to Be Resolved

Apart from the normal preoperative assessments and issues involved, Angela's case poses additional concerns. She has had multiple medical problems leading to motor difficulties, general developmental delay, and possible intellectual deficits. We must be concerned about the effect of Angela's multiple handicaps on her ability to learn to use auditory information. Motor problems may impact on the potential for speech development. To a large extent, such effects are obscured by the profound deafness, which in itself prevents assessment of auditory processing and produces language and speech delays. Nonverbal cognitive testing may provide useful information but an accurate

prediction of benefit from implantation is difficult. Again, it would appear to be important to address these issues with the parent and attempt to ensure realistic expectations if an implant is performed.

Investigations

Audiometry showed a total bilateral hearing loss (see Figure 6–3). This was confirmed by objective testing. Aided speech perception testing was not possible due to the degree of hearing loss. CT scans showed no abnormality of the cochlea on either side. Angela had no spoken language at preoperative evaluation. She had a signing vocabulary of approximately 50 signs. She had attended an oral preschool but this center had advised that Angela move to a total communication setting. Psychological evaluations were inconsistent, with some reports suggesting below normal functioning on cognitive tasks, and others reporting age-appropriate performance. Teachers at Angela's school were openly opposed to cochlear implantation in her case. Medical evaluation showed no contraindication to implant surgery and there was no history of middle ear problems.

Discussion

In cases such as Angela's, a first approach may be to review all available information and decide whether she has any chance of benefiting from an implant. If Angela was considered to be unable to function at a level that would allow programming of the device, then it would seem ill-advised to proceed. On the other hand, it could be argued that a multiply handicapped child deserves as much help as possible and Angela is clearly profoundly deaf. Expectations from a cochlear implant may be limited, but if Angela is capable of cooperating with programming of the device and has some learning potential, she may show significant bene-

UNAIDED AUDIOGRAM

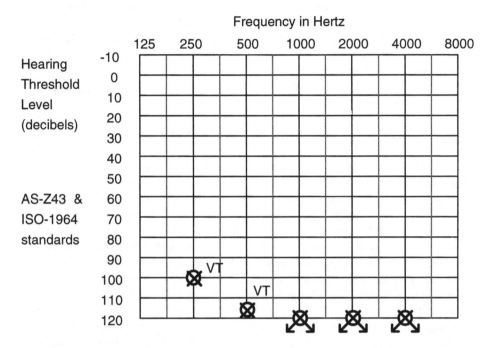

AIDED THRESHOLDS

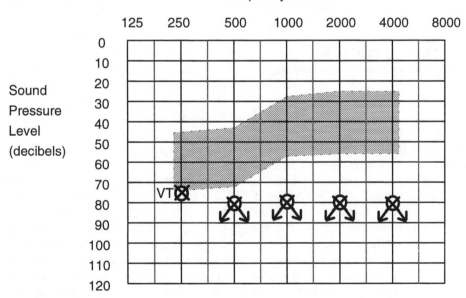

FIGURE 6–3. Unaided and optimal aided audiometric thresholds for Case 3. Crosses denote left ear results, and circles denote right ear results. The shaded area of the aided audiogram chart represents the long-term average 70 dB SPL speech spectrum.

fit. The issues raised by this case become particularly difficult at many clinics where the funding for implant devices is limited. Does one provide implants only for children who, based on preoperative assessment, have the best chance of success, or should one assess the individual needs of each child and attempt to provide help where it is most needed?

Outcomes

Angela was implanted after lengthy discussion among clinicians and many couseling sessions with her mother. She has progressed slowly but steadily with use of the implant and has achieved some open-set speech perception at a single word level. Her speech has also improved slowly but has not progressed past a single word stage. She uses some sign language for communication at home and at school. Although Angela will probably always rely on some sign language and will struggle to interact independently in the hearing world, there is no doubt that the implant has provided significant benefit.

CASE 4: GEOFFREY (AGE: 16 YEARS 2 MONTHS)

History

Geoffrey was born with a bilateral, moderate to severe hearing loss and had been fitted with hearing aids from the age of 2 years. He made good use of his hearing aids, attended regular school, and developed normal speech and language except for a few speech production errors. His hearing deteriorated to a severe to profound loss when he was 10 years old, although he could still make good use of more powerful hearing aids. He was now attending a high school which had a special unit for hearing-impaired students using total communication. Next year he will be in his final year of high school and his results will determine his later study or career opportunities. He and his parents would like him to have the cochlear implant so as to give him the best possible chance in his studies.

Main Issues to Be Resolved

Based on the predictive factors for which there is some information, Geoffrey's hearing history makes him an excellent candidate for cochlear implant. Despite having a hearing loss early in his life, he can be considered to be postlinguistically deafened, as he has developed essentially normal speech and language through use of his hearing. His residual hearing must be assessed carefully to ensure that he does stand to benefit from implantation. Geoffrey's motivation is also important. Many hearing-impaired teenagers of his age are beginning to assert their independence, which can take the form of a move toward the Deaf culture and sign language despite good oral skills. If these issues are resolved, the choice of when to have the implant becomes important. Is it advisable to have the procedure at this crucial time in his education? Most children and many adults take several months or years to reach their full potential. Would this be more disruptive than helpful for his final high school year?

Investigations

Audiometry showed a severe to profound loss bilaterally, which was worse in the left ear (see Figure 6–4). Aided threshold testing with his current aids showed useful hearing to 2000 Hz in the right ear and to 1000 Hz in the left. Aided speech perception testing showed the following results. Open-set (BKB) sentences: audition alone—18% (R), 6% (L), 20% (BIN); lipreading alone—74%; lipreading with audition—98% (R), 96% (L), 92% (BIN).

UNAIDED AUDIOGRAM

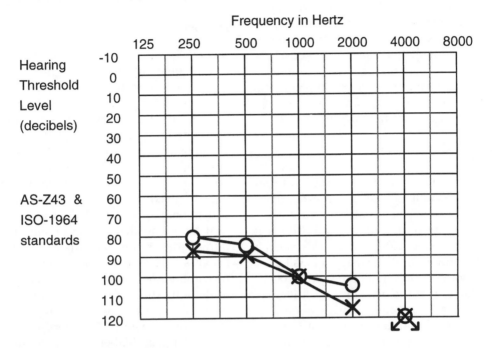

AIDED THRESHOLDS

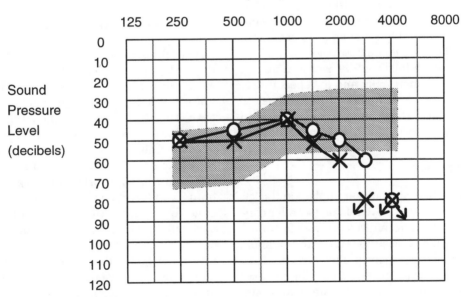

FIGURE 6-4. Unaided and optimal aided audiometric thresholds for Case 4. Crosses denote left ear results, and circles denote right ear results. The shaded area of the aided audiogram chart represents the long-term average 70 dB SPL speech spectrum.

Promontory testing gave a good positive result on both sides. CT scans showed no abnormality of the cochlea on either side. Medical evaluation showed no contraindications to implant surgery and there was no evidence of middle ear disease. Discussions with Geoffrey showed that he was enthusiastic about having the cochlear implant, and was unconcerned that some of his hearing-impaired peers may be opposed to implants.

Discussion

As already mentioned, it is important that Geoffrey is well motivated. The other main issues in this case are the residual hearing and the timing of implantation if it goes ahead. Although Geoffrey's speech perception with his hearing aids is better than some children achieve with a cochlear implant at the present time, it is more appropriate to compare his speech perception performance with adult implant scores. With improvements in speech processing, mean performance for postlinguistically deafened adults is at least 50% for open-set sentences. In this light, Geoffrey stands to improve his speech perception considerably if the surgery goes well. The left ear would be the choice for implantation as it has slightly worse hearing, both audiometrically and for speech perception, but it is important for Geoffrey to understand that the residual hearing in this ear will be lost following implantation.

Outcomes

Geoffrey had his cochlear implant in the left ear prior to his last year at school after considering the alternatives. He was fortunate to have a successful result within a short time period. Six months after surgery, Geoffrey was able to score over 90% for open-set sentence testing using the implant alone. He found the improved speech perception helpful for his studies and went on to study at a university.

CASE 5: MABEL
(AGE: 5 YEARS 3 MONTHS)

History

Mabel was diagnosed with a profound bilateral hearing loss at 12 months and aided soon after this. Later investigations showed the cause of deafness to be maternal rubella. She was referred to the cochlear implant clinic due to a lack of progress with her speech production and language at the age of 5 years. At this stage, she was attending a preschool for hearing-impaired children that used an oral educational approach. There was concern that Mabel needed a visual communication mode as she had made very little progress despite relatively good aided hearing. Mabel's parents were desperate to do something about these problems, particularly the lack of progress with speech and language. Teachers at the preschool felt that Mabel was a "visually oriented child" and did not attend well to auditory input.

Main Issues to Be Resolved

This child provides a typical example of the cochlear implant as the "last hope" for a hearing-impaired child following the failure of a particular approach, in this case, the use of residual hearing in an oral/aural preschool. One issue here is why the failure has occurred. This could be due to poor central processing of auditory input, inappropriate management at home and/or at the preschool, a preference for visual input over auditory (as suggested by teachers), or a combination of these factors. If poor central processing is a major factor then a cochlear implant may show similar poor results. This may or may not be determinable from preoperative assessments. Additionally, this child now has very delayed speech and language development. A successful result with the implant in terms of speech perception may not guarantee that speech production and language will catch up. The amount of residual hearing is again important in this case, but in an unusual way. The audiometric results may show relatively good thresholds that make the decision for an implant difficult. On the other hand, reports suggest that this hearing is not being used effectively for communication. The dilemma is that to not perform an implant because the hearing is "too good" would probably close off the oral/aural approach for this child.

Investigations

Audiometry showed a severe to profound hearing loss with better thresholds in the left ear. Aided assessment showed thresholds within the speech spectrum to 2000 Hz in the left ear and to 1000 Hz in the right (see Figure 6–5). Aided speech perception was very poor initially, with no clear discrimination of suprasegmental aspects of speech. Due to this poor speech perception, retrocochlear pathology was suspected, but further investigations did not reveal any neurological or central abnormalities. Mabel underwent 6 months of intensive auditory training with a clinician from the implant clinic, and at the end of this time, speech perception testing showed results more consistent with her aided hearing (for instance, discrimination of vowels differing in first formants). CT scans were normal. Mabel had a history of chronic middle ear infection and the right ear had a large central perforation. Medical investigations did not reveal any other contraindications for implant surgery.

Discussion

The investigations have indicated that, with appropriate habilitation strategies, this child was able to use her residual hearing effectively. Her lack of progress in an oral setting may well have been due to a preference for or reliance on visual information. Provided the middle ear problems can be resolved satisfactorily (this may require surgery), the question remains as to whether a cochlear implant will provide additional help. It can be argued that an implant would provide access to high frequency speech sounds that Mabel is unable to detect at present. It is possible that the improvement in auditory abilities will be minimal. As the hearing is slightly worse in the right ear, this would be the first choice for implantation following otological management of the middle ear disease.

Outcomes

Following extensive discussion, Mabel's parents decided to proceed with implantation in the right ear. Mabel showed good progress in speech and language areas almost immediately. Her speech perception improved over a number of years to current scores (5 years postimplant) of approximately 50% for open-set sentences. Mabel has attended a normal primary school for the last 3 years, although speech and language abilities remain significantly delayed.

CASE 6: PAUL (AGE: 2 YEARS 1 MONTH)

History

Paul was a normal hearing baby who contracted bacterial meningitis at the age of 18 months. A profound bilateral hearing loss was diagnosed soon after his recovery. The parents were referred to the cochlear implant clinic 2 months later. At this stage Paul was having severe behavioral problems and they expressed a lack of confidence in the medical profession. Paul had normal speech development

UNAIDED AUDIOGRAM

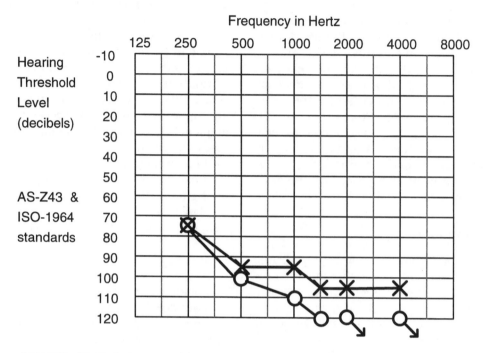

AIDED THRESHOLDS

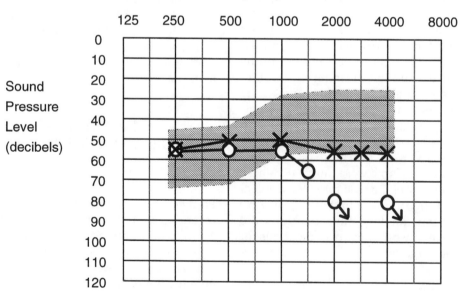

FIGURE 6–5. Unaided and optimal aided audiometric thresholds for Case 5. Crosses denote left ear results, and circles denote right ear results. The shaded area of the aided audiogram chart represents the long-term average 70 dB SPL speech spectrum.

prior to his illness, but had been virtually silent since leaving the hospital.

Main Issues to Be Resolved

One important issue raised by this case is the distress and anger that may be present for parents whose child has been through meningitis. The loss of speech and communication skills is also devastating to parents and behavioral problems due to frustration and/or neurological damage are common. In terms of the hearing loss, there is some possibility of recovery of hearing thresholds following meningitis although there are no documented cases where a total loss has recovered to a significant degree. It has been suggested that there should be a wait of 12 months or more before implantation is considered in case of hearing recovery. Conversely, there is an urgent need to restore hearing, if possible, to regain lost ground in speech and language development. In addition, there is evidence that ossification of the cochlea following meningitis is progressive over time and in many cases it is important to proceed with surgery as soon as possible. Ossification may be present soon after the meningitis so it is important that the otological review and radiological investigations are performed early in the program. Thus, there are a number of competing issues in these cases. The need for the parents to come to terms with their child's problems and overcome the behavioral difficulties requires some time, but the loss of speech and language skills and the possibility of cochlear ossification creates some urgency about proceeding with an implant.

Investigations

Audiometry (visual reinforcement testing) suggested a total hearing loss, bilaterally (see Figure 6–6). Objective audiometric assessment was also consistent with a total

hearing loss. Aided assessment did not show any useful thresholds within the speech spectrum with powerful aids. CT scans showed the right cochlea to be obliterated with new bone formation and unsuitable for implant surgery. The left cochlea showed signs of new bone formation in the basal turn but appeared to be implantable. Attempts to assess speech and language met with a lack of cooperation and aggressive behavior from Paul. There were no medical contraindications to implant surgery, but there was a history of middle ear infections during the previous winter.

Discussion

Careful pediatric audiological assessment has shown that Paul is an implant candidate in terms of hearing. The total hearing loss and degree of ossification in both cochleae would make a recovery of useful hearing extremely unlikely. The remaining issues center around the timing of the procedure. As already mentioned, proceeding immediately with an implant may be best for avoiding additional ossification but this may not give adequate time to resolve Paul's behavioral problems and allow his parents to be comfortable with the decision. The fact that only the left ear is suitable for implantation and that an optimum surgical result may not be possible in this ear due to the ossification is important information for his parents to understand. They may also need to understand that even a good result is unlikely to restore Paul's communication in the short term.

Outcomes

Paul's parents decided to proceed with the implant as soon as possible. A good surgical result was obtained in the left ear. The immediate postoperative programming and habilitation was difficult due to continuing behavioral problems, but Paul

UNAIDED AUDIOGRAM

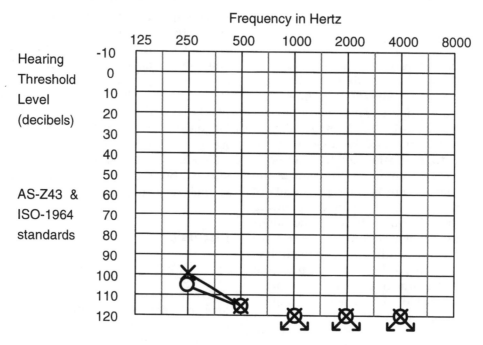

AIDED THRESHOLDS

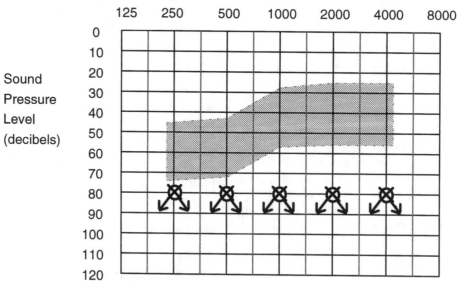

FIGURE 6-6. Unaided and optimal aided audiometric thresholds for Case 6. Crosses denote left ear results, and circles denote right ear results. The shaded area of the aided audiogram chart represents the long-term average 70 dB SPL speech spectrum.

slowly began to make some progress and as some communication was restored his behavior improved. Five years after implantation, Paul shows scores of 70% for open-set sentences but still has some degree of speech and language delay. His parents hope he will be fully integrated at a regular school within the next year.

CONCLUSION

The basic audiological questions that must be addressed in the selection of children for cochlear implantion have been introduced here and illustrated in practical examples. Many of the issues are complex, particularly in young children, but an attempt has been made to formulate guidelines for the selection process based on preoperative information and consideration of individual characteristics. A careful approach to the preoperative audiological evaluation will provide reliable information that can be used in deciding whether a child has potential to benefit from a cochlear implant. Additional information is provided by comparison of preoperative evaluations with predictive factors determined from long-term results. Speech and language assessment can also provide useful information for pre- and postoperative management and confirmation of audiological and medical findings. It remains difficult to predict accurately whether a child will maximize his or her auditory potential in the long term, but a careful informed consent process involving the child's family should provide a realistic and positive framework for the long-term communication development of the child.

REFERENCES

Balkany, T. (1993). A brief perspective on cochlear implants. *New England Journal of Medicine, 328,* 281–282.

Bench, R. J., & Bamford, J. (Eds.). (1979). *Speech-hearing tests and the spoken language of hearing-impaired children.* London: Academic Press.

Boothroyd, A. (1991). Assessment of speech perception capacity in profoundly deaf children. *American Journal of Otology, 12*(Suppl.), 67–72.

Brookhauser, P. E., Gorga, M. P., & Kelly, W. J. (1990). Auditory brainstem response results as predictors of behavioral auditory thresholds in severe and profound hearing impairment, *Laryngoscope, 100,* 803–810.

Busby P. A., Dettman, S. J., Altidis, P. M., Blamey, P. J., & Roberts S. A. (1990). Assessment of communication skills in implanted deaf children. In G. M. Clark, Y. C. Tong, & J. F. Patrick (Eds.), *Cochlear prostheses* (pp. 223–236). Edinburgh: Churchill Livingstone.

Byrne, D., & Dillon, H. (1986). The National Acoustic Laboratories' new procedure for selecting the gain and frequency response of a hearing aid. *Ear and Hearing, 7*(4), 257–265.

Byrne, D., Parkinson, A., & Newall, P. (1990). Hearing aid gain and frequency response requirements for the severely/profoundly hearing-impaired. *Ear and Hearing, 11*(1), 40–49.

Dettman, S. J., Barker E. J., Dowell R. C., Dawson P. W., Blamey P. J., & Clark G. M. (1995). Vowel imitation task: Results over time for 28 cochlear implant children under the age of eight years. *Annals of Otology, Rhinology and Laryngology, 104*(9), (Suppl. 166), 321–324.

Dowell, R. C., Blamey, P. J., & Clark, G. M. (1995). Potential and limitations of cochlear implants in children. *Annals of Otology, Rhinology and Laryngology, 104*(9), (Suppl. 166), 324–327.

Fryauf-Bertschy, H., Tyler, R. S., Kelsay, D. M., & Gantz, B. J. (1993). Performance over time of congenitally deaf and postlingually deafened children using a multichannel cochlear implant. *Journal of Speech and Hearing Research, 35,* 186–203.

Haskins, J. (1949). Kindergarten Phonetically Balanced Word Lists (PBK). St Louis: Auditec.

Ling, D., & Nienhuys, T. G. (1983). The deaf child: Habilitation with and without a cochlear implant. *Annals of Otology, Rhinology and Laryngology, 92,* 593–598.

McCormick, B. (Ed.). (1993). *Paediatric audiology 0–5 years.* London: Whurr Publishers.

Northern, J. L., & Downs, M. P. (1991). *Hearing in children.* Baltimore: Williams & Wilkins.

Osberger, M. J., Robbins, A. M., Todd, S. L., Riley, A. I., & Miyamoto, R. T. (1994). Speech production skills of children with multichannel cochlear implants. In I. J. Hochmair-Desoyer & E. S. Hochmair (Eds.), *Advances in cochlear implants* (pp. 503–508). Vienna: Manz.

Plant, G., & Spens, K-E. (Eds.). (1995). *Profound deafness and speech communication.* London: Whurr Publishers.

Rance, G., Rickards, F. W., Cohen T., DeVidi, S., & Clark G. M. (1995). The automated prediction of hearing thresholds in sleeping subjects using auditory steady-state evoked potentials. *Ear and Hearing, 16,* 499–507.

Rickards, F. W., Dettman, S. J., Busby, P. A., Webb, R. L., Dowell R. C., Dennehy, S. E., &

Nienhuys, T. G. (1990). Preoperative evaluation and selection of children and teenagers. In G. M. Clark, Y. C. Tong, & J. F. Patrick (Eds.), *Cochlear prostheses* (pp. 135–152). Edinburgh: Churchill Livingstone.

Staller, S. J., Dowell, R. C., Beiter, A. L., & Brimacombe, J. A. (1991). Perceptual abilities of children with the Nucleus 22-channel cochlear implant. *Ear and Hearing 12*(4) (Suppl.), 34–47.

Tait, D. M. (1993). Video analysis: A method of assessing changes in preverbal and early linguistic skills after cochlear implantation. *Ear and Hearing, 14*(6), 378–389.

Tobey, E. A., & Hasenstab, S. (1991). Effect of a Nucleus multichannel cochlear implant upon speech production in children. *Ear and Hearing 12*(4 (Suppl.), 48–54.

Tyler, R. S. (Ed.), (1993). *Cochlear implants: Audiological foundations.* San Diego: Singular Publishing Group.

7

SURGERY

GRAEME M. CLARK
BRIAN C. PYMAN
ROBERT L. WEBB

Cochlear implant surgery should be undertaken only after the cochlear implant team has established that the child is not achieving useful communication with a hearing aid. This can be difficult because of poor language development in deaf children in this age group, or because the child is at a preverbal stage and too young for the use of formal assessment tests. The child's unaided and aided thresholds, however, are important for assessment, as are his or her communication skills. These need to be evaluated by an experienced pediatric audiologist. Their assessment is discussed in detail in Chapter 6.

In addition, surgery should only be undertaken if there are no medical contraindications. The most important of these are uncontrolled otitis media, autism, severe mental retardation, and possibly, central nervous system disorders affecting the auditory pathways so that speech perception is likely to be poor. In addition, middle ear effusion will delay surgery, and the status of the middle ear will need to be confirmed with tympanometry and otoscopy.

The surgery for infants and children has evolved in the first instance from the procedures developed for adults. The surgery for the implantation of the first prototype multiple-channel cochlear implant and banded electrode array (fabricated by The University of Melbourne) was outlined by Clark, Pyman, and Bailey (1979). The claw used for its insertion was described in this paper. The modifications to the procedure for implanting the first Nucleus receiver-stimulator and banded electrode for clinical trial were outlined by Clark et al. (1984). The surgery for the safe insertion and reinsertion of the banded array was discussed by Clark et al. (1987). In 1990 there was a description of the surgery for multiple-channel cochlear implantation using the CI-22M receiver-stimulator, now part of the Nucleus-22 system. The use of the platinum electrode tie was outlined by Webb et al. (1990). The modifications of the surgical procedure required for implanting the Nucleus CI-22M receiver-stimulator in children 2 years of age and older were outlined by Clark, Cohen, and Shepherd (1991). The following text provides more details for the surgery for the receiver-stimulator in the Nucleus-22 system for children and outlines the surgery for the thinner receiver-stimulator (CI-24M) in the Nucleus-24 system that can be used for infants and young children as well as for older children and adults.

ANESTHETIC AND PREOPERATIVE PREPARATION

During the preoperative medical assessment for the anesthetic the anesthetist will find it is difficult to communicate with the deaf child verbally, and should use an open, friendly approach with the parents, as this will help establish rapport with the child, and gain the family's confidence. If the preoperative assessment reveals a temperature greater than 38°C, due to, for example, an upper respiratory tract infection, not only does this predispose to a postoperative chest infection, but the elevated temperature can render a child susceptible to poor temperature control intraoperatively. The operation should be postponed under these circumstances.

The anesthetist should be aware that the child may also have a syndrome associated with deafness that could lead to anesthetic difficulties. Enquire specifically if the child has had a history of fainting or seizures as this may indicate the presence of Jervell and Lange-Nielsen syndrome. An ECG is needed to exclude this syndrome, which can lead to fatal cardiac irregularities developing during surgery. Certain musculoskeletal abnormalities such as Klippel-Feil syndrome may result in difficulties with intubation, and an X-ray is required to determine the degree of fusion of the cervical vertebrae. As children having a cochlear implant will have had a general anesthetic for the CT scan and steady state evoked potential (SSEP) testing, any difficulties associated with these procedures need to be reviewed.

There is no need to routinely obtain a hemoglobin level, and as blood loss is minimal, crossmatching of blood is not required, unless a large mastoid emissary vein is seen on the X-ray. Premedication should be given 30–45 minutes prior to induction to render the child docile and easily managed. This is not required if the child is under 12 months of age.

At the induction of the anesthetic it is very desirable to have a parent present, especially for children aged 1–6 years. Either gaseous or intravenous induction can be used. As access to the head and body in general will be limited during surgery the endotracheal tube should be taped firmly in place, and the foot is a convenient site for the intravenous line. Some surgeons use a stimulator to help locate the facial nerve, in which case there should be minimal or no relaxant used. If, at the end of the operation, brain stem evoked potentials are to be recorded to check the integrity of the implant, the inhalation agents must be kept below a certain limit, and no great fluctuations in the blood carbon dioxide level should occur.

The length of the operation is normally from 2 to 3½ hours, and the total time taken up to 5 hours. Fluid replacement will be needed over this period. Intravenous antibiotics are administered during and after the procedure and then orally when tolerated. The body temperature is usually well maintained as the child is completely draped except for the wound, so no active heating is required unless the ambient temperature is low. In this case, forced air warming is preferred. Finally, to reduce bleeding during surgery, maintain an adequate depth of anesthesia, mild hypotension, and mild hypocapnia using controlled ventilation.

After the child has been induced in the anesthetic room the hair is clipped and shaved over an area to provide a margin of at least 25 mm around the incision to ensure sterility. The child is then taken to the operating room.

The cochlear implant surgery should be done with care to prevent infection. This requires good aseptic procedures and routine. When implanting a foreign body there is an increased risk of postoperative infection, and with cochlear implants this has occurred in 1.2% of adults and 0.73% of children (Hoffman & Cohen, 1995). In the operating room electrodes for recording facial muscle stimulation and EABRs are applied if required. The shaved area is then sterilized with antiseptic solution. After a change of gown and gloves, the drapes are applied to the patient, and the operating microscope and other surgical items put in place. The anterior limit of the receiver-stimulator antenna coil is then marked on the skin. To allow for an ear level speech processor or the microphone assembly used with a body-worn speech processor, this anterior limit is a posterosuperior arc approximately 45 to 50 mm from the external auditory meatus (Figure 7–1.) This ensures there is enough space between the ear level speech processor (ESPrit™) or microphone case for the SPrint™, and the receiver coil, so the transmitter coil can be easily aligned. This anterior limit should be the same in both adults and young children to allow for subsequent growth and reorientation of the pinna.

A dummy package is next placed on the skin so the antenna coil lies behind the arc. It is then moved upward and downward and rotated so that it is optimally placed flush against the skull. In infants where the skull is smaller and the curvature greater, it may have to be orientated so its posterior end is more superior than in an adult. When the dummy package is optimally placed its outline is marked on the skin. The skin incision, which is an inverted-J, is then delineated (Figure 7–1). It commences at the inferior limit of the postauricular sulcus, and passes superiorly to a point just below the superior limit of the attachment of the pinna to the scalp. From there it sweeps posterosuperiorly at

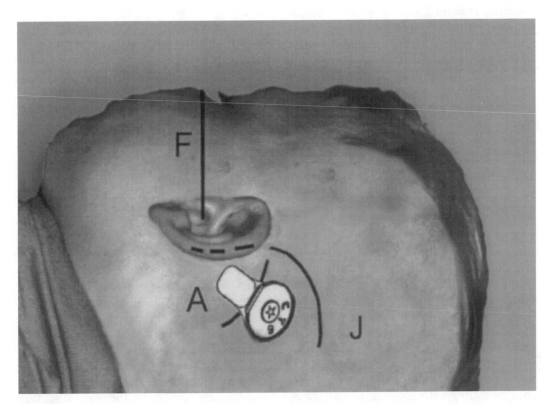

FIGURE 7–1. A diagram showing the location of the posterosuperior arc 45–50 mm from the external auditory meatus for the anterior limit of the receiver-stimulator coil, and the siting of the inverted-J incision. F - Frankfurt's line; A - posterosuperior arc; J - incision.

an angle of approximately 30° to the infra-orbital/meatal line (Frankfurt's line) for a distance of up to 80 mm. This will appear relatively large on the infant's scalp, but it is important not to compromise the size of the incision, otherwise it may lie near the edge of the package. This would predispose to wound breakdown. The incision should lie 20 mm from the margins of the receiver-stimulator. Other incisions have been used for cochlear implantation. These include a C-incision and one similar to the inverted-J but commencing as an endaural incision with extension posteriorly (Lehnhardt & Hirshorn, 1986). The C-incision is now not appropriate as the posterior margin of the multiple-channel implant is further back than the single-channel implant the C-incision was first used for, and the limbs of the C cannot be brought far enough forward to obtain a good view of the round window without compromising the blood supply of the flap. The C-incision does not have good dependent drainage like the inverted-J, and also cuts branches of the occipital artery. The extended endaural and inverted-J incision may be preferred if the middle ear needs to be explored, for example, following the treatment of a middle ear effusion.

INCISION AND CREATION OF FLAPS

After demarcating the incision, the skin and deeper tissues are injected with a solution containing a vasoconstrictor to reduce bleeding. A steridrape is applied over the exposed skin and side drapes. The incision is made through the steridrape, skin, and subcutaneous tissue down to the deep fascia. This is preferably done with a scalpel rather than cutting diathermy in line with good plastic surgical principles to facilitate skin healing. The flap of skin and subcutaneous tissue is dissected inferiorly to expose the deeper

tissues overlying the mastoid and inferior portions of the parietal and occipital bones. An anteriorly based flap of deep fascia and periosteum is then created and dissected anteriorly to the external auditory meatus. In elevating the deep fascia and periosteal flap, special care should be taken in dissecting inferiorly to avoid cutting the facial nerve in very young children and the occipital artery or a mastoid emissary vein. Some mastoid emissary veins can cause marked blood loss, and should always be looked for in the preoperative X-ray. Some surgeons prefer to elevate the skin and superficial and deep fascia together as a single flap. We prefer to raise the two flaps, as the deeper flap can be sutured separately over the package at the completion of the operation to provide better stabilization.

MASTOIDECTOMY AND POSTERIOR TYMPANOTOMY

When the landmarks of the mastoid bone are exposed and identified, and the cartilaginous auditory canal dissected forward, the cortical mastoidectomy is commenced. Using a large cutting burr, the cortex of the mastoid superior and posterior to the external meatus is removed. The excavation is deepened and air cells are removed superior and posterior to the meatus. Be careful when drilling superiorly not to expose dura when there is a low lying middle fossa. Drilling close to the posterior and superior walls of the bony meatus will ensure the safest approach to the mastoid antrum, by minimizing the risk of damaging the facial nerve, especially when there is a poorly pneumatized mastoid. When the mastoid antrum is exposed, identify the horizontal semicircular canal and the short process of the incus, which are the superior landmarks for the vertical section of the facial nerve. Extend the excavation of mastoid air cells inferiorly initially to the floor of the ear canal.

It is preferable to approach the facial nerve from behind and deliberately define the position of the nerve within its bony canal (Fallopian) before making the posterior tympanotomy. It is important to identify the facial nerve for two reasons. First, it can swing laterally in a third of cases where it is at risk when extending the posterior tympanotomy inferiorly, and second, the chorda tympani may be taken as the facial nerve, in which case the dissection will enter the ear canal. When identifying the facial nerve ensure the drilling is always parallel to its anticipated line. Preoperative CT scans of the facial nerve will also indicate whether there are any anomalies such as a sharply posteriorly angled genu that could put the nerve at risk of injury. If the bone is sclerotic and the nerve is not readily identified a diamond paste burr should be used as it is less likely to damage the nerve if it is inadvertently exposed. However, good irrigation is important to prevent overheating of the nerve.

Having exposed the facial nerve, drill anterolaterally to identify the chorda tympani. This can arise at various points along the facial nerve, and if arising high can compromise the tympanotomy. In this case, the chorda may need to be cut. It can be helpful with difficult posterior tympanotomies to drill the bone at the junction of the bony meatus and floor of the antrum to expose a small posterosuperior segment of the annulus of the tympanic membrane. This landmark will assist in defining the boundaries of the facial recess for the completion of the posterior tympanotomy. The boundaries are the fossa incudis superiorly, the chorda tympani laterally and anteriorly, and the facial nerve medially and posteriorly. Identifying these boundaries will help ensure the middle ear is exposed without damaging the facial nerve or entering the external auditory canal. Commencing the posterior tympanotomy and entering the middle ear is best done by following "sentinel" air cells lying inferior to the floor of the mastoid antrum into the middle ear. However, these cells are not always present, especially when the mastoid is sclerotic. In this case, having identified the facial nerve, drill anterior to it, and medial to the chorda tympani. Once the middle ear is entered, enlarge the opening. In doing so be careful not to have the heel of the burr placed posteriorly where it may injure the facial nerve. Also ensure that the shaft does not rotate on the facial nerve, particularly if it is exposed, as the heating may cause a palsy.

When the posterior tympanotomy is partially completed, identify the round window niche. This may be facing posteriorly and difficult to see unless the view through the microscope is directed more medially, and any bone overlying the facial nerve anteriorly removed. Sometimes the niche is obliterated due to adhesions or with new bone following meningitis, in which case the center of its superior margin can be located on average 1.5 mm below the center of inferior margin of the oval window. Note that an air cell inferior to the cochlea (hypotympanic air cell or tunnel of the cochlea) may appear very similar to the round window, and has been implanted on occasions by mistake. This can be avoided if the surgeon is aware of the characteristic anatomy of the first part of the scala tympani with its curvature passing anteroinferiorly. When the posterior tympanotomy has been completed an adequate view should be obtained of the round window and the promontory anterior to this, so that a cochleostomy can be completed. The surgery then proceeds with the completion of a bed for the receiver-stimulator package.

CREATION OF A BED FOR THE RECEIVER-STIMULATOR

With the receiver-stimulators for both the Nucleus-22 (Figure, 7–2) and Nucleus-24

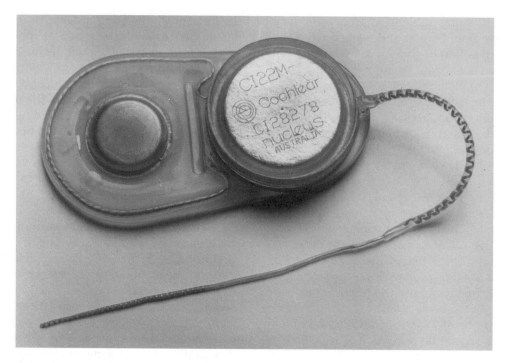

FIGURE 7–2. A photograph of the receiver-stimulator (CI-22M) for the Nucleus-22 system.

(Figure, 7–3) systems there is a need to drill a round or an ovoid bed, respectively. The bed is made in the mastoid bone and mastoid angle of the parietal bone in the region of the asterion. Drill the bed so the anterior limit of the coil lies posterior to an arc 45–50 mm posterosuperior to the external auditory meatus, as illustrated in Figure, 7–1. The bed is created to accommodate either the circular electronics package of the CI-22M receiver-stimulator which has a diameter of 21.5 mm (Figure, 7–4), or the ovoid protuberance on the under surface of the CI-24M receiver-stimulator which has a minimum diameter of 10 mm and maximum of 15 mm. The bed is fashioned initially with a cutting burr, and then completed with a diamond paste burr. A template provided with the device assists in making this the right size. A diamond paste burr should be used when approaching dura and when dura is exposed to minimize the risk of tearing it. Meticulous hemostasis is needed with bipolar electrosurgical diathermy on dura to avoid any risk of an extradural hemorrhage or hematoma. After the bed is created, drill a gutter anteriorly into the mastoid cavity to accommodate the lead wire assembly. The retractors should then be released, hemostasis obtained, and the wound irrigated to remove bone dust.

COCHLEOSTOMY AND ELECTRODE INSERTION

After completing the bed for the receiver-stimulator, preparations are then made for making the cochleostomy and inserting the electrode array. It is our practice to change gowns and gloves and irrigate the site with a dilute antibiotic solution to minimize the risk of introducing infection into the cochlea. Before commencing the cochleostomy it is important to understand that the orientation of the cochlea within the temporal bone is slightly differ-

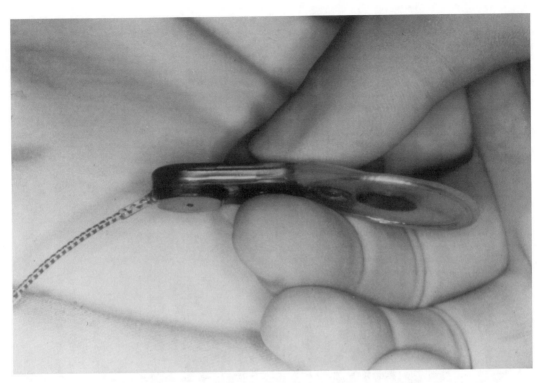

FIGURE 7-3. A photograph of the receiver-stimulator (CI-24M) for the Nucleus-24 system. (From Surgical considerations for the placement of the new Cochlear Pty Limited micro-multiple-channel cochlear implant for research studies by G. M. Clark et al., 1995, p. 408. *Annals of Otology, Rhinology and Laryngology, 104*(Suppl. 166). Reprinted by permission.)

ent in the infant and young child from that in the older child or adult. As a result, the round window will appear higher than usual, lying closer to the short process of the incus and the floor of the mastoid antrum. This may be due to the orientation of the head of a child where the occiput is large and the shoulders small. This should be compensated for by a small towel under the shoulders.

At this stage of the operation the sealed package containing the receiver-stimulator is opened, and the fixation device removed. This can be either a platinum wire tie placed around the floor of the antrum (Webb et al., 1990) or a titanium clip (Cohen, 1995) for clamping to the floor of the antrum. With the platinum wire tie, it is passed as a loop around the floor of the antrum, and one free end is inserted through the loop. The loop is pulled tight against bone and the free ends twisted. The free ends will be twisted later around a sleeve slid over the electrode using a special instrument.

It is now more usual to carry out a cochleostomy rather than incise the round window membrane and insert the electrode through it. The cochleostomy is made 1 mm anteroinferior to the round window (Figure, 7-4). In making the cochleostomy it is preferable to use a small diamond paste drill and drill from below upward. In this way there is less risk of any trauma to the spiral lamina which would lead to loss of auditory nerve fibers. In making the opening, if possible, the endosteal lining should be preserved until the last moment, and then opened with a perforating needle. This is described in more detail by

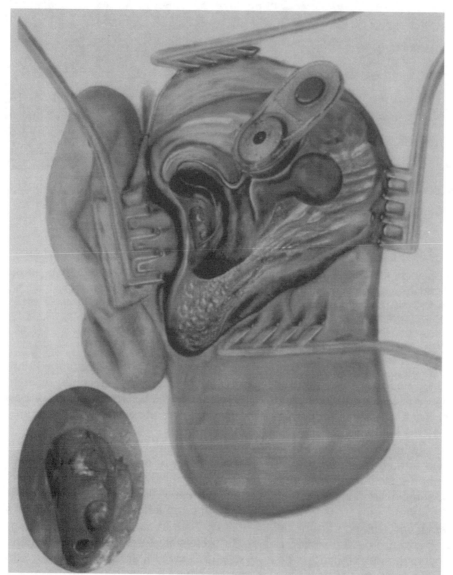

FIGURE 7-4. A drawing of the surgical implantation of the Cochlear Limited (CI-22M) receiver-stimulator showing the mastoid exenteration, posterior tympanotomy, bed for receiver-stimulator, electrode array inserted, and receiver-stimulator package about to be placed in its bed. Insert shows the posterior tympanotomy exposing the head of stapes, round window niche, and promontory with a cochleostomy created 1 mm anteroinferior to the round window niche (Clark, in press).

Professor Dr. E. Lehnhardt, and referred to as a "soft" insertion aiming to minimize trauma and preserve residual hair cells (Lehnhardt, 1993).

When the scala tympani is affected by new bone following labyrinthitis, it is often soft enough to remove with a needle and sucker but may require some burring. The removal of the bone should continue for up to 8 mm from the round window region, not the cochleostomy, otherwise any further penetration could risk entering the internal carotid artery. After making this cavity, it is still not possible to have the electrode pass around freely, an opening should then be attempted into the scala vestibuli. The drilling should be commenced 2.5 mm anteroinferior to the oval window. A patent scala vestibuli may be present postlabyrinthitis and not visible on the CT scan. If the scala vestibuli has been involved with new bone formation and the electrode will not pass, then the canals in the scala vestibuli and tympani should be joined and the electrode placed in the cavity (Balkany, Gantz, & Nadol, 1988; Gibson, 1995). The bone over the scala tympani can also be drilled to make a gutter in which the electrode is laid, but in this case it is more difficult to stabilize the array.

After making the cochleostomy the receiver-stimulator is removed from its package and the Silastic sheath slid over the array to protect the electrode when the tie is made. When inserting the electrode array in an infant also remember the orientation of the cochlea within the temporal bone may appear different from that of the adult. The basal turn will often appear to pass more superiorly, and be rotated more medially than in the adult. Prior to inserting the electrode check hemostasis, as it is best not to use diathermy once the electrode has been inserted. If this is necessary it must be bipolar and not monopolar. The package is then taken in one hand, and a specially designed claw (Clark et al., 1979) in the other hand is used to direct the tip to the cochleostomy opening, and then to ease the electrode along the scala tympani by stroking it gently forward. The electrode should be inserted to the point where slight resistance is felt. If it is pushed too hard the tip may penetrate the basilar membrane or buckle in the basal turn near the round window which could cause a fracture of the spiral lamina. In the uncomplicated case the electrode array can usually be inserted for a distance of 21 mm on average. The range is 15 mm to 27 mm. If an adequate depth of insertion has not been obtained before resistance is felt, this can often be rectified by slightly withdrawing the electrode and rotating it 90° counterclockwise in the right ear or clockwise in the left, before further advancing it. A deeper insertion has also been reported if the electrode array is coated with Healon (Donnelly et al., 1995; Laurent, Anniko, & Hellstrom, 1991; Lehnhardt, 1993), which reduces the friction between the array and the outer wall of the scala. When the electrode insertion is completed it is stabilized, and the platinum tie twisted around the protecting sheath to hold it in place or it is inserted into the titanium clip. A small fascial graft taken from the temporalis region is placed around the electrode entry point, as studies by Clark and Shepherd (1984) and Dahm et al. (1995) have shown that this can provide significant protection from an infection from otitis media passing around the electrode entry point.

FIXATION OF PACKAGE AND WOUND CLOSURE

The CI-24M receiver-stimulator can be flexed and bent at its center so that it can lie flat against the skull of an infant or young child as illustrated in Figure, 7–5. This is a distinct advantage over packages that are completely rigid. Prior to the fixation of the package (Figure, 7–6) some surgeons will

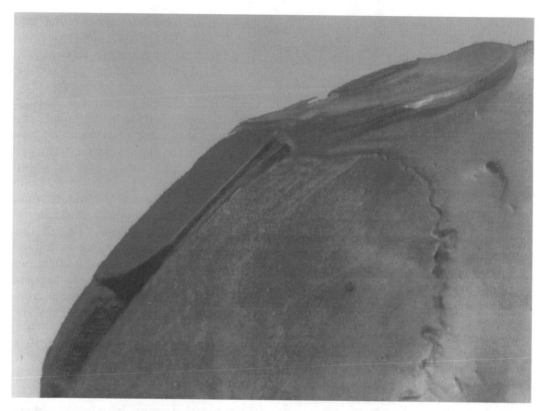

FIGURE 7–5. A diagram showing the Nucleus CI-24M superimposed on the temporal bone indicating how it can accommodate the curvature of the skull.

have drilled small tunnels in the bone on either side of the package bed to place ties to hold the receiver-stimulator in place. In an infant this is not a good procedure as the bone is thin, the drill may abrade the dura, and bleeding could occur and be difficult to control. In children it is best to tie the package down with ligatures that are placed through the temporalis and deep fascia, and also to stitch the anteriorly based fascial flap back over the package. It is important to release the retractors before this is done.

When the package has been fixed in its bed, it is useful to stimulate the package and record compound action potentials (CAPs), EABRs, and electrode impedances. This will indicate the placement is satisfactory, the auditory nervous system is being stimulated, and provide some baseline data on the thresholds that may be appro-

priate when the child is stimulated postoperatively. EABRs can be recorded using the Nucleus CI-22M receiver-stimulator. The telemetry system for the Nucleus CI-24M receiver-stimulator also allows the recording of CAPs and electrode impedances. In addition, it is necessary to take a lateral or Stenver's plain X-ray view in the operating room to see if the electrode has been placed satisfactorily within the cochlea. The wound is then closed in layers and a firm dressing applied. It has not been our practice to use a drain.

SPECIAL PROBLEMS DURING SURGERY

Hemorrhage is likely to be a problem only if there is a large mastoid emissary vein.

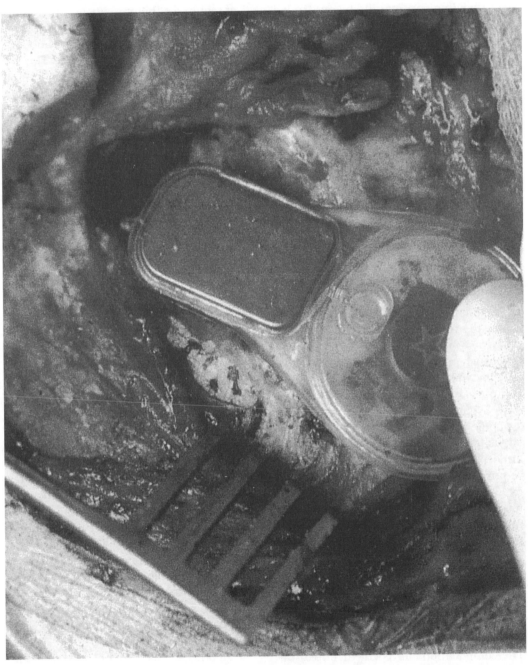

FIGURE 7–6. The CI-24M receiver-stimulator placed in its bed. (From Surgical Considerations for Placement of the New Cochlear Pty. Limited Micro-Multiple-Channel Cochlear Implant for Research Studies by G. M. Clark et al., 1995, p. 408 *Annals of Otology, Rhinology and Laryngology, 104*(Suppl. 166). Reprinted with permission.)

This should always be looked for on the X-rays. Bleeding can usually be controlled with bone wax, crushed muscle, or absorbable packing. In a severe bleed, absorbable gauze may have to be stitched in place to apply compression and the operation abandoned.

A perilymph gusher is managed by letting fluid drain off before inserting the electrode and then sealing around the entry point with fibrous tissue or absorbable packing. Perforation of the tympanic membrane or tearing of dura should be repaired at the time of surgery with fascia.

POSTOPERATIVE MANAGEMENT

The patient is normally discharged 3 days postoperatively. The wound should be inspected daily, and a tight bandage maintained to avoid a hematoma. If this develops it may need aspiration. An aerocele arising when air is forced up the Eustachian tube will also normally resolve with a compression bandage maintained for 5 days. Wound infection will require further systemic antibiotics according to the sensitivity of the organism, as well as topical antiseptics. In some cases the wound will require exploration, especially if there is exposure of the receiver-stimulator. In most cases the surgical outcome is uneventful and the receiver-stimulator can be "fired up" when the scalp is healed, 2 to 3 weeks postoperatively.

POSTOPERATIVE COMPLICATIONS

The complications for cochlear implantation in 309 children were analyzed (Clark et al., 1991) and divided into major and minor complications. Major complications that required either surgery or intravenous antibiotics occurred in 12 patients (3.9%). There were six flap complications and four of these required revision surgery. The flap complications were more common in children under age 7 due to their smaller heads and thinner tissues. Receiver-stimulator migration occurred in two, a perilymph gusher in two, a delayed facial nerve palsy in one, and hypotympanic electrode insertion in one. Subsequently, in a total of 548 children an additional four facial nerve palsies were reported. One was due to operative trauma to an anomalous facial nerve, and three were due to heating of bone. There were nine (2.9%) minor complications. Facial nerve stimulation occurred in four, flap problems in two, resolved dizziness in two, and electrode migration in one.

Most of the complications can be avoided by attention to the details of the surgical technique described previously. The C-incision was predominantly associated with the wound breakdowns reported, and the incidence should be much less with the inverted-J or extended endaural incisions. If a wound breakdown is not controlled with systemic and/or local antibiotics then wound debridement and a rotation flap may result in healing and save removal of the package. Long-term antibiotics will be required in addition. If there is widespread infection or a recurrence then the package will need to be removed. In this case it is usually preferable to cut the lead near the round window so that another electrode with a new package could be reinserted at a later date when complete healing had taken place.

Another sequela, but not a surgical complication, is package failure. This occurred more commonly in children and increased in incidence over time. It was due to an early design weakness in the CI-22M receiver-stimulator, where the entry of the antenna to the package was prone to injury when the child hit his or her head. This is discussed in more detail in Chapters 8 and 13. The design fault has been corrected, and results of analyses (von Wallenberg, Brinch, & Parker, 1996) show that the reliability of the new design is high, with no evidence of higher failure rate in children than for adults. This experience has emphasized the importance of having a robust coil and connection with the receiver-stimulator package so damage will not occur. This is particularly important for cochlear implants in children as they are frequently bumped during play. The receiver-stimulator coil of the CI-24M has been made robust for this reason. Injury to the child was also a consideration by Cochlear Limited in deciding whether to develop a titanium or ceramic package for the new implant. As outlined in Chapter 8 the ceramic package without supporting flange could be more easily driven inward with damage to the electrode as well as to the brain and other intercranial structures. This is not as likely to occur with the titanium package because it has the receiver-stimulator coil attached posteriorly to provide support. These points are illustrated in Figure, 7–7, where drawings of titanium and ceramic package profiles are made over the axial CT scan of the temporal bone of a 2-year-old child.

ACKNOWLEDGMENTS

We thank Dr. Linda Cass for helpful comments on anesthesia, Mr. Trevor Carter and Mr. Tony Stephens for the Figures, and Mrs. Sue Davine and Ms. Jacky Gray for secretarial support.

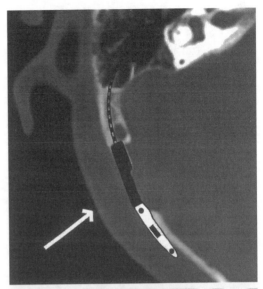
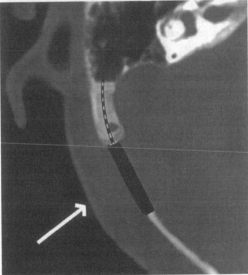

FIGURE 7–7. A diagram showing the placement of the CI-24M titanium receiver-stimulator package with external coil *(Top)*, and ceramic package *(Bottom)* superimposed on a CT scan of the skull of a 12-month-old child. The arrow indicates the direction of a blow to the head which could more easily force the ceramic package inward, unless it has a flange to protect it. The coil of the Nucleus-24 provides support for the titanium package.

REFERENCES

Balkany, T., Gantz, B., & Nadol, J. B. (1988). Multichannel cochlear implants in partially ossified cochleas. *Annals of Otology, Rhinology and Laryngology, 97*, 3–7.

Clark, G. M. (in press). Cochlear implants. In H. Ludman & A. Wright (Eds.), *Diseases of the ear*. London: Edward Arnold.

Clark, G. M., Cohen, N. L., & Shepherd, R. K. (1991). Surgical and safety considerations of multi-channel cochlear implants in children. *Ear and Hearing*, (Suppl. 12), 15–24.

Clark, G. M., Pyman, B. C., & Bailey, Q. R. (1979). The surgery for multiple-electrode cochlear implications. *Journal of Laryngology and Otology, 93*, 215–223.

Clark, G. M., Pyman, B. C., Webb, R. L., Bailey, Q. R., & Shepherd, R. K. (1984). Surgery for an improved multiple-channel cochlear implant. *Annals of Otology, Rhinology and Laryngology, 93*, 204–207.

Clark, G. M., Pyman, B. C., Webb, R. L., Franz, B. K-G., Redhead, T. J., & Shepherd, R. K. (1987). Surgery for the safe insertion and reinsertion of the banded electrode array. *Annals of Otology, Rhinology and Laryngology, 96*(Suppl. 128), 10–12.

Clark, G. M., & Shepherd, R. K. (1984). Cochlear implant round window sealing procedures in the cat. *Acta Otolaryngologca (Stockholm)*, Suppl. 410, 5–15.

Cohen, N. L. (1995). Medical and surgical perspectives: Issues in treatment and management of severe and profound hearing impairment. *Annals of Otology, Rhinology and Laryngology, 104*(Suppl. 166), 149–150.

Dahm, M. C., Clark, G. M., Franz, B. K-H, Shepherd, R. K., Burton, M. J., & Robins-Browne R. (1995). Cochlear implantation in children: Labrynthitis following pneumococcal otitis media in unimplanted and implanted cat cochleas. *Acta Otolaryngologica, 114*, 620–625.

Donnelly, M. J., Cohen, L. T., Xu, J., Xu, S.-A., Clark, G. M. (1995). Investigations on a curved intracochlear array. *Annals of Otology, Rhinology and Laryngology, 104*(Suppl. 166), 409–412.

Gibson, W. P. R. (1995). Surgical technique for inserting the cochlear multielectrode array into ears with total neo-ossification. *Annals of Otology, Rhinology and Laryngology, 104*(Suppl. 166), 414–416.

Hoffman, R. A., & Cohen, N. L. (1995). Complications of cochlear implant surgery. *Annals of Otology, Rhinology and Laryngology, 104*(Suppl. 166), 420–422.

Laurent, C., Anniko, M., & Hellstrom, S. (1991). Hyaluronan applied to lesioned round window membrane is free from cochlear ototoxicity. *Acta Otolaryngologica, 111*, 506–514.

Lehnhardt, E. (1993). Intracochleäre plazierung der cochlear-implant elektroden in soft surgery technique. *HNO, 41*, 356–359.

Lehnhardt, E., & Hirshorn, M. S. (1986). *Cochlear implant*. Berlin: Springer-Verlag.

von Wallenberg, E. L., Brinch, J., & Parker, J. (1996, June). The reliability of the nucleus electrode array. *Proceedings of the Third European Symposium on Paediatric Cochlear Implantation*. Hannover, Germany.

Webb, R. L., Pyman, B. C., Franz, B. K-HG., & Clark, G. M. (1990). The surgery of cochlear implantation. In G. M. Clark, Y. C. Tong, & J. F. Patrick (Eds.), *Cochlear prostheses* (pp. 153–179) Edinburgh: Churchill Livingstone.

8

ENGINEERING

JAMES F. PATRICK
PETER M. SELIGMAN
GRAEME M. CLARK

The last two decades have seen major advances in cochlear implants for profoundly deaf people. Implants are now used by severely to profoundly deaf adults and children in almost every phase of daily life. They have become an established treatment, and today's expectations for all aspects of the cochlear implant system are much greater than they were for the experimental devices of the early 1980s. Hardware designs have improved to meet clinical and research demands, technological developments have made the devices smaller and more reliable, and speech processing research has yielded a series of improvements in patient benefit.

The cochlear implant characteristics that are now widely anticipated are summarized in Table 8–1. In planning the development of a more advanced implant system, it is important for it to meet or exceed these characteristics. It must deliver the best performance available for every recipient, and have the potential for future enhancement, both in speech understanding and appearance. These improvements should preferably occur through change to the external components (the speech processor), while still using the same implant and electrode array. Finally, the implant and electrode array should be replaceable without trauma to the cochlea, either for a future device upgrade or in the unlikely instance of device failure.

The multiple-channel cochlear implant is of value to people who have severe to profound sensorineural hearing loss. As illustrated in Figure 8–1, the Nucleus systems have an array of 22 electrodes placed in the scala tympani, stimulating the residual auditory nerve fibers and causing the perception of sound. The place of stimulation is used to code frequency on a place basis, and a fixed frequency range is associated with each electrode position. Stimulus amplitude is used to code intensity, with the amplitude envelope providing temporal information. The stimuli are generated by a small receiver-stimulator implanted in the temporal bone. Outside the body, sounds are picked up by a microphone. A speech processor translates the spectral energy into a pattern of stimuli to be delivered by the implanted stimulator, and encodes this into a combined data/power signal that is transmitted across the skin to the implant.

SPEECH PROCESSING FOR COCHLEAR IMPLANTS

Nucleus (Cochlear Limited) initially developed The University of Melbourne's prototype receiver-stimulator industrially, and it was first trialed in 1982. The receiver-stimulator was designed to allow the speech processing strategy coding the fundamental (F0) and second formant

Table 8–1. Anticipated characteristics of cochlear implant systems.

Surgery:

The electrode will be easy to insert.

Device function will be confirmed intraoperatively.

There will be minimum drilling.

The electrode will be easily removable, should this be necessary.

The incidence of complications and side-effects will be low.

Device Adjustment:

Programming software will be "friendly."

The Program will be flexible to optimize patient benefit.

The default parameter settings will provide a good starting point.

There will be responsive support from the manufacturers for clinical problems.

There will be simple diagnostic procedures to identify device problems.

Patient Benefits:

The implant will provide a useful benefit, compared with present hearing.

The implant will be reliable.

The speech processor will be compatible with assistive devices, such as FM systems.

There will be access to future product improvements.

(F2) frequencies (Tong et al., 1981) to stimulate auditory nerve fibers, and to ensure the stimulus parameters would be safe and not damage the nerve fibers (Clark et al., 1987). Safety was achieved by means of an electronic design that minimized charge imbalance for the bi-phasic pulses and provided shorting between pulses. The custom-designed integrated circuit for this receiver-stimulator was hermetically sealed inside a rugged titanium capsule (Patrick et al., 1990). This technology had been pioneered by Nucleus for the pacemaker industry, but further advances were needed to develop the high density ceramic/platinum feed- through and connector that was used to connect to each of the 22 lead wires from the electrode array. Outside the capsule, a platinum receiver coil was enclosed in flexible, biocompatible, silicone rubber. The electrode lead was helically wound for reliability under repeated flexing, and contained 22 separately insulated platinum/iridium wires. The electrode array (Clark, Patrick, & Bailey, 1979) contained 22 cylindrical platinum electrodes at a pitch of 0.75 mm, and tapered in diameter from 0.4 mm at the tip to 0.6 mm for the basal 12 electrodes. An additional 10 isolated rings with the same spacing allowed easy, atraumatic insertion to 25 mm. Finally, the speech processor was designed to not only enable the F0/F2 strategy to be used, but incorporated an EPROM chip that could be interfaced to a programming unit for a patient's "map" to be written in (Patrick et al., 1990). This "map" provided informa-

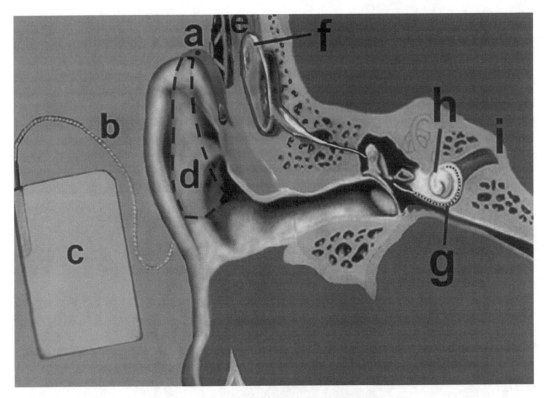

FIGURE 8–1. A diagram of the Nucleus-22 multiple-channel cochlear implant systems: a - microphone; b - cable; c - body-worn speech processor; d - ear level speech processor; e - transmitter coil; f - receiver stimulator; g - electrode array; h - cochlea; i - auditory nerve (From Cochlear Implants by G. M. Clark, 1996. In A. Wright & H. Ludman, Eds., *Mawson's Diseases of the Ear.* Copyright 1997 Edward Arnold. Reprinted with permission.)

tion about the patient's stimulation levels between the threshold and maximum comfortable level for each electrode, so that the speech processing strategy could be set for individual variations in sensitivity. Different levels were required for the bipolar or common ground stimulus modes. In bipolar stimulation, the current flows between one electrode and a neighboring one. In common ground stimulation, the current flows between one electrode and the others connected together electronically. Both modes provide localized stimulation for place coding of frequency with the banded array, and the one that is required for best results depends on the effects of pathology and anatomy on current flow within the cochlea.

After the Nucleus F0/F2 device was approved by the U.S. Food and Drug Administration (FDA) in 1985 for use in postlinguistically deaf adults, work commenced to develop the device for children. This meant making it smaller and developing a better method of holding the transmitter coil in place without having to rely on a headband. The package depth was reduced by dispensing with the connector, as our biological and surgical studies had shown that the electrode array could be removed easily from the cochlea, should replacement of the implant be necessary. The alignment of the transmitting and receiving coils was improved by incorporating a rare earth magnet in both (Dormer et al., 1980). This receiver-stimulator, called the Mini 22 (CI-22M), has a flexible receiver coil that is easily formed to the shape of a small child's head.

The speech processor (Seligman et al., 1984) for the CI-22M was also made smaller, and it incorporated our next improvement in speech processing, which was a strategy presenting F2 and the first formant (F1) as place of stimulation, as well as coding F0 as rate of stimulation (Dowell et al., 1987). This cochlear implant system was tested in clinical trials on children, and approved by the FDA on June 27, 1990. The system subsequently incorporated a further improvement in speech processing developed by The University of Melbourne, in co-operation with Cochlear Limited, called "Multipeak" (Dowell et al., 1990). This strategy not only coded F0/F1/ F2, as described before, but also presented the level of high frequency energy measured by bandpass filters in the regions 2.0–2.8 kHz; 2.8–4.0 kHz; and >4.0 kHz on a place coding basis.

NUCLEUS-22 SYSTEM

The Nucleus-22 system includes the Mini-22 (CI-22M) and Mini-20+2 receiver-stimulator implants, and the Spectra-22 speech processor, illustrated in Figure 8–2. The Spectra-22 processor provides excellent performance using its normal

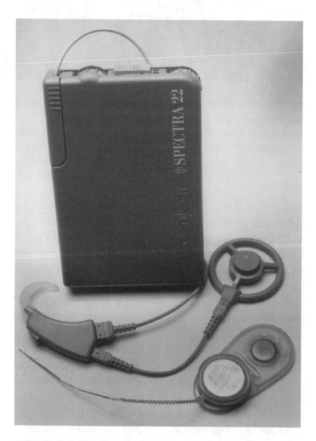

FIGURE 8–2. The Nucleus-22 system showing the CI-22M receiver-stimulator and the Spectra-22 speech processor.

directional microphone, and can also be used with assistive devices such as FM systems and the Audallion beamformer (Lindemann, 1994) in difficult acoustic environments. The Audallion beamformer has shown promising results in preliminary clinical studies, with about half of the group receiving speech comprehension improvements of greater than 15% at signal to noise ratios of 5 dB. The Spectra-22 incorporates the Spectral Maxima Sound Processor by the University of Melbourne (the Spectral Maxima Sound Processor), (McDermott, McKay, & Vandali, 1992; McKay, McDermott, & Clark, 1991), which has been implemented by Cochlear Limited as the SPEAK strategy. With SPEAK, the 6–10 maximal outputs from 20 bandpass filters are coded as place of stimulation, but instead of using rate of stimulation to code voicing frequency, a randomized stimulus rate is used, and the amplitude envelopes from the outputs of the filters then provide voicing information. This strategy is illustrated in Figure 8–3. The strategies just described have resulted in significant improvements in speech perception scores as shown in Figure 8–4 (Clark, 1996; in press). The average SPEAK result for open-set CID sentence scores for electrical stimulation alone in postlinguistically deaf adults is 70% (Skinner et al., 1994), while the mean was 86% for a group of nonselected patients at the Royal Victorian Eye and Ear Hospital, as shown in Figure 8–4. The improvement in scores is in large part due to the better presentation of spectral information on a place coding basis. This can be seen in the outputs to electrodes (electrodograms) for the Multipeak and SPEAK speech processing strategies that are illustrated in Figure 8–5.

This SPEAK strategy incorporated in the Spectra-22 speech processor has been shown to provide significant improvements in speech perception not only for adults, but also for children, as reported by Cowan et al. (1995) for 12 children who changed from the Multipeak to SPEAK strategies.

The CI-22M receiver-stimulator has now been implanted in a sufficiently large number of patients over a period of time long enough to permit an accurate assessment of its reliability. Device reliability is commonly measured by the percentage of devices that survive beyond a defined period. This defined period should be as long as possible, but the number of "survivors" also needs to be large for the cumulative survival figure to be meaningful. For the CI-22M receiver-stimulator, some 98.04% of all units that have ever been implanted in adults have survived more than 42 months. For children, the total 42 month cumulative survival is 94.56% (Figure 8–6). From this large implanted base, two predominant causes of failure have been identified and eliminated. The first failure mode was damage to the antenna coil caused by a blow to the head. Additional stress relief was built into the antenna, and since then there have been no failures of this type. The second mode was damage due to electrostatic discharge (ESD), and implant recipients and their parents were warned of this potential problem, and advised how to minimize the risk of ESD damage. An unusual mechanism of ESD was identified, whereby static electricity would discharge through the headset coil, producing an electromagnetic pulse that would damage the implant electronics. A protective coil has been since developed which suppresses the pulse and so protects the implant from ESD. All CI-22M patients can benefit from this coil and the immunity it provides. Since these changes were implemented in 1992, the 42 month cumulative survival has risen to 99.26%, with no difference between adults and children (Figure 8–6).

The first CI-22M recipients were implanted in 1986. By September 1996 some 14,000 units had been implanted with the 22-electrode implant. It offers excellent flexibility for different stimulus regimes, and has been the basis for a sequence of improvements in speech processing.

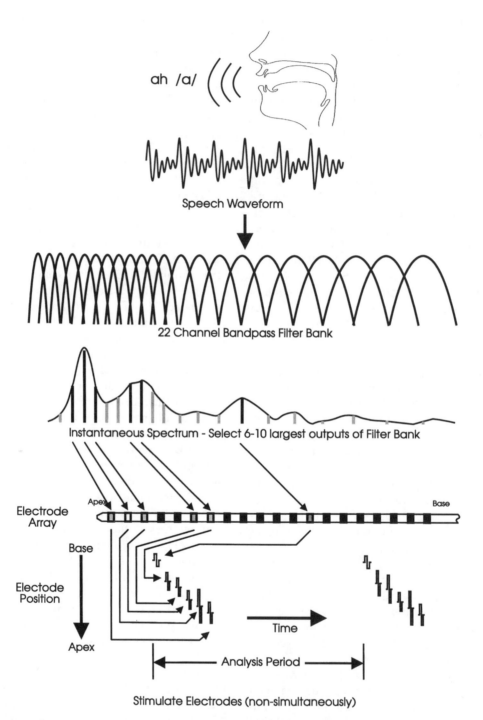

ah /a/

Speech Waveform

22 Channel Bandpass Filter Bank

Instantaneous Spectrum - Select 6-10 largest outputs of Filter Bank

Electrode Array

Apex   Base

Base

Electrode Position

Time

Apex

Analysis Period

Stimulate Electrodes (non-simultaneously)

FIGURE 8–3. A diagram of the SPEAK strategy. The speech waveform in the time domain is filtered by 20 band-pass filters. The 6–10 maximum outputs are selected and stimulate appropriate electrodes according to a frequency place coding representation.

CID Open-Set Sentence Scores
Electrical Stimulation Alone

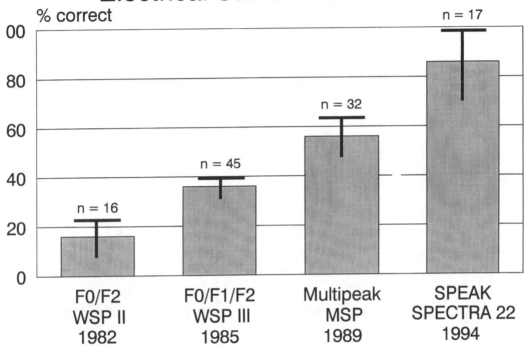

FIGURE 8–4. CID open-set sentence scores for electrical stimulation alone for the F0/F2,F0/F1/F2, Multipeak, SPEAK strategies on unselected patients at The Royal Victorian Eye and Ear Hospital, Cochlear Implant Clinic less than 6 months postoperatively. The speech processor that presents the strategies is shown following the strategy (From Cochlear Implants by G. M. Clark, in press-b. In A. Wright & H. Ludman, Eds., *Mawson's Diseases of the Ear.* Copyright 1997 Edward Arnold. Reprinted with permission.)

NUCLEUS-24 SYSTEM

The SPEAK and Continuous Interleaved Sampler (CIS) strategies are the two strategies presently used worldwide. With CIS, sequential (interleaved) pulsatile outputs are applied in turn to up to eight sites (Wilson et al., 1991), whereas in the SPEAK strategy sequential stimuli are applied to 6–10 of 22 electrodes on the basis of the incoming energy distribution. The amplitude envelope in the incoming signal is represented as variations in the current of the stimulating signal for both these strategies. CIS uses a high stimulus rate

to each of a small number of electrodes, whereas SPEAK stimulates roving clusters of closely spaced electrodes, with each electrode being stimulated at a much lower rate. The overlap of the stimulus fields of nearby electrodes, and the similarity in amplitude envelopes of adjacent frequency bands, means that SPEAK will have high regional stimulus rates, as well as a detailed spectral representation. On the other hand, CIS provides a constant stimulation rate, whereas for SPEAK, the effective rate will vary with the number of electrodes in the cluster. Thus, SPEAK might be expected to be more effective at transmitting

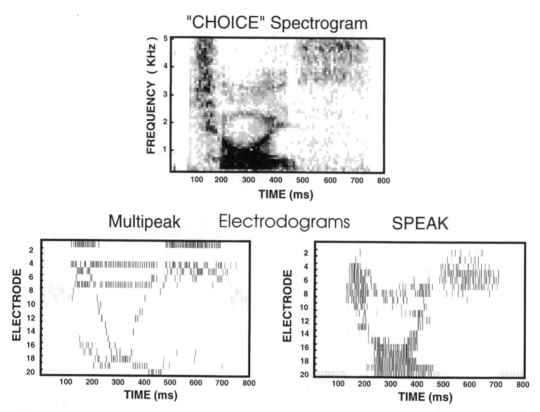

FIGURE 8–5. Spectrogram for the word "choice" and the electrode representations (electrodograms) for this word using the Multipeak and SPEAK strategies (From Cochlear Implants by G. M. Clark, in press-b. In A. Wright & H. Ludman, Eds., *Mawson's Diseases of the Ear.* Copyright 1997 Edward Arnold. Reprinted with permission.)

spectral information, and CIS at transmitting temporal information.

Performance data reported to the FDA for these two strategies has been surprisingly similar, as shown in Figure 8–7. However, because no implant system has previously been able to stimulate a large number of electrodes at a high rate, it has not been possible to combine the potential benefits of a high electrode density with the capacity for a high pulse rate.

Although the speech perception results with the SPEAK strategy are good in both adults and children, and compare more than favorably with CIS, they are still significantly below normal hearing, and there is considerable variation in per-

formance with both strategies. There is, therefore, a need for a receiver-stimulator that can use new strategies to provide more information through the interface with the nervous system, or electroneural bottleneck. This may be achieved in part by high stimulus rates, now that we have shown (Xu et al., in press) that these high rates are safe. The receiver-stimulator also needs to provide more place coding of frequency. This will occur in the first instance through alternative electrode designs, which position the electrode array close to the spiral ganglion cells in the modiolus.

Not only have the Nucleus-24 receiver-stimulator (CI-24M) electronics been designed to allow the SPEAK and CIS strate-

COCHLEAR CI-22M Implant Reliability

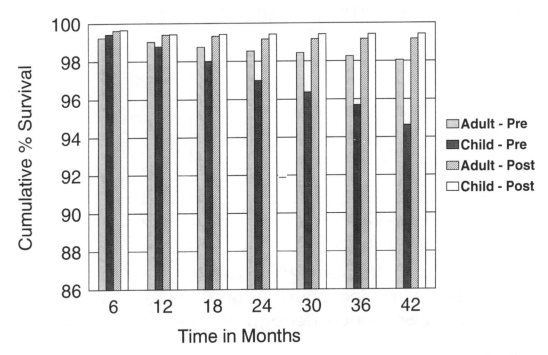

FIGURE 8–6. Accumulative survival of the CI-22M (Mini) receiver-stimulator in adults and children before and after the antenna coil design was amended to prevent device failure caused by a blow to the head of a child.

gies to be presented safely at higher stimulus rates, but other alternative strate-gies can be used as well. The device (Figure 8–8) will not only allow bipolar and common ground stimulation, as occurs in the Spectra-22 system, but monopolar stimulation as well. Studies have shown that, although monopolar stimulation was originally found to give widespread stimulation of auditory nerve fibers, if the electrode lies close to the ganglion cells localized stimulation will occur, especially when there is tissue rather than fluid between the array and the modiolus. The stimulus current levels required for neural excitation will also be lower with monopolar stimulation.

The receiver-stimulator for the SPrint™ and ESPrit™ speech processors (CI-24M)

has also been designed for use in infants, because research in children indicates that operating at a young age is important. Just how young a child should be for optimal results has not yet been established. It can be deduced, however, from results with deaf children fitted with hearing aids, that hearing restoration should occur before 2 years of age and even as young as 6 months. To allow for this need, the receiver-stimulator needs to be smaller and to have telemetry to transmit externally information on compound action potentials (CAPs), (Figure 8–9), so that these could be used, as well as EABRs, for setting thresholds and maximum comfortable levels. Other benefits of telemetry are the ability to determine if the electrodes are functioning,

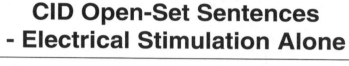

CID Open-Set Sentences
- Electrical Stimulation Alone

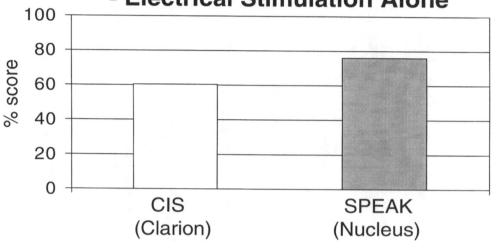

Nucleus 22 vs Clarion
Performance Distribution Comparison
Open Set Sentence Recognition Listening Alone

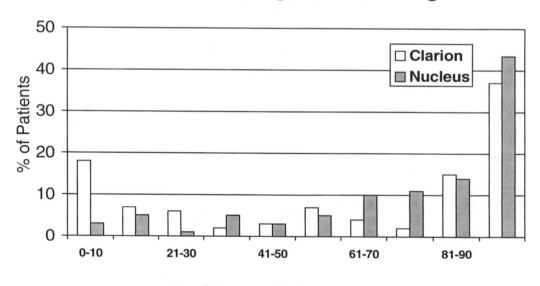

% Score Correct

FIGURE 8–7. The mean open-set CID sentence score of 71% for the SPEAK (The University of Melbourne/ Nucleus) strategy on 51 patients (data presented by Cochlear Limited to the U.S.A. Food Drug Administration, January, 1996) and 60% for the CIS (Advanced Bionics) strategy on 64 patients (Graphs constructed from data presented by Cochlear Limited and reported by Kessler, Loeb, and Barker, 1995.)

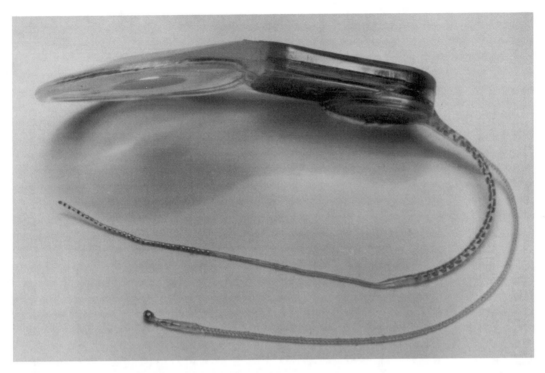

FIGURE 8–8. The CI-24M receiver-stimulator for use with the SPrint™ body-worn speech processor or ESPrit™ ear-level speech processor.

and precise measurements of the impedances of the electrode tissue interfaces to assess the extent of pathology within the cochlea.

In making the receiver-stimulator suitable for infants, the shape of the titanium capsule has been changed so that only a small amount of drilling is required in the thinner bone of an infant skull.

The CI-24M Cochlear Implant

With the CI-24M receiver-stimulator (Figure 8–8) the coil and top thin section of the titanium housing are designed to lie above the skull, and a cavity just 1.7 mm deep and 15 mm in width is needed for the locating stud. A 1 mm deep channel is also cut to protect the exit of the electrode lead.

During the design of the CI-24M a ceramic packaging technology was also developed, but this approach was rejected for two reasons. First, the ceramic would need to be thicker than the titanium version to provide the same measure of mechanical protection, and second, for young children where the package bed is down to dura, the electrode lead from the ceramic package could be vulnerable to impact, with potential shear if the package is displaced relative to the bone. The shape of the titanium capsule, however, would prevent such shearing, even in children. The titanium package, with attached coil lying external to the skull, is also less likely to be forced intracranially with a severe blow to the head. Figure 8–10 shows both designs. Thus, we elected to continue with the titanium/Silastic approach, despite its marginally lower power efficiency (and correspondingly lower battery life) compared with a ceramic package and internal copper coil.

Neural Response Telemetry

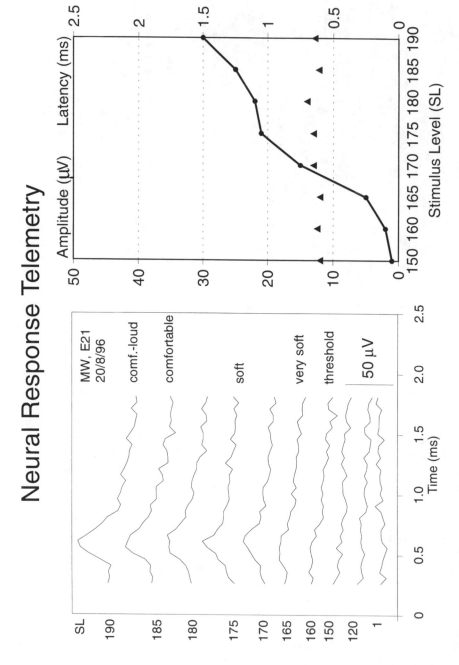

ENT-Department, University Hospital Zürich

FIGURE 8–9. Compound action potential (CAP) recorded from auditory nerve using the CI-24M telemetry system (Dillier, personal communication)

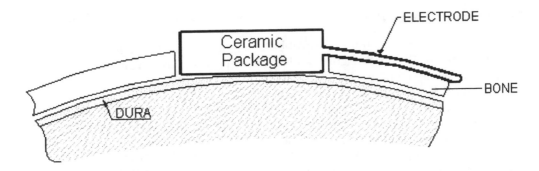

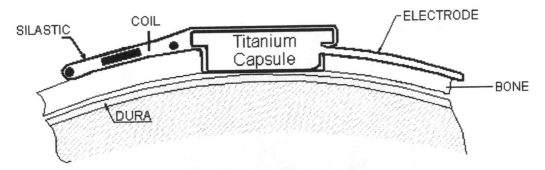

Surgical Placement of
Ceramic and Titanium/Silastic Packages

FIGURE 8–10. Comparison of titanium and ceramic design for receiver-stimulator.

Key design features for the CI-24M implant are:

- Stimulus rates of up to 14,250 pulses/s
- Intracochlear electrodes
- Extracochlear electrodes: one ball electrode to be placed under the temporalis muscle and a set of four interconnected plate electrodes on the medial surface of the receiver/stimulator body
- Choice of monopolar, bipolar, or common ground stimulation
- Normal telemetry, to signal internal stimulator voltages and electrode characteristics
- Unique, high sensitivity Neural Response Telemetry (NRT) to measure the CAP of the auditory nerve

- Output currents amplitude between 10 µA and 1750 µA, with a logarithmic current law
- Output pulse widths 7 µs, 13 µs, and variable 25 µs and above
- MRI compatibility, having a magnet that can easily be removed, should MRI be necessary
- Amplitude modulated combined power/data link at 5 MHz, with error detection, stimulus shut down for 200 ms following data corruption
- Coupling capacitors to extracochlear electrodes to allow for potential differences between intra-and extracochlear electrodes
- Slow turn on of shorting between intra-and extracochlear electrodes at startup.

The SPrint™ Speech Processor

The Nucleus-24 system has a wearable speech processor SPrint™ (Figure 8–11A, 8–11B) that allows standard and high rate SPEAK and CIS strategies to be presented safely, as well as alternative strategies. The SPrint™ speech processor includes a custom analog circuit, with preamplifier and signal conditioning circuitry. This front-end chip is digitally controlled, and includes extensive options for mixing from other audio sources, such as FM systems, TV, telecoils, and telephone adaptors. A low power, custom DSP chip then analyzes the incoming signals and implements a wide range of processing options under program control. SPrint™ features include:

■ Choice of SPEAK, CIS, and other enhanced algorithms as they become available
■ Enhanced noise reduction programs
■ Choice of four different program options immediately available
■ Sensitivity and loudness controls available

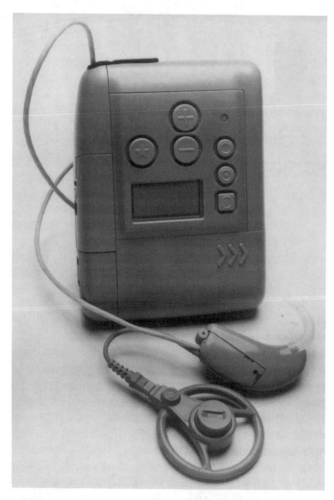

FIGURE 8–11. A. The body-worn SPrint™ speech processor in the Nucleus-24 system speech processing strategy.

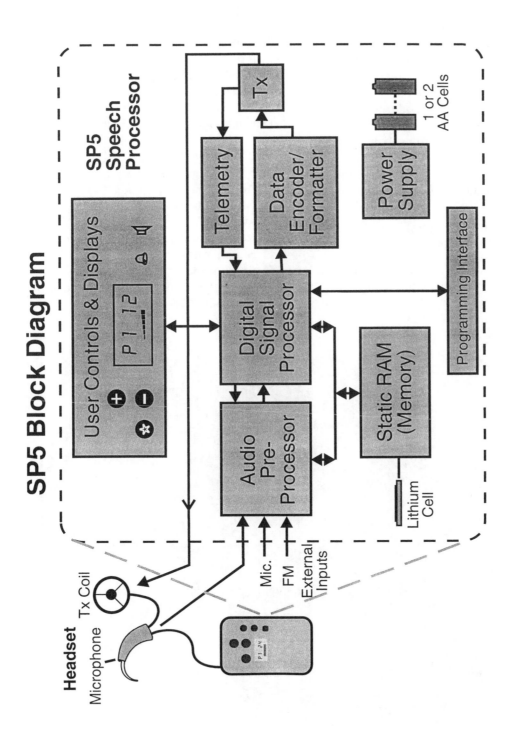

FIGURE 8-11. *(continued)* **B.** A block diagram of the SPrint™ speech processor.

- Automatic sensitivity control for noisy environments
- Telemetry link back to the Clinical Programming System
- Liquid crystal display of program settings, signal levels, and diagnostics
- Push button controls, with a disable feature for young children
- Data logging, to monitor usage
- Compatibility with assistive devices
- Single and double battery packs, depending on individual usage; weight 114 g (single) and 146 g (double battery pack).

The ESPrit™Ear Level Speech Processor

The Nucleus-24 system has an ear level speech processor (ESPrit™), (Figure 8–12A, 8–12B). The ESPrit™ headset processor is a flexible, very low power speech processor. Initially, it will be programmed with SPEAK, and used with the CI-24M implant. The custom integrated circuit (IC) used in the ESPrit™ has evolved from the best aspects of the SPECTRA design, and uses the high-rate communications link of the CI-24M.

Features of the ESPrit™ include:

- 22 channel filter bank
- SPEAK signal processing
- Autosensitivity circuit
- Choice of two programs immediately available
- Choice of sensitivity or loudness control
- Simple rotary and in-line switches
- Compatibility with assistive devices
- 50 to 100 hours typical battery life from dual 675 zinc-air cells

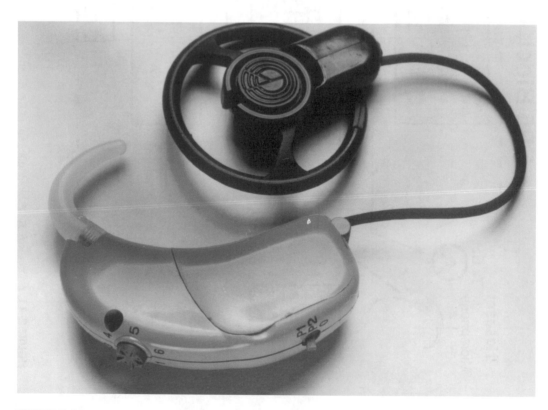

FIGURE 8–12. A. The "ear level" ESPrit™ speech processor in the Nucleus-24 system.

SP7 Block Diagram

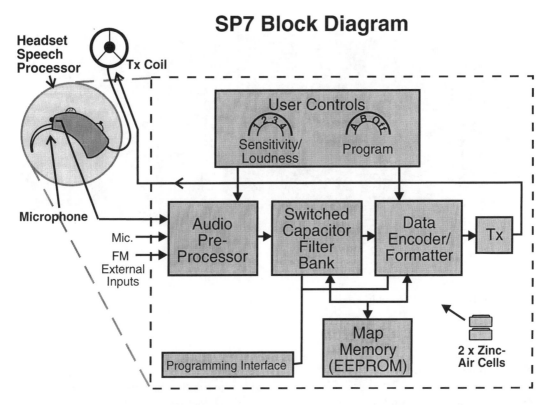

FIGURE 8–12. *(continued)* **B.** A block diagram of the ESPrit™ speech processor.

■ Daily running costs around 25 to 50 cents
■ Permanent, fast EEPROM memory for patient data.

The ESPrit™ will also be available to use with the CI-22M receiver-stimulator and be part of the Nucleus 22 system. It will incorporate a novel power control system that will improve the efficiency of the RF link to the implant, and should make this processor available to almost all Mini-22 (CI-22M) users.

Programming Systems

The SPrint™ and ESPrit™ processors are programmed with a Windows® program on an IBM-compatible PC or laptop computer. The computer is connected to the speech processor through either the fully optioned Patient Clinical Interface (PCI, Figure 8–13) for the Clinical Programming System option (CPS) or the small Portable Programming System option (PPS). The PCI includes an light emitting diode (LED) display of electrodes in use and Neural Response Telemetry (NRT); the PPS is designed for portable use in schools, and does not have these features, although it is otherwise fully equipped for normal programming and troubleshooting.

Features of the program system running under the Windows® are:

■ Support for clinical and portable configuration
■ Single screen mapping
■ Icon driven

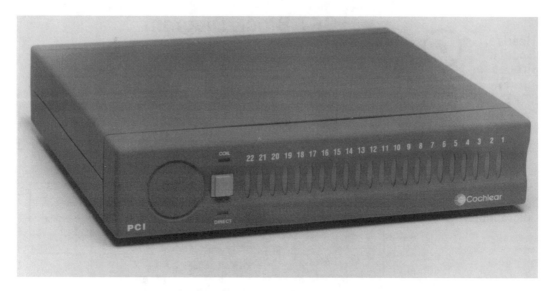

FIGURE 8–13. Patient Clinical Interface and PCI programming systems.

- Database patient records instead of separate disks
- Modular and expandable design
- Interaction with third party programs capability
- NRT with the CPS configuration.

Neural Response Telemetry

Neural Response Telemetry (NRT) has the potential to develop into a clinical tool, allowing the objective setting of stimulus levels. At this early stage, however, the technique must be considered a research tool. NRT measurements can be made using the CPS running under Windows®. This program was developed by Professor Norbert Dillier and his colleagues from Zurich (Dillier, personal communication), and an example of its output is shown in Figure 8–9.

Peri-Modiolar Electrodes

To improve the place and temporal coding of frequency for cochlear implants it may be necessary to place electrodes closer to the spiral ganglion cells, which are situated in the modiolus. This will not only allow the more localized stimulation of neurons at low current levels, but permit the use of an increased number of electrodes. Some of these peri-modiolar electrode designs are precurved prior to insertion, but held straight during the initial insertion, and then allowed to curl so they can be advanced around the modiolus (Figure 8–14). A second group is constructed straight with bilaminar layers of material. The outer layer lengthens when it absorbs water, and so causes the array to curl and lie close to the modiolus (Figure 8–15). The third design has a strip of material attached to the tip of the array, and at the end of its introduction, force is applied to the strip, causing the array to move to the center of the spiral (Figure 8–16). These approaches to electrode design are now being studied, first to identify the best design approach, and then to determine the perceptual benefit provided by modiolar electrode placement. These results will influence future implant designs.

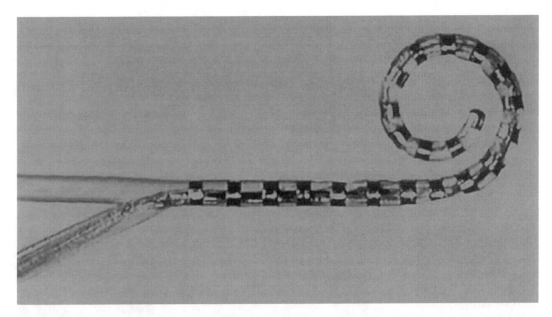

Figure 8–14. A precurved banded array being loaded into the insertion tool.

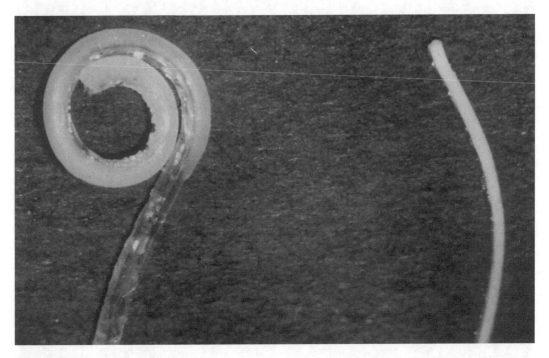

FIGURE 8–15. An electrode array fabricated from two layers of Silastic. The outer layer is mixed with polyacrylic acid, which makes it lengthen and curl when it absorbs water. (From Cochlear Implants: Future Directions by G. M. Clark. *Annals of Otology, Rhinology and Laryngology, 104* [Suppl. 166]. Reprinted 1995, p. 408 with permission.)

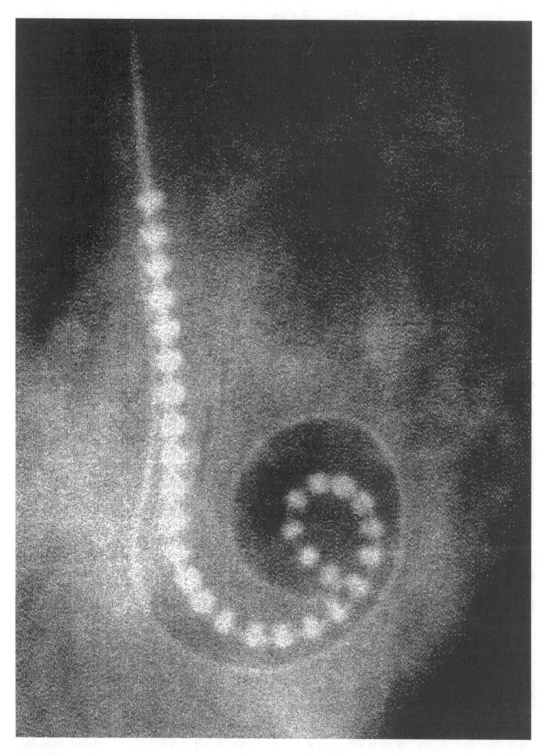

FIGURE 8–16. An X-ray of an array with a leader strip attached to its tip in place in a temporal bone (Kuzma, personal communication).

REFERENCES

Clark, G. M. 1996. Electrical stimulation of the auditory nerve, the coding of frequency, the perception of pitch and the development of cochlear implant speech processing strategies for profoundly deaf people. *Journal of Clinical Physiological, Pharmacological Research 23*, 766–776.

Clark, G. M. (in press). Cochlear implants. In A. Wright & H. Ludman (Eds.), *Mawson's Diseases of the Ear*. London: Edward Arnold.

Clark, G. M., Blamey, P. J., Brown, A. M., Busby, P. A., Dowell, R. C., Franz, B. K.-G., Pyman, B. C., Shepherd, R. K., Tong, Y. C., Webb, R. L., Hirshorn, M. S., Kuzma, J., Mecklenburg, D. J., Money, D. K., Patrick, J. F., & Seligman, P. M. (1987). The University of Melbourne—Nucleus multi-electrode cochlear implant. *Advances in Oto-Rhino-Laryngology, 38*. Basel: Karger.

Clark, G. M., Patrick, J. F., & Bailey, Q. R. (1979). A cochlear implant round window electrode array. *Journal of Laryngology and Otology, 93*, 107–109.

Cowan, R. S. C., Brown, C., Whitford, L. J., Galvin, K. L., Sarant, J. Z., Barker, E. J., Shaw, S., King, A., Skok, M., Seligman, P. M., Dowell, R. C., Everingham, C., Gibson, W. P. R., & Clark, G.M. (1995). Speech perception in children using the advanced SPEAK speech-processing strategy. *Annals of Otology, Rhinology and Laryngology, 104*(Suppl. 166), 318–321.

Dormer, K. J., Richard, G., Hough, J. V. D., & Hewett, T. (1980). The cochlear implant (auditory prosthesis) utilizing rare earth magnets. *American Journal of Otology, 2*, 22–27.

Dowell, R. C., Seligman, P. M., Blamey, P. J., & Clark, G. M. (1987). Speech perception using a two-formant 22-electrode cochlear prosthesis in quiet and in noise. *Acta Otolaryngologica (Stockholm), 104*, 439–446.

Dowell, R. C., Whitford, L. A., Seligman, P. M., Franz, B. K.-G., & Clark, G. M. (1990). Preliminary results with a miniature speech processor for the 22-electrode Melbourne/Cochlear hearing prosthesis. Otorhinolaryngology, Head and Neck Surgery. *Proceedings of the XIV Congress of Oto-Rhino-Laryngology, Head and Neck Surgery* (pp. 1167–1173). Madrid, Spain.

Kessler, D. K., Loeb, G. E., & Barker, M. J. (1995). Distribution of speech recognition results with the Clarion cochlear prosthesis. *Annals of Otology, Rhinology and Laryngology, 104*(Suppl. 166), 283–285.

Lindemann, E. (21 January 1994). Subject of published PCT Patent Application 95\20305-A1, Inventor-Eric Lindemann, Assigned to Audiologic Incorporated.

McDermott, H. J., McKay, C. M., & Vandali, A. E. (1992). A new portable sound processor for The University of Melbourne/Nucleus Limited multi-electrode cochlear implant. *Journal of the Acoustical Society of America, 91*, 3367–3371.

McKay, C. M., McDermott, H. J., & Clark, G. M. (1991). Preliminary results with a six spectral maxima speech processor for The University of Melbourne/Nucleus multiple-electrode cochlear implant. *Journal of the Otolaryngological Society of Australia, 6*, 354–359.

Patrick, J. F., Seligman, P. M., Money, D. K., & Kuzma, J. A. (1990). Engineering. In G. M. Clark, Y. C. Tong, & J. F. Patrick (Eds.), *Cochlear prostheses*. (pp. 99–124). Edinburgh: Churchill Livingstone.

Seligman, P. M., Patrick, J. F., Tong, Y. C., Clark, G. M., Dowell, R. C., & Crosby, P. A. (1984). A signal processor for a multiple-electrode hearing prosthesis. *Acta Otolaryngologica (Stockholm)*, (Suppl. 411), 135–139.

Skinner, M. W., Clark, G. M., Whitford, L. A., Seligman, P. M., Staller, S. J., Shipp, D. B., Shallop, J. K., Everingham, C., Menapace, C. M., Arndt, P. L., Antognelli, T., Brimacombe, J. A., Pijl, S., Daniels, P., George, C. R., McDermott, H. J., & Beiter, A. L. (1994). Evaluation of a new spectral peak coding strategy for the Nucleus 22 channel cochlear implant system. *The American Journal of Otology, 15*, 15–27.

Tong, Y. C., Clark, G. M., Dowell, R. C., Martin, L. F. A., Seligman, P. M., & Patrick, J. F. (1981). A multiple-channel cochlear implant and a wearable speech processor. An audiological evaluation. *Acta Otolaryngologica (Stockholm), 92*, 193–198.

Wilson, B. S., Finley, C. C., Lawson, D. T., Wolford, R. D., Eddington, D. K., & Rabinowitz, W. M. (1991). Better speech recognition with cochlear implants. *Nature, 352*, 236–238.

Xu, J., Shepherd, R. K., Millard, R. E., & Clark, G. M. (in press). Chronic electrical stimulation of the auditory nerve at high stimulus rates: A physiological and histopathological study. *Hearing Research.*

9

SPEECH PROCESSOR PROGRAMMING

GARY RANCE
RICHARD C. DOWELL

For cochlear implant users to perceive the desired range of acoustic signals from their environment, the features of these sounds must control the electrical stimulation within the cochlea in an appropriate way. Low amplitude speech sounds of different spectral structure should elicit soft percepts and higher amplitude acoustic signals should elicit louder percepts while avoiding uncomfortably loud stimulation. As the useful dynamic range for electrical stimulation is relatively narrow and varies across patients and electrodes, there is a need to individually tailor the amplitudes of electrical stimulation for each patient. Simple psychophysical measurements establish the useful range for each electrode, and this information is stored digitally in the patient's speech processor. This process of programming or "mapping" is crucial to providing maximum speech information through the multiple-channel cochlear implant. The "mapping" process is a key part of the postoperative management of all cochlear implantees and occupies a significant proportion of the postoperative clinical time.

In adult cochlear implant users, programming is a relatively straightforward task as the psychophysical measure-

ments can be explained, and patients quickly understand the link between the mapping process and the output of their system. Young children and infants, on the other hand, require special care for a number of reasons if this process is to be successful. It is not possible to explain the requirements of the mapping procedure to young children. The stimulus-response and judgment tasks involved may be beyond their cognitive abilities, and the cooperation of young children for long sessions of testing can be variable.

This chapter briefly describes the technical framework for the mapping process in terms of basic physiology and electrical stimulation parameters and their relevance to auditory percepts and speech processing. It then outlines how modifications of standard pediatric audiological techniques can provide the necessary measurements for mapping of cochlear implants for young children and infants. Some of the problems encountered in programming implants in children are discussed along with approaches to their solution, and the chapter concludes with a discussion of the ongoing management of young implantees.

THE NUCLEUS-22 COCHLEAR IMPLANT

Damage to the basilar membrane or cochlear hair cells impedes or prevents the transduction of acoustic information into neural firing patterns in the auditory nerve. Cochlear implants offer a means of overcoming this signal breakdown, bypassing the normal cochlear mechanisms and providing artificial electrical stimulation directly to the auditory nerve. The most widely used cochlear implant system has been the Nucleus-22 device.

The Nucleus CI-22M Cochlear Implant

The Nucleus CI-22M multiple channel cochlear implant is a transcutaneous device. Information and power are passed to the system via radio frequency (RF) induction from an externally worn transmitting coil. The implant package consists of a coil that receives the RF signal, electronics that decode this signal and convert it into patterns of electrical stimulation, and an array of electrodes that presents these patterns to the auditory nerve.

The electrode array comprises a series of 32 platinum bands which are supported by a flexible Silastic carrier (Figure 9–1). The 22 bands located in the distal portion of this carrier are connected to the system's electronics via Teflon coated platinum-iridium wires. These bands are the implant's stimulating or "active" electrodes. The array is inserted into the scala tympani of the cochlea through a cochleostomy opening made near the round window. Insertion depths of at least 17 mm are desirable so that each of the active electrodes will be located within the cochlea. This objective is now routinely achieved in anatomically normal ears. Cases of congenital abnormality or cochlear damage resulting from pathologies such as labyrinthitis or cochlear otosclerosis can present a surgical problem, and occasionally result in "incomplete insertions" where active electrodes remain outside the cochlea. This situation has implications for the programming process which are discussed in later sections.

The New CI-24M Implant System

Cochlear Limited has recently developed a more advanced multiple-channel implant. This device, known as the CI-24M, contains a number of design modifications that affect the mapping process. The most obvious difference between this and the previous system can be seen in the configuration of the stimulating electrodes (Figure 9–2). In addition to the intracochlear array available with the Nu-

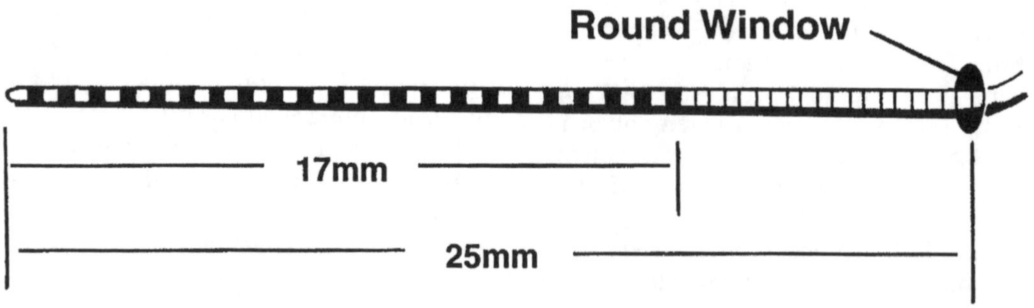

FIGURE 9–1. The intracochlear implant array (Nucleus–22).

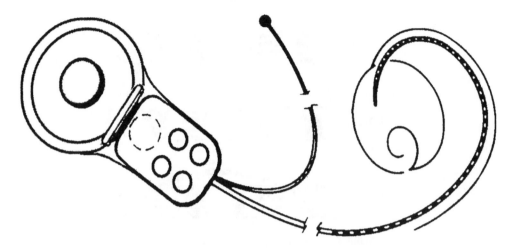

FIGURE 9–2. Diagram of the Nucleus CI-24M receiver/stimulator.

cleus-22 system, the CI-24M also offers the option of monopolar stimulation through either a ball electrode (placed in the temporalis muscle) or a series of four disk electrodes that are situated on the receiver/stimulator package.

ELECTRICAL STIMULATION OF THE COCHLEA

Stimulation Mode

Bipolar Stimulation

Auditory sensations arise when a flow of electrical current between electrodes stimulates auditory neural tissue in the cochlea. This current flow can be produced in a number of ways. The stimulation configuration most commonly used for adult implantees with the Nucleus 22 system is referred to as the "bipolar" mode (Figure 9–3). In this case, the current passes from one active electrode to one reference electrode. The physical separation of these electrodes determines the spread of the current, thereby controlling the area over which the spiral ganglion cells are stimu-

lated and the amount of current required to elicit a hearing sensation. In the true bipolar mode of stimulation where the active and reference electrodes are next to each other on the array (i.e., only 0.75 mm apart), there are often too few ganglion cells stimulated to create a sufficiently loud percept within the output limits of the system. Wider stimulation modes can be employed to overcome this problem. In the bipolar + 1 (BP+1) mode, for example, the stimulation distance is doubled as the active and reference electrodes are separated by an intermediate band. (See Figure 9–3 for details.) The amount of current required to produce a hearing sensation is subsequently reduced.

The optimal bipolar mode of stimulation for a particular subject is that which provides a sufficiently loud auditory percept, with the smallest distance between the stimulating electrodes. The BP+1 stimulation mode is appropriate for most cases. For some patients (particularly those with cochlear malformation), however, high threshold levels are often found with this strategy, and wider modes such as BP+2 or BP+3 may be necessary to provide a percept that is sufficiently loud.

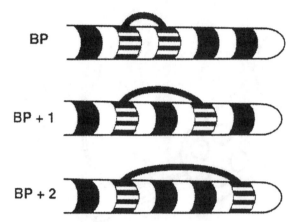

FIGURE 9–3. Schematic representation of bipolar stimulation modes.

Common Ground Stimulation

A flow of electrical current can also be generated within the cochlea using a technique referred to as "common ground" stimulation. In this mode, when an active electrode has been designated, all of the other electrodes are connected together electronically to constitute a single reference electrode. As a result, current spreads from the active channel to each of the others in the array. Figure 9–4 shows a simplified description of current flow for the bipolar, common ground and monopolar stimulation modes.

The representation of frequency information with multiple-channel implants is contingent on the ability of the electrode array to stimulate different groups of nerve fibers when the current is sent to different electrodes. Intuitively, bipolar modes of stimulation with their comparatively localized current distributions would seem better suited to this purpose. In practice, however, the common ground mode, in spite of its wider current spread, offers electrode discrimination equivalent to that provided by bipolar modes (Lim, Tong, & Clark, 1989). This occurs because the concentration of the current or the "charge density" is greatest in the vicinity of the active electrode (see Figure 9–5). The spiral

ganglion cells in this region therefore receive the most stimulation, and the pitch of the resulting auditory sensation relates to the position of this electrode within the cochlea. As such, there appears to be no disadvantage in employing the common ground mode for young implantees with complete electrode insertions.

Monopolar Stimulation

The CI-24M device, in addition to the bipolar and common ground modes, can also offer the option of monopolar stimulation. The monopolar mode is similar to the bipolar in the sense that a current flow is generated between a pair of electrodes. It does however differ from bipolar stimulation in that the current passes between an intracochlear and an extracochlear electrode. This stimulation paradigm offers a number of advantages over the previously described methods. The wide current spread can produce auditory percepts using much lower current levels than would be possible with common ground or even wide bipolar modes. This improvement in the efficiency of the stimulation means that information can potentially be presented at a faster rate and that the power consump-

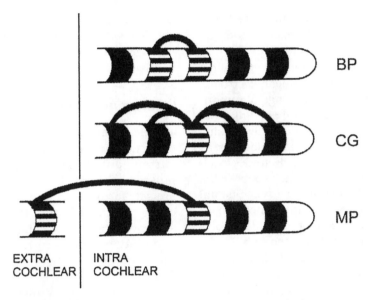

FIGURE 9–4. Diagram of current flow for bipolar (BP), common ground (CG), and monopolar (MP) stimulation modes.

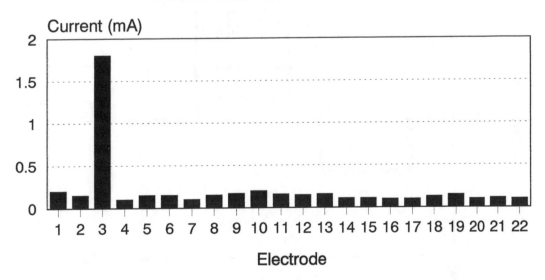

FIGURE 9–5. Current distribution for the common ground stimulation mode.

tion of the system can be minimized. The tonotopic pitch order of the electrode percepts is maintained with monopolar stimulation as the current density is greatest around the active intracochlear electrode.

The possible disadvantage of a monopolar system is that some current flows external to the cochlea, potentially causing stimulation of other structures. However, as the size of the extracochlear electrodes is relatively large, the current density outside the cochlea is small and unlikely to elicit neural stimulation. In practice, unwanted sensations are no more common for monopolar stimulation than for bipolar modes.

Although the Nucleus CI-22M implant does not have an extracochlear electrode, it is possible in cases of incomplete insertion to use extracochlear active channels in a "pseudomonopolar" paradigm. Typi-

cally electrode 1, which is outside the cochlea, will be used as the common reference electrode and paired sequentially with bands that are within the scala tympani.

Stimulation Parameters

The electrical stimuli presented by the Nucleus devices are in the form of biphasic current pulses (see Figure 9–6). These pulses are charge-balanced, and as such are safe for biological systems, preventing charge build-up within the cochlear tissues or the electrode bands as a result of stimulation. The perceived loudness of these pulses is related to the total charge delivered (Shannon, 1983), with louder sounds produced by higher levels. The total charge is determined by two pulse parameters: the pulse height and the pulse

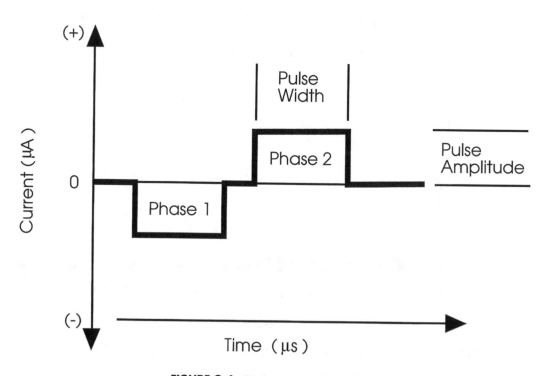

FIGURE 9–6. Biphasic stimulus pulse.

width. The pulse height is the level of current and ranges from 20 μA to 1750 μA (Nucleus CI-22M), and from 10 μA to 1750 μA (CI-24M). The pulse width is the stimulus duration and ranges from 19.2 μs to 400 μs (Nucleus CI-22M), and from 7 μs to 400 μs (CI-24M).

These parameters are manipulated to produce sufficiently loud stimuli in the shortest possible time. This allows the highest possible stimulation rates for signal processing. These considerations have resulted in the "stimulus level" scale used within the programming software, which provides a logarithmic scale of "charge delivered" by varying current and pulse width.

FROM ACOUSTIC TO ELECTRICAL INFORMATION

It is now well established that multiple-channel implant systems such as the Nucleus devices can efficiently and effectively provide stimulation to the auditory nerve. Improvements in signal coding engineering over the last 10 years have resulted in implant systems that provide significant open-set speech perception abilities to the majority of users. This level of performance is achieved through provision of accurate, encoded representations of the major features of the acoustic signal.

Spectral Coding

In the normal ear the mechanics of the basilar membrane and the active process of the outer hair cells allow a fine spectral analysis of the acoustic signal by transposing acoustic frequency into position on the basilar membrane. This place/frequency or "tonotopic" organization, which is maintained throughout the auditory system to the level of the cortex, forms the basis for the transmission of frequency information with multiple-channel cochlear implants. Psychophysical studies have es-

tablished that, by varying the site of electrical stimulation within the cochlear partition, different pitch percepts can be elicited (Tong et al., 1982; Tong et al., 1983). Furthermore, the relationship between the site of electrical stimulation and pitch has been shown to be similar to that seen for acoustic signals. As a result, spectral information can be represented by arranging the stimulation channels in accordance with the natural tonotopic organization of the cochlea.

In the current signal processing scheme (SPEAK) for the Nucleus 22 and 24 systems, the incoming signal undergoes a spectral analysis using a set of 20 band-pass filters covering the main audible frequency range (100 to 10,000 Hz). Each of the 20 filters is assigned to an electrode channel based on the tonotopic arrangement of the cochlea. In the simplest situation, where 20 intracochlear electrode channels are available, there is a one-to-one correspondence. For each stimulation sequence, the filters with the maximum amplitudes (between 6 and 10) determine which electrode channels are to be stimulated. The outputs of these filters then control the stimulation level for each of these channels. The channels are then stimulated sequentially. Once the sequence is completed, the filters are scanned again and a different sequence of electrode channels will be stimulated. With the CI-24M system, overall stimulation rates of 12,000 pulses per second are possible allowing a rate of 2,000 Hz for cycling through six electrodes.

Temporal Coding

Along with the fine spectral analysis provided by the cochlea, temporal patterns in the firing of auditory nerve fibers are also related to the incoming acoustic signal. For low and mid frequencies, the action potentials within the nerve fibers can be shown to be phase-locked to the acoustic signal. Electrical stimulation has been shown to precisely control the firing of auditory nerve fibers. As such, cochlear implant systems can effectively represent temporal information.

Intensity Coding

The loudness of auditory signals in the normal auditory system is related to the overall rate of firing of individual nerve fibers as well as the number of fibers actually firing above threshold. The dynamic range of this system exceeds 100 dB. This poses something of a problem in the case of electrical stimulation of the auditory nerve, where dynamic ranges of only 12 dB to 15 dB are typical (Shannon, 1983). As a result, precise control of the levels of electrical stimulation that are provided to the subject is required to ensure that uncomfortably loud signals are prevented.

A degree of signal compression is also required so that the loudness differences within the acoustic signal can be represented within the implantee's electrical dynamic range. Loudness is encoded via stimulus amplitude using variations of pulse height and width as described previously. The current speech processors have a working acoustic dynamic range of approximately 30 dB. Under normal operating conditions, this range will encompass sounds from approximately 40 dB SPL to 70 dB SPL across the speech frequencies. This acoustic range is set by the user with the sensitivity control on the speech processor which determines the gain of the preamplifier. An Automatic Gain Control operates when the acoustic amplitude reaches the high end of this dynamic range (~70 dB under normal conditions). The low point of the operating range (nominally 40 dB) is mapped to just above the threshold level for the electrode to be stimulated, and the high point and any sounds exceeding this level are mapped to the maximum comfort level.

IMPLANT PROGRAMMING

An early observation with cochlear implants was that the amount of current required to elicit a hearing sensation was different for each patient and for each stimulation channel. As such it is impossible to build a system that will automatically suit all patients. Each speech processor must be individually tailored to suit the particular implantee. This task, referred to as "programming" or "mapping," is typically performed by an audiologist operating a diagnostic programming system (DPS).

The diagnostic programming system is essentially an interface, providing a link between a computer and the patient's speech processor (see Figure 9–7). It allows bursts of electrical pulses (pulse trains) to be presented at precisely determined levels to the implant. These stimuli can be used to establish the function of each channel individually, providing information that can be programmed into the memory of the speech processor.

The basic aim of programming is to determine the useful dynamic range of electrical stimulation for each electrode channel. The dynamic range is bounded by the threshold level (T-level) and the maximum comfort level (C-level). Threshold level refers to the smallest amount of current that can consistently elicit a hearing sensation. It has a clear psychophysical definition and is usually established by passing threshold twice using an ascending method.

C-level is the upper limit of stimulation that is allowable for a particular channel. As such, it is analogous to the maximum power output (MPO) level in a hearing aid. It can be described as the maximum stimulation level that does not produce an uncomfortably loud sensation.

Once the dynamic range has been established for each channel, the processor can be programmed to present the encoded speech and environmental sounds at

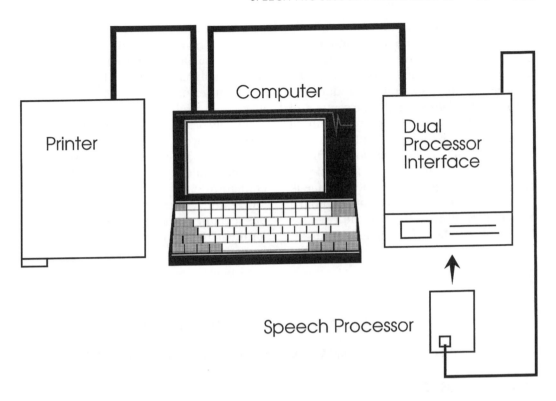

FIGURE 9–7. Block diagram of the programming hardware.

stimulus levels between the threshold and C-level. The overall loudness of this signal, although influenced by the threshold levels, is primarily determined by the C-levels. C-levels set too low will restrict the stimulation to levels close to the patient's threshold, resulting in an overall percept that is too soft. C-levels set too high, on the other hand, will result in stimulation that may be uncomfortable or even painful.

Before the First Programming Session

The timing of the first programming session varies from one clinic to the next, from as early as 10 days to 6 weeks after surgery. Readers should refer to Chapter 4 on the Melbourne Cochlear Implant Program and Surgery for a discussion of the relevant issues.

The audiologist should be aware before the first postoperative programming session of the location of the implanted electrode array, and the possibility that some active channels may be outside the cochlea. This will usually be clear from the surgical report, and can be confirmed by postoperative X-ray. This information is useful in determining both the number of channels that are likely to be available for speech processing and the most appropriate stimulation mode.

Stimulation Mode (Nucleus CI-22M)

The common ground stimulation pattern is currently the most used configuration for young implantees who have all of their active electrodes within cochlea. This approach offers a number of practical advantages over bipolar modes. First, the common ground mode allows comparatively easy identification of electrode anomalies. Occasionally, the wires linking the electrodes to the implant electronics can be damaged during the surgery, producing a range of effects such as short circuits and open circuits. The specific programming consequences of these anomalies are discussed in detail in a later section. Suffice it to say at this stage that, with common ground stimulation, electrode damage is far more obvious during the standard mapping procedure than is the case for bipolar stimulation. As it is difficult to ob-

tain accurate information in the early stages of programming for young children, the common ground mode reduces the risk that such damage will remain undetected.

Another major advantage of common ground stimulation relates to the predictability of stimulation levels for channels across the array. Only minor T- and C-level differences are usually seen between adjacent electrodes with this mode. The typical configuration of stimulation levels shows low T- and C-levels on the most apical and basal channels, and slightly higher levels for the midrange channels (Figure 9–8).

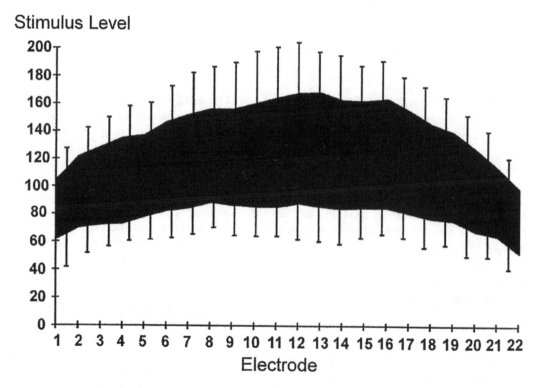

COMMON GROUND MODE

Average T-Levels and C-Levels for a group of implanted children

FIGURE 9–8. Mean thresholds amd maximum comfortable levels for 28 implanted children in the common ground mode.

The stimulation level predictability provided by the common ground mode can be of assistance when establishing threshold levels with children, as their limited concentration span prevents detailed assessment of every channel within a test session. It is therefore necessary to estimate the levels of at least a few untested channels. As significant level differences between adjacent channels are quite unusual with common ground stimulation, assessment of every second or third channel across the array can provide sufficient information for the intermediates to be predicted.

With common ground stimulation, estimates of C-level can also be made for channels that have not been thoroughly investigated during the test session. A degree of caution is however necessary in this case as the child could potentially be presented with unpleasantly loud stimuli. It is therefore essential that the child be tested with at least one stimulus at the proposed C-level to ensure that it is not uncomfortable.

One situation in which common ground stimulation may be considered inappropriate for use with young implantees is where the electrode array has been only partially inserted into the cochlea. Each of the 21 nonactive electrodes when using the CG paradigm are connected, and therefore receive a small amount of current. This is the case even for electrodes that have been deactivated using the programming software. As a result, current spread to extracochlear electrodes can occur, producing unusual (nontonotopic) hearing sensations, or tactile sensations if the electrodes are in contact with structures in the middle ear.

Identification of extracochlear electrodes is also more difficult with the common ground mode. Current spread from an active electrode in the cochleostomy, or in the middle ear to electrodes inside the cochlea, can result in T-levels and C-levels that are similar to those seen for intra-cochlear channels. The point at which the electrode array leaves the cochlea is more obvious when bipolar stimulation is used. In this case, the localized current spread results in sharp T- and C-level increases for active electrodes beyond the cochlear partition.

Stimulation Mode (CI-24M)

The monopolar mode offers the same stimulation level predictability as the common ground mode. As the reference electrode (extracochlear) remains fixed in this case, the electrical stimulation levels needed for threshold and maximum comfortable levels are relatively similar across the array. This allows estimation of threshold levels for untested channels, which can save time in programming young children.

Unlike the common ground mode, electrode shorts between active electrodes may be difficult to identify in the monopolar mode as normal percepts are likely on the affected channels. The use of the electrode telemetry available with the CI-24M system does, however, make shorted electrodes easy to isolate. Damaged electrodes should be conspicuous by their low impedance levels.

Objective Test Techniques and Speech Processor Programming

Averaged Electrode Voltages

Measurement of the electrical artifact of stimulation pulses from surface electrodes is easily accomplished with modern evoked potential equipment (Shallop et al., 1995). This type of testing can be performed at the time of surgery, after surgery using sedation, or in awake children who will accept the measuring electrodes. This can provide valuable information about overall function of the device, electrode anomalies, and confirmation of electrode positioning (Mahoney & Proctor, 1994). Many clinics use this procedure during surgery to ensure that the implant is functioning. Postoperatively, this technique is helpful in cases of suspected device failure or in identifying problem electrodes. This information, along with surgery reports, radiology findings, and psychophysical measurements can be valuable for the managing audiologist in deciding which electrode channels and mode of stimulation to use. It would appear essential for implant centers to have access to this technique, particularly for young children and infants.

Electrically Evoked Auditory Brainstem Response (EABR)

Auditory potentials evoked by pulsatile electrical signals delivered within the cochlea have been measured in many adult and child implant users (Kileny, 1991; Shallop et al., 1990). The potentials arising within the first 5 ms following the stimulus correspond in latency to the well-known click-evoked auditory brainstem response. In the case of electrical stimulation the latencies are shortened by around 1.5 ms due to the direct stimulation of the auditory nerve. This removes the delays associated with basilar membrane and hair cell processes. In addition, latencies show little change with intensity, again due to the removal of the normal cochlear processes. The relatively large amplitude of the electrical signals produced by the implant can make recording of the EABR difficult. For this reason, it is important for audiologists attempting to measure these responses to have good engineering support. Further problems can arise when attempting to record in operating theaters due to external electrical interference. If the technical problems are dealt with adequately, measurement of the EABR can provide useful guidance for programming young children. On the other hand, results obtained during the surgical procedure are typically different from those obtained postsurgery (Brown et al., 1994). Although EABR thresholds correlate with T- and C-levels obtained from behavioral testing, they do not provide enough reliable information for accurate programming (Shallop et al., 1991). The EABR has been useful in developmentally delayed or disabled children where behavioral testing has been difficult and poor responses suggest possible device failure or retrocochlear pathology.

Electrically Evoked Stapedial Reflexes

The stapedius reflex has been measured in response to electrical stimulation within the cochlea by direct observation during surgery (Battmer, Laszig, & Lehnhardt, 1990) or using standard acoustic impedance measurement techniques in the contralateral ear (Jerger et al., 1986). This technique has also been used to estimate C-levels for speech processor programming. The stapedial reflex thresholds were found to be acceptably close to behavioral C-levels in some adults and children but to over- or underestimate these levels in others (Spivec & Chute, 1994). In addition, the stapedial reflex could not be elicited in 40% of subjects, presumably due to middle ear pathology or abnormalities. As with the EABR, these measurements can provide some guidance for programming but do not replace the need for careful behavioral assessment.

Measurement of Auditory Nerve Compound Action Potential Using Implant Telemetry

This technique incorporated into the Nucleus CI-24M system may offer the best possibility of providing automatic speech processor programming for young children and infants (see Chapter 8). The intracochlear electrodes are used as recording electrodes between stimulus pulses giving a near-field recording of the activity of the auditory neurons in the vicinity. The growth function of the compound action potential may provide a reliable relationship with behavioral T- and C-levels for children.

Although these nonvolitional techniques can provide technical information about device function and electrode placement, and can give a rough guide to programming for some children, we would suggest that behavioral test techniques are essential for the optimal setting of the implant system.

Behavioral Programming Techniques

Behavioral testing with young implantees can be a long and complicated process. The limited auditory experience that most of the children have had prior to implantation means that, in the early stages of programming, their responses to the implant signal can be subtle and inconsistent. As such, it is essential the audiologists dealing with the child have as much experience with pediatric assessment as possible.

It is also useful to have two audiologists working together to identify and interpret the child's reactions. The first audiologist is involved with the DPS equipment and is responsible for the presentation of the test stimuli. This tester is usually not in the direct view of the child, reducing the risk of responses arising from visual, rather than auditory, cues. The second audiologist works more closely with the child, ensuring that there is an appropriate response state, watching for behavioral responses, and preparing the child for conditioned listening tasks. Both testers should be involved in decisions of response validity. Thus, the test room should be set up in such a way that both can have a clear view of the child at all times (see Figure 9–9).

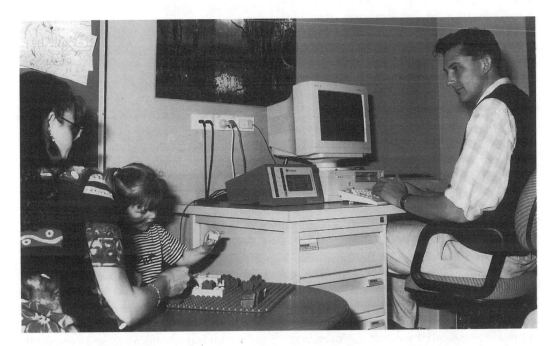

FIGURE 9–9. Photograph of room configuration for behavioral testing.

First Stimulation

Although nonvolitional tests of implant function can offer evidence of signal audibility, currently, available techniques can provide only estimates of stimulation levels. For the vast majority of children, the most effective way to initially determine the amount of current that can elicit an auditory sensation is through observation of behavior. If the child is calm and settled, short duration stimuli (such as a 500 ms train of pulses) can be presented at increasing intensity levels until a response is observed. The changes in behavior suggesting that the child has become aware of the signal include alterations in facial expression, momentary stilling, and touching of the stimulating coil. For a child in a good response state, the novelty of the implant signal usually allows responses to be observed at near threshold levels. This "novelty period" can be used to obtain clear responses for a number of channels until the child begins to habituate to the signal. Once a clear response has been obtained for the stimulus at a particular level, this signal can be used as a basis for conditioned audiometric testing.

Measuring Threshold Levels

Techniques for measuring thresholds to acoustic stimuli in young children are well established. These same test methods can be employed to assess the thresholds for electrical stimulation in young implantees.

Visual Reinforcement Audiometry (VRA)

This technique is appropriate for assessment of children as young as 5 months of age. In the initial stages of the testing, a visual reward such as the illumination of a concealed puppet is paired with an audible stimulus (classical conditioning). The sound is subsequently presented in isolation and the child, if properly conditioned, should anticipate the reward and turn to the puppet (operant conditioning). A response is accepted and a reward provided only if the child responds at the appropriate time. Once reliable responses have been obtained at the conditioning level, the intensity of the stimulus is reduced to determine the softest signal to which the child can respond. Results obtained using this test technique suggest that, provided the child is in a reasonable response state and is sufficiently rewarded by the visual reinforcer, responses can be obtained at threshold levels (Moore, Thompson, & Thompson, 1975; Moore & Wilson, 1978).

Play Audiometry

From the age of approximately 2 years, children can be trained to wait for a stimulus and then to respond to it with a simple task (Wilson & Thompson, 1984). Test materials that lend themselves to this technique involve simple, repetitive play activities such as placing a peg in a board or a candle on a cake. As with VRA testing, the child is initially trained using a suprathreshold stimulus before responses to threshold level stimuli are sought.

Conditioned audiometric testing using either the VRA or play audiometry techniques is one of the bases for preoperative assessment of cochlear implant candidates. As such, all young implantees should be familiar with these procedures when the time comes for their devices to be programmed. Whether or not this familiarity is an advantage or a disadvantage depends to an extent on the creativity of the clinicians involved. It can certainly help the testing process if the children understand what is expected of them. Practice with play activities similar to those used in audiometric testing can often form an important part of the preoperative training program. Children who have been assessed repeatedly with the same activities, on the other hand, can quickly lose interest. A wide range of test materials is desirable.

Maximum Comfortable Levels (C-Levels)

C-levels in initial programming sessions are usually arbitrarily set slightly above threshold to minimize the risk of device rejection. As the child becomes more confident with the system over the next few weeks or months, the levels can be increased to give "appropriate" signal loudness.

The setting of the upper limits of stimulation in children is a complicated task. C-levels in adult implantees are set subjectively by users to suit their tastes. As such, they are not psychophysically definable in the same sense as thresholds. This variability poses a problem with implant programming for young children who cannot make, or at least express, subjective judgments on the tolerability of a particular level of stimulation.

Older children (from the age of around 5 years) can be trained to give estimates of stimulus loudness using written scales or pictorial representations of comfort (Staller, Beiter, & Brimacombe, 1991), but a significant number will not be able to carry out these types of tasks before the age of 7 years without extensive training and experience with the device (MacPherson et al., 1991).

The only practical way of establishing loudness estimates for young children is through behavioral observation. The level of the stimulus on a particular channel can be gradually increased until a loudness discomfort level (LDL) is obtained. Once this point has been reached the C-level can be set below it. Recent clinical studies at The University of Melbourne have been carried out to investigate the relationship between LDL and C-level in a group of experienced adult implant users. The results, shown in Figure 9–10, varied slightly among patients, but suggested that maximum comfort levels were typically preferred at about 70% of the T-level to LDL range (L. Whitford, personal communication). In accordance with these findings, C-levels for children at the authors' center are typically set at levels around 30% of the dynamic range below the point at which an LDL is observed.

Loudness discomfort levels in children can be established using different types of stimuli. One such stimulus is the "single electrode map" (Mecklenberg et al., 1990). Speech and environmental inputs in this case are programmed onto a particular channel, and the child's behavior is monitored while the C-level and/or T-level is gradually increased. The advantages of this stimulus are that it can provide a "natural" sound over which the child may be able to exert some control (with toys, noisemakers, etc.) and the signal is continuous and, as such, similar to the stimulation that would be presented in the normal listening environment. The usefulness of the single electrode map in C-level estimation has, however, proven to be limited. Because the stimulus is constant, it can be difficult to correlate the implant signal with changes in child's behavior. Responses also tend to be difficult to identify, and may be as subtle as slight changes in facial expression or an increase in the aggressiveness of the child's play. Furthermore, the continuous input usually results in the child adapting to the signal. When this occurs, the stimulus tends to be completely ignored until it becomes unbearably loud, at which point the child becomes distressed.

Clinical experience has shown that behavioral responses are more clearly seen to discrete stimuli such as the 500 ms pulse trains used to set thresholds. This signal offers a number of advantages for the setting of C-levels in young children. First, the clinician can control the timing of the stimulus presentation, choosing a moment when the child is still and calm, and

C-level as a Percentage of the Threshold to LDL Range

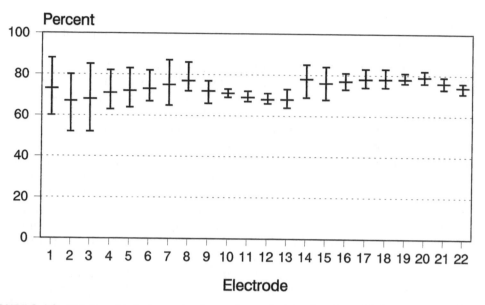

FIGURE 9–10. Relationship between loudness discomfort level and useful dynamic range for adult implant patients. The C-levels are shown as a percentage of the range from threshold to loudness discomfort level.

thereby increasing the chances of response identification. Second, by employing inter-stimulus times of sufficient length, the audiologist can avoid the adaptation problems seen with frequent or constant inputs. Third, the pulse train stimulus allows precise control of the presentation level. This is in contrast to the situation with single electrode maps, where the exact level of stimulation is contingent on the level of the environmental input. The final major benefit afforded by the brief stimulus relates to the type of response that it elicits. Where constant signals produce minor changes in the child's affect, the rapid onset of the pulse train usually elicits an aural palpebral reflex (APR). This eye blink response is identical to that which can be clearly and reliably seen in normally hearing subjects to sudden acoustic stimuli such as a drum beats and bursts of narrow band noise (Taft & Cohen, 1967). As with the acoustic case,

the electrically evoked APR can be consistently elicited by stimuli at loud, but not distressingly loud, levels. It can therefore provide a useful guide to C-level estimation in young implantees.

Interchannel Loudness Balancing

To ensure that the cues available in the speech signal are faithfully conveyed by the implant, it is desirable to have the implantee match the relative loudness of stimulation for each of the channels. The benefits of providing a signal that is loudness balanced across the frequency range have been demonstrated in a number of hearing aid studies and have been reported anecdotally for implant users (Byrne & Tonisson 1976; Skinner et al., 1981). Furthermore, a recent study of speech perception abilities in 10 postlinguistically deafened adult implantees showed that optimal results were obtained when the implant signals at C-level for each channel were considered to be of equal loudness. When this loudness equilibrium was disrupted by a random alteration of the patient's C-levels by as little as 0 to ± 20% of the dynamic range, significant deteriorations in performance were obtained in most cases (Dawson, Skok, & Clark, in press). The authors of this study felt that the observed decrease in perception ability was likely to be the result of both a disruption of the amplitude cues within the speech signal and a loss of spectral information presented to the softer channels. These results suggest that attempting to obtain loudness balanced maps for our young implantees is a worthwhile objective.

Interchannel loudness balancing tasks can be structured in a variety of ways. The task requires that the implantee manipulate the stimulation levels in order to match the loudness across a number of channels. Testing with adult subjects has shown loudness balancing to be a perceptually difficult task, requiring comparison of stimuli that differ in pitch as well as loudness. For young children, particularly those with limited listening experience and language development, it is often impossible to obtain meaningful results. For these children we must rely on the loudness discomfort measures used to set the maximum comfort levels. By setting the C-level for each channel a standard percentage of the dynamic range below the loudness discomfort level, an approximate loudness balance across the array should arise if the growth of loudness is similar for each channel.

Problem Electrodes

Damage to the Electrode Array

Electrode problems due to mechanical trauma during the implant surgery are rare with the Nucleus CI-22M and CI-24M arrays. They do however occur from time to time, producing complex and potentially unpleasant effects, particularly in bipolar modes of stimulation. As such, it is essential that audiologists be aware of the symptoms of these anomalies so that the affected electrodes can be identified and removed from the speech processor map.

Open Circuit

An open circuit arises when the platinum-iridium wire leading to a particular electrode is broken. This situation can be detected relatively easily, as stimulation using that electrode will produce no sensation. In bipolar modes, each electrode is involved in two stimulation channels (once as the active electrode, and once as the reference electrode). Both of these channels will be affected in the case of an open circuit. In the common ground and monopolar modes, only the channel that employs the broken electrode as the active will be involved.

Short Circuit Between Active Electrodes

A short circuit between two active electrodes can occur when the insulation coating surrounding a number of electrode wires is damaged, but the wires themselves are not broken. As was mentioned previously, stimulation using these electrodes can still occur, but the short circuit produces unusual current distributions affecting the stimulation levels.

In the case of bipolar stimulation four channels are usually affected, with two showing lower T- and C-levels than the channels around them and two showing higher T- and C-levels. This pattern can be seen in Figure 9–11 which shows the map obtained for an adult subject programmed in BP+1. In this case, the abnormal current distribution patterns produced by a short circuit between electrodes 5 and 10,

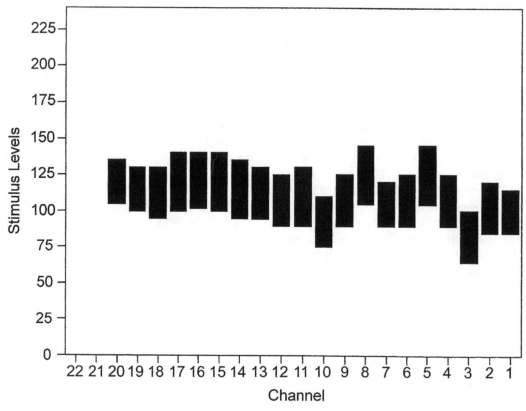

FIGURE 9–11. Graph of T- and C-levels for a subject with a short between electrodes 5 and 10 (bipolar+1 mode).

have resulted in significantly reduced levels for channels 3 and 10 and elevated levels for channels 5 and 8.

Identification of shorted electrodes is often difficult in bipolar modes even with cooperative adult subjects. In young children for whom the setting of stimulation levels may be based on conservative estimation, it can be almost impossible. It is partly for this reason that the common ground mode is recommended for all children with complete electrode insertions. In the CG mode only channels employing the shorted bands as the active electrode will be affected (see Figure 9–12). These channels are relatively easy to isolate in that they typically show higher threshold levels and no growth in loudness with increases in stimulus level

(in the example, C-levels will not be obtainable for channels 5 and 10).

Another important reason for not using the BP+1 mode with children relates to the potential for unpleasantly loud stimulation with intermittent short circuits. As can be seen in the bipolar example, where the short was present during the programming session, elevated levels have been obtained for channels 5 and 8. If the electrode wires in this case were subsequently to move out of contact, the current distributions would return to normal. The appropriate T- and C-levels for these channels would drop to levels more like those seen for the others in the map. Stimulation within the limits set while the short was present would then be uncomfortable for the implantee.

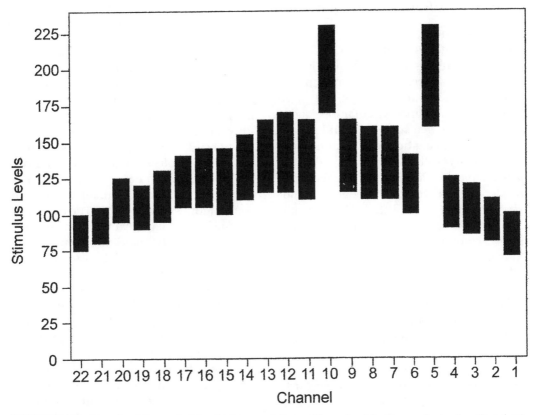

FIGURE 9–12. Graph of T- and C-levels for a subject with a short between electrodes 5 and 10 (common ground mode).

A short between two active electrodes in the monopolar mode results in normal percepts for the affected channels. The current is in this case split between the two, typically resulting in elevated stimulation levels.

Short Circuit Between an Active and a Nonactive Electrode

Short circuits can also occur between the wires leading to active electrodes and the stiffening rings (nonactive electrodes), which are found at the electronic package end of the array. In this case, two electrode channels are affected in the bipolar mode. These channels may experience changes in the pitch and loudness of the hearing sensation and may produce a tactile sensation through current flow to the nonactive band at or outside the cochleostomy. The effect will be similar in the common ground and monopolar modes.

Electrode shorts and open circuits are almost always the result of damage to the array at the time of the implant surgery. As such, these anomalies are usually present at the time of the first programming session. The effects of the damage may, however, be intermittent and may not become obvious in the short term. An intermittent problem should be suspected if large changes in C-level are seen for isolated channels. The appropriate action when an anomaly has been identified is to deactivate the affected electrode(s).

Nonauditory/Painful Sensations

Electrical stimulation can occasionally produce nonauditory percepts. Certain patients (particularly those with otosclerosis or unusually shaped cochleas) may notice a tactile rather than auditory sensation with stimulation on particular electrodes or may experience some unusual sensations in the face, such as twitching near the eye as a result of current spread to the facial nerve. The latter of these effects can be identified in children through close observation at the time of stimulus presentation. In the case of a feeling sensation, however, young implantees may be unable to express the nature of their percept to the audiologist. As a result, identification of electrodes producing nonauditory sensations can be difficult. The most obvious indication of a problem channel can usually be found in its dynamic range. Clear aversive reactions to the stimulus are most commonly obtained at levels quite close to threshold (within 10 stimulus levels) in these cases. If large differences in dynamic range between adjacent electrodes are observed, nonauditory stimulation should be suspected, and the questionable channels should be deactivated.

Creating a Map

Once threshold and C-level measurements have been made for some or all of the channels, the speech processor can be programmed with the dynamic ranges for stimulation. These and other parameters that control the presentation of encoded speech information through the implant are typically referred to as the "map." They are stored in the memory of the speech processor, controlling its function during normal use. The thresholds and, most importantly, the C-levels obtained for individual electrodes clearly have a bearing on the loudness of the speech signal. There are, however, two major reasons why the

levels set in psychophysical testing may not necessarily produce a level of speech that is comfortable for the implantee. First, the speech signal may be continuous whereas the test stimuli are transient (usually lasting only 500 ms). Stimulation at a particular level may be tolerable for a limited time, but could potentially become uncomfortable over a longer period.

Second, the presentation of speech information involves stimulation on a number of channels in quick succession. This quasi-simultaneous stimulation results in some loudness summation. The number of channels stimulated varies with encoding system, but with the SPEAK strategy, for example, there could be as many as 10 channels involved.

It is essential that the child be observed wearing the device in speech mode before the completion of the test session. This observation can take the form of a structured listening task, such as a phoneme detection test, or can be carried out with the child involved in a free-play activity. In either case, it is important that the acoustic stimuli be loud enough to reach C-level (70 dB SPL) on each of the channels. As with testing of individual channels, reactions to a map with levels set too high can be idiosyncratic. The child may, for example, become quiet and withdrawn while listening to the stimulus, or he or she may become aggressive during play. As these reactions can also be the result of the strangeness of the signal, particularly in the first session(s), the best way to establish if a map is too loud is to present the child with a number of loud, sudden speech stimuli. If the child becomes upset or shows an eye-blink response, then the map or certain channels in the map may be too loud.

The appropriate action in this case is to reduce the levels of stimulation. The C-levels can be lowered on a channel by channel basis or by employing a global modification across the whole array. The most efficient approach depends on the circumstances. If, when testing the child with individual phonemes, it is possible to isolate certain sounds, and as a result, certain groups of channels that are causing the discomfort, it may be sufficient to reduce only the C-levels in that part of the array. Otherwise, the C-levels on each of the channels can be reduced by a percentage of the dynamic range (up to 30%) until a comfortable map is obtained.

Follow-up Mapping Sessions

Regular programming sessions are typically required for children in the weeks following the start-up. The limitations of clinical assessment with infants and young children usually mean that it is not possible to obtain threshold level responses for every channel in a single session. As such, it is necessary to test the child on a number of occasions before a clear picture of the stimulation levels begins to emerge.

The need for gradual increases in dynamic range also requires that the child be seen regularly in the initial period. The major programming aim in the first few weeks of implant use should be to create a signal that the child is prepared to tolerate. Device rejection can occasionally occur if the child is uncertain about the implant and the "foreign" sounds it produces. It is for this reason that a degree of caution in the setting of C-levels is required. Clinical experience has shown that, for the first map, C-levels are best set arbitrarily at a level slightly above threshold (with a dynamic range of perhaps 10–15 stimulus levels). This range should then be increased slowly over a number of sessions until the child is confident enough to tolerate a map with levels set using the behavioral observation techniques discussed previously.

Another reason for regular programming sessions in the initial period relates to the effects of postsurgical physiological changes. Healing mechanisms within the cochlea such as the formation of a fibrous tissue sheath around the electrode array can affect the current flow induced by the implant and can result in significant changes in both T- and C-levels up to 6 months after implantation. The presence of these clinically observed changes is consistent with telemetric evidence that has shown significant variations in electrode impedance in the initial postimplant period (Swanson, Seligman, & Carter, 1995). Careful and regular monitoring of the progress of young children is therefore required for a number of months after the surgery as initially appropriate maps could potentially become inaudible or uncomfortably loud.

Map Fluctuations

After an initial adjustment period, stimulation levels usually stabilize, allowing the implantee to listen to a consistent signal for extended periods. Level fluctuations can however arise, even in long-term users of the system. Minor T- and C-level variations are not necessarily cause for concern, often occurring gradually without the patient noticing any loss of signal clarity. Stimulus level fluctuations can however be more dramatic, with significant changes to T- and C-levels arising over a short period of time. Such fluctuations can be distressing to the implantee, and may be the result of some problem with the implant device or a change in the status of the patient's ear.

The clearest indication of stimulus level fluctuations in children can usually be obtained from threshold testing. Unlike C-levels, which are based on subjective estimates of loudness or on behaviorally observed responses, threshold levels are psychophysically well defined. Significant variations in threshold levels therefore reflect a change in the function of the system rather than a change in the percept. The amount of stimulus level variation that constitutes a "significant" change depends to an extent on the dynamic range of the channel. A shift of 20 stimulus levels in a range of 100 stimulus levels is less of a concern than if the dynamic range was only 30 stimulus levels. As a general rule, changes of greater than 20% of the dynamic range should be treated as abnormal.

Clues to the cause of extreme level fluctuations can often be found in the pattern of the changes. In cases where there is a trend in the threshold shifts (a decrease or an increase in the thresholds for a group of channels), for example, some pathological changes in the vicinity of the array should be suspected. Changes to the composition of the cochlear fluids or tissue in the cochlea may affect the flow of current from the implant to the spiral ganglion cells, resulting in changes to stimulation levels. Such variations have been observed in conjunction with active middle ear disease for a number of child and adult cases (Donnelly, Pyman, & Clark, 1995).

Stimulus level shifts affecting groups of channels can also be the result of movement of the electrode array. The risk of this occurring is very low with current surgical techniques, but in some cases it may be prudent to obtain an X-ray to confirm electrode position within the cochlea. Immediate referral to the otologist is the appropriate course of action when a significant shift in stimulus levels is observed across a number of implant channels.

Level fluctuations on isolated channels are more likely to be the result of electrode anomalies. Electrode damage usually occurs at the time of the surgery, but its effects, particularly if they are intermittent, may not present themselves for some time.

If no response can be obtained to stimulation on some or all of the channels, some form of implant failure should be suspected. Although the Nucleus CI-22M receiver/stimulator has over the past 15 years proven itself to be a resilient and highly reliable device, problems with the implant package do occasionally occur. Objective confirmation of such a problem can be obtained from analysis of averaged electrode voltages (described previously). An absent or unusually shaped stimulus artifact can be evidence of implant abnormality.

Ongoing Management

Optimizing a child's use of the cochlear implant system is an interactive process that is most effective when it involves input from a number of parties. The audiologist is an important part of this process, programming the child's speech processor and thus determining the access that the child will have to auditory information. Responsibility for maintaining this access must rest in part with the teachers, habilitationists, and parents who are involved with the child on a daily basis.

As a young implantee may not be able to indicate when a problem has arisen, it is essential that the people around him or her be able to detect significant changes. Observation of the child's behavior can often reveal a change in implant function, particularly if the sound has become too loud for the child. In such cases, the child may blink, become upset, or perhaps even remove the transmitter coil upon hearing a loud sound. Behavioral observation is less effective in situations where the signal has become too soft or the sound quality has been affected. In such cases the only indication of a problem may be a tendency for the child to withdraw from communication or perhaps behave badly.

Regular listening checks are the best way to monitor the child's hearing through the implant. A simple phoneme detection task that can be quickly carried out at various times during the day can easily identify a problem. The child should be able to hear and respond to each of the speech sounds at levels around 40 dBA. If the child is unable to do so, a problem with either the device hardware (cables, microphone, speech processor, etc.) or with the levels in the map should be suspected.

SUMMARY

The basic elements of speech processor programming have been discussed in relation to the management of young children and infants with cochlear implants. With the careful use of established pediatric audiological techniques and information provided by objective assessments, reliable programming is possible in children as young as 5 months. At this stage, objective measures cannot substitute for behavioral information but telemetry provided by the latest implant system may assist this process.

REFERENCES

Battmer, R. D., Laszig, R., & Lenhardt, E. (1990). Electrically elicited stapedius reflex in cochlear implant patients. *Ear and Hearing, 5*, 370–374.

Brown, C. J., Abbas, P. J., Fryauf-Bertschy, H., Kelsay, D., & Gantz, B. J. (1994) Intraoperative and postoperative electrically-evoked auditory brainstem responses in Nucleus cochlear implant users: Implications for the fitting process. *Ear and Hearing, 15*, 168–176.

Byrne, D., & Tonisson, W. (1976). Selecting the gain of hearing aids for persons with sensorineural hearing impairments. *Scandinavian Journal of Audiology, 5*, 51–59.

Dawson, P. W., Skok, M., & Clark, G. M. (manuscript in preparation). The effect of loudness imbalance between electrodes in cochlear implant users.

Donnelly, M. J., Pyman, B. C., & Clark, G. M. (1995). Chronic middle ear disease and cochlear implantation. *Annals of Otology, Rhinology and Laryngology, 104*(9, Suppl. 166), 406–408.

Jerger, J., Jenkins, H., Fifer, R., & Mecklenberg, D. (1986). Stapedius reflex to electrical stim-

ulation in a patient with a cochlear implant. *Annals of Otology, Rhinology and Laryngology, 95*, 151–157.

Kileny, P. R. (1991). The use of electrophysiologic measures in the management of children with cochlear implants: Brainstem, middle latency and cognitive (P300) responses. *American Journal of Otology, 12*(Suppl.), 37–42.

Lim, H. H., Tong, Y. C., & Clark, G. M. (1989). Forward masking patterns produced by intra-cochlear electrical stimulation of one and two electrode pairs in the human cochlea. *Journal of the Acoustical Society of America, 86*(3), 971-980.

MacPherson, B. J., Elfenbein, J. L., Schum, R. L., & Bentler, R. A. (1991). Thresholds of discomfort in young children. *Ear and Hearing, 12*, 184–190.

Mahoney, M. J., & Proctor, L. A. R. (1994). The use of averaged electrode voltages to assess the function of Nucleus internal cochlear implant devices in children. *Ear and Hearing, 15*, 177–183.

Mecklenberg, D. J., Blamey, P. J., Busby, P. A., Dowell, R. C., Roberts, S., & Rickards, F. W. (1990). Auditory (re)habilitation for implanted deaf children and teenagers. In G. M. Clark, Y. C. Tong, & J. F. Patrick (Eds.), *Cochlear prostheses* (pp. 207–221). London: Churchill Livingstone.

Moore, J. M., Thompson, G., & Thompson, M. (1975). Auditory localization of infants as a function of reinforcement conditions. *Journal of Speech and Hearing Disorders, 40*, 29–34.

Moore, J. M., & Wilson, W. R. (1978). Visual reinforcement audiometry (VRA) with infants. In S. Gerber & G. Mencher (Eds.), *Early diagnosis of hearing loss* (pp. 177–213). New York: Grune & Statton.

Shallop, J. K., Beiter A. L., Goin D. W., & Mischke, R. E. (1990). Electrically-evoked auditory brainstem responses (EABR) and middle latency responses (EMLR) obtained from patients with the Nucleus multi channel implant. *Ear and Hearing, 11*, 5–15.

Shallop, J. K., Kelsall, D. C., Caleffe–Schenck, N., & Ash K. R. (1995). Application of averaged electrode voltages in the management of cochlear implant patients. *Annals of Otol-*

ogy, Rhinology and Laryngology, 104(9, Suppl. 166), 228–230.

Shallop, J. K., VanDyke, L., Goin, D. W., & Mischke, R. E. (1991). Prediction of behavioral threshold and comfort values for Nucleus 22–channel implant patients from electrical auditory brainstem response test results. *Annals of Otology Rhinology and Laryngology, 100*, 896–898.

Shannon, R. V., (1983). Multichannel electrical stimulation of the auditory nerve in man: I. Basic psychophysics. *Hearing Research, 11*, 157–189.

Skinner, M. W., Pascoe, D. P., Miller, J. D., & Poelka, G. R. (1981). Measurements to determine the optimal placement of speech energy within the listener's auditory area: A basis for selecting amplification characteristics. In G. A. Studebaker & F. H. Bess (Eds.), *The Vanderbuilt report; State Art—Research Needs.* Monographs in Contemporary audiology, Upper Darby, PA: Instrumentation Associates.

Spivec, L. G., & Chute, P. M. (1994). The relationship between electrical acoustic reflex thresholds and behavioral comfort levels in children and adult cochlear implant patients. *Ear and Hearing, 15*, 184–192.

Staller, S., Beiter, A. L., & Brimacombe, J. A. (1991). Children and multichannel cochlear implants. In H. Cooper (Ed.), *Cochlear implants: A practical guide* (pp. 283–321). London: Whurr.

Swanson, B., Seligman, P., & Carter, P. (1995). Impedance measurement of the Nucleus 22–electrode array in patients. *Annals of Otology, Rhinology and Laryngology, 104*(9, Suppl. 166), 141–144.

Taft, L. T., & Cohen, H. J. (1967). Neonatal and infant reflexology. In J. Hellmuth (Ed.), *Exceptional infant. Vol. 1: The normal infant.* New York: Brunner–Mazel.

Tong, Y. C., Clark, G. M., Blamey, P. J., Busby, P. A., & Dowell, R. C. (1982). Psychophysical studies for two multiple channel cochlear implant patients. *Journal of the Acoustical Society of America, 71*, 153–160.

Tong, Y. C., Dowell, R. C., Blamey, P. J., & Clark G. M. (1983). Two–component hearing sensations produced by two-electrode stimulation in the cochlea of a totally deaf patient. *Science, 219*, 993–994.

Wilson, W. R., & Thompson, G. (1984). Behavioral audiometry. In J. Jerger (Ed.), *Pediatric audiology* (pp. 1–44). San Diego: College-Hill Press.

10

HABILITATION: INFANTS AND YOUNG CHILDREN

ELIZABETH J. BARKER
SHANI J. DETTMAN
RICHARD C. DOWELL

Habilitation is a teaching/learning process in which the clinician guides the parent to facilitate development in the child. The key to successful use of the cochlear implant lies in vigilance in the technical management of the device and provision of an optimal environment to stimulate the development of listening as a learning tool for the child.

This chapter describes the historical development of the various educational and habilitation approaches now in use for hearing-impaired children. The impact of cochlear implants on these approaches is then discussed. Also outlined is a practical approach to the development of listening and comprehension in implanted children. Examples of habilitation activities and goals are provided.

LISTENING

Listening develops as a result of the search for meaning (Ling & Ling, 1978). The hearing or hearing-impaired infant will actively engage in this search in order to understand and influence the events in his or her environment. As early as 6 months,

the hearing infant can come to realize which acoustic cues are important for meaning (Kuhl et al., 1992; Ling & Ling, 1978). Language emerges to meet the ever more complex and developing needs of the child to make choices, reject offerings, and share experiences with those around him or her. The essential problem in the case of the hearing-impaired child is to determine whether an amplified or processed signal is sufficient for this process to occur. Habilitation attempts to address this problem.

HABILITATION

The role of the clinician providing an habilitation program is to facilitate acquisition of listening, speech, and language in a normal developmental order. This differs from providing rehabilitation, which aims to encourage reacquisition of lost communication skills (Dettman et al., 1996). For the adult with acquired hearing loss, the cochlear implant might be expected to assist rehabilitation by restoring an auditory percept. This should facilitate speech perception and provide the adult with a speech feedback loop. In this case, the linguistic and auditory processing systems are largely intact and provide a framework for dealing with an incomplete auditory signal.

For the child receiving a cochlear implant, the habilitation aims are more complex and holistic. The device needs to provide auditory abilities to facilitate the development of the entire linguistic system, to develop a range of speech sounds, to enable speech monitoring via auditory feedback, and therefore access shared knowledge of the world. Linguistic elements of language such as pragmatic skills, semantic concepts, vocabulary, and syntactic, morphological, and phonological systems must develop adequately to allow social, conversational interaction to take place. The framework for the processing and effective use of oral language must be created from the beginning.

The habilitation program must address the need for parent guidance, therapy, and informational and affective counseling. It may incorporate all of these aspects but, in dealing with preschool children, should be primarily parent focused. Sessions may be carried out in the clinical setting, the home, or a preschool environment. Parents who elect to proceed with a cochlear implant for their young child should be made aware of the importance of the habilitation program to optimize the result for the child.

Preoperative Habilitation

If possible, a regular routine of attending the clinic for habilitation sessions preoperatively will help the parent to know what to expect. The child will also become familiar with the clinic staff and environment, and will therefore be more likely to cooperate with programming and use of the device postoperatively. Preoperative habilitation sessions also provide opportunities to develop optimal use of the child's current device, hearing aids, or tactaid. Preoperative evaluations of the child's communicative

performance using these devices can prompt discussion of expectations of performance with the cochlear implant.

Some families are unable to attend the clinic regularly for habilitation sessions due to distance from the clinic. In this situation, liaison with local professionals who are qualified in early intervention with hearing-impaired children is essential to ensure adequate monitoring of device use. Meetings with both the professional and family will help to outline the role of each person. Families should still be aware of the need to attend the clinic regularly for programming the speech processor and medical monitoring, and these visits can be utilized also to review and discuss the child's progress in habilitation.

Educational Approaches and Communication Mode

Until the 1940s, oral approaches to the education of deaf children involved primarily the teaching of lipreading due to the inability to accurately measure or improve the residual hearing of the child. As a result of improvements in technology it became possible to assess the hearing of infants and fit wearable hearing aids. Up to 95% of children who had previously been labeled as "deaf" were found to have had useful residual hearing (Pollack, 1984). At this time the *oral* approach became known at the *oral/aural* approach, taking into consideration the use of the hearing aid to facilitate communication. Pollack began a program in 1948 to determine how infants could be educated to use their residual hearing and the guidelines for her "Acoupedic" program were formulated (Pollack, 1984). Further improvements to hearing aids and the advent of cochlear implants in the 1980s allowed greater numbers of young profoundly deaf children to access spoken language through audition.

The development and use of *signing* as a gestural code for language, used either alone or in combination with spoken language, has a long history (Clark et al., 1991). Whether choosing to use an oral/aural or a signing approach there are different emphases on visual or auditory elements. These may be considered along a continuum from visual to auditory perception (see Figure 10–1).

Sign Language of the Deaf is a gestural system that has a unique syntactic structure and no spoken correlate. *Signed English* encodes language with a specific sign for every individual word and morphological marker. *Total Communication* involves the use of Signed English, lipreading, and listening for the hearing-impaired person to perceive language. *Cued speech* employs a series of hand signals to indicate certain phonetic features (e.g., tongue position for vowels) which are not visible when lipreading. The *Oral/Aural* approach emphasizes the optimum use of residual hearing in conjunction with lipreading cues. The *Auditory/Verbal* approach emphasizes learning language and speech through the exclusive use of residual hearing and the deemphasis of lipreading cues.

Sign Language of the Deaf

Sign Language of the Deaf is a signing system that is totally visual and gestural (Clark et al., 1991). As it has no spoken syntactic equivalent it is difficult to speak in English

and use Sign Language of the Deaf simultaneously. As this system provides no auditory input and does not stimulate the use of residual hearing, the educational choice of Sign Language of the Deaf does not appear to be compatible with the choice of a cochlear implant for a child.

Total Communication

Total Communication aims to utilize gestural, lipreading, and auditory components of speech by combining Signed English and spoken English (Ling, 1984). The speaker must match every morpheme of spoken English with a sign or fingerspelled marker. The child is then exposed simultaneously to several cues indicating the same word or concept. Skilled users of this method are able to sign quickly enough to maintain normal prosody while speaking and signing. However, for many parents this method results in either a compromise of the complexity of the language used due to inadequate knowledge of the sign needed or a marked slowing of the rate of speech causing unnatural prosodic cues to be presented to the child.

The implant does offer improvement in the loudness and quality of the auditory component presented to the child, so for some children whose parents have chosen the total communication method, the implant allows for the input to become more

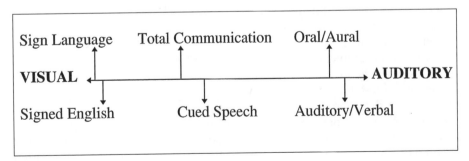

FIGURE 10–1. Habilitation approaches used with hearing-impaired children range along a continuum from highly visual to highly auditory.

truly total. Children vary in their ability to focus on the auditory component, which is competing with the equally accessible visual component. If the child is to maximize use of the auditory input provided by the cochlear implant then at least some time each day should be spent focusing on the auditory signal. As this divides the child's learning into separate skills, it is difficult to predict how well any individual child can combine these elements into a total comprehension of spoken language.

Oral/Aural Method

Cole (1992) provided an introduction to the differences behind visual versus auditory intervention for hearing-impaired children. One view is that the hearing-impaired child has a reorganized cognitive and psychological system due to the hearing loss, and therefore requires a visual code for language. A differing view is that the hearing-impaired child has normal cognitive function (unless shown otherwise by additional developmental delay), but requires "adequate" auditory and enriched linguistic experiences to develop optimally. The latter approach, which has been described as Oral/Aural habilitation, makes use of "embellishments" to normal interaction as suggested by Cole (1992). These include sitting close to the child, using an interesting voice, and increasing the frequency and consistency of interactions. Parents naturally begin to reward and reinforce the infant's first communicative attempts and tend to reward vocalizations. The child reacts to this and increases vocal behavior, thus commencing the process of oral language acquisition. The profoundly deaf child using an implant may evidence vocal and phonological errors. However, if internal oral language is developed as a first priority, formal therapy to correct some of the speech errors can be carried out later in the child's development.

Auditory/Verbal Method

Auditory/Verbal therapy is an habilitation method currently in use that was developed from the Acoupedic program (Pollack, 1984) described earlier. With only limited access to sounds in the range of speech, many children are not able to interpret the speech signal adequately unless direct steps are taken to develop this skill. Thus, the concept of helping children to "learn to listen" emerged (Beebe, Pearson, & Koch, 1984). It has been observed that some children with only limited access to speech via audition can learn to make certain discriminations when encouraged to process spoken input by listening only.

The deemphasis of lipreading cues can initially be achieved by covering the speaker's mouth with the hand or a screen. However, as the child develops and experiences some success with listening, the speaker should need only to be positioned next to the child, who would be less likely to look for visual cues once used to the method. Training is carried out in such a way that the child gradually moves from making very broad discriminations (e.g., /ba ba ba/ versus /ba:/) to progressively finer discriminations such as formant discrimination (e.g., /bi/ versus /ba/) or listening for the vowel transitions that may indicate the presence of certain consonants. Language goals can also be introduced using this method, and the child is expected to gradually learn to process longer and more complex strings of linguistic information.

Cued Speech

Cued speech was developed in the 1960s out of a recognition that hearing aids at the time could not provide enough information for some profoundly deaf children to adequately discriminate speech and learn oral language efficiently (Cornett, 1974–1975). Hand cues were used to visually inform the child of the presence of inaudible information. This method served as an aid to lipreading. The implant offers the possibility that children whose parents are encouraging oral development can now access a much wider range of speech sounds and therefore not require such visual supports for speech development.

Choosing a Method

Educational approaches in deaf education today continue to divide along this visual versus auditory continuum. Parents of recently diagnosed hearing-impaired children are faced with making a decision that may have far-reaching consequences for the long-term communication skills of their child. The decision regarding choice of communication mode is complex and often emotional and may be raised again by parents at the time of implantation. The clinician then has a role in discussing what is known in the research about the influence of educational approach on the performance of children with implants.

Parental decisions are often highly influenced by first contacts with professionals soon after diagnosis of the child's hearing loss and may not be based on knowledge of current research. Personal differences among parents also play a part. A parent whose personal values emphasize language and culture may choose a system that provides ready access to these things, such as signing. A parent whose personal values and goals emphasize an ability to speak may tend to favor an oral approach (Musselman, Lindsay, & Wilson, 1988).

Although recognizing the right of the parent to make these decisions, cochlear implant clinicians and other professionals cannot ignore the responsibility to make a careful and informed recommendation. Results detailed elsewhere (Dowell, & Clark, 1994; Reid & Lehnhardt, 1993) give strong support to the argument that for many children an oral habilitation program is most effective in optimizing performance with a multichannel cochlear implant.

When the choice is an oral method, the authors would recommend an approach that combines aspects of the oral/aural and auditory-verbal methods. That is, most of the clinical session time is spent using natural auditory-visual input with some embellishments, such as sitting close to the child and using increased repetition. However, in order to maximize the listening development of the child, some unisensory input is used. A hierarchy of auditory challenges is highlighted in each clinical session. Overall, the approach is described as one that is synthetic but takes into consideration the components of an analytical approach and attempts to apply these components to natural parental input as much as possible.

LISTENING AND PREVERBAL DEVELOPMENT

Current theories of communication development propose that spoken language emerges within the context of conversations between the caregiver and the child (Bruner, 1975; Owens, 1992). Three facets of early communication may be described: joint attention, turn taking, and information exchange.

Joint Attention

To initiate and maintain communication, the parent and child must share the same topic or focus. The clinician working with the cochlear implanted child may assist the parent to achieve such joint focus. For example, the structure inherent in repetitive daily routines helps the infant to determine what the parent is attending to, and subsequently what the parent is talking about. The importance of establishing joint attention was discussed by Tomasello and Todd (1983), who first correlated effective joint focus with the child's subsequent language growth. Extended joint attention episodes between the parent and child appear to provide important nonlinguistic scaffolding for the child's early linguistic development.

Tait and Wood (1987) further elaborated on joint attention skills, describing the child as "engaged" or "disengaged" from the interaction. The input provided by the cochlear implant may initially assist in the development of joint attention and allow the child to become "engaged" in the communicative exchange. Preimplant children may have developed some of these skills to various degrees. Those who would be considered "disengaged" from the adult and interaction should be monitored closely to look for the emergence of visual regard patterns suggesting progress.

Turn Taking

Researchers have proposed that turn taking in early interaction is a prerequisite to language development (Bruner, 1975, Kaye & Charney, 1981; Snow, 1972). That is, turn taking has a role far greater than merely providing structure; it also provides context and facilitates learning. Within the context of daily routines, rituals, and game playing, the parent's assist the cochlear-implanted child to enter into the dialogue more frequently. The clinician may suggest strategies such as those described by Schaffer (1977) that parents use to monitor and modify their interactional behaviors: phasing, adaptive, facilitative, elaborative, initiating, and control strategies.

Information Exchange

Finally, with a shared focus of attention and a set of turn-taking conventions the young cochlear-implanted child sets out to signal a range of communication intentions. The clinician and parent may encourage a broad range of communication contexts. For example, the clinical room may be set up to promote commenting, acknowledgment, negation, requesting action, or requesting objects.

Tait and Lutman (1996) studied the relationship between preoperative preverbal skills and performance on formal speech perception measures postoperatively. It was found that children who responded to adult speech during interaction (when not in eye contact with the adult) and used vocal rather than gestural responses preoperatively also performed best on the speech perception tests carried out postoperatively. This finding supports the use of listening for preverbal development in the habilitation program for children with cochlear implants. This process should also be encouraged preoperatively using hearing aids if possible.

In summary, the recently implanted child using a cochlear implant learns to respond to spoken input from parents, which is an important part of formal language development. The clinician aims to provide access to a range of auditory experiences and guides parents to actively develop communication with their child. Bloom and Lahey (1978, p. 573) stated "the facilitator's task is to provide experiences that clearly demonstrate certain concepts while providing the linguistic forms that code these concepts, at a time when the child is attending to both." First, the child's attention needs to be engaged by the parent or the parent should follow the child's lead. Second, the child and parent need to share a common topic or referent. This will ensure that what the child hears is related to what the child sees or experiences. Third, play activities that have maximum auditory contrasts need to be selected. In this way, the child is likely to be successful in discriminating the differences between sounds during play.

Linguistic input to the child may need to be controlled initially to ensure success. For example, the choice of toys may be limited so that specific auditory contrasts are presented. By carefully managing these auditory contrasts, the child will experience success more easily and begin to listen for meaning habitually. The clinician assists the parents in observing responses from the child and guides the parents to gradually increase the level of auditory challenge for the child. When the child is listening well, he or she will teach himself or herself language and become a more independent learner. At this point the need for structured input is much reduced.

Clinical experience indicates that some young implanted children are able to extract the relevant auditory cues which are meaningful from normal language models. For these children, there is no need to influence the auditory content of parental input. Only encouragement of normal "motherese" (Snow & Ferguson, 1977) input and numerous opportunities for a range of pragmatic communicative experiences is required to result in a normal pattern of oral language acquisition. The parent's use of motherese may include a higher than normal pitch, a slower overall rate of speech, an emphasis on key content words, reduced syntactic complexity, some exaggeration of facial expression and body gesture, and the offering of "turns" to the child. The parents treat the child as a hearing child and stimulate development in the normal way.

In these cases, the clinician takes on a monitoring role, providing feedback to the parent on the progress of the child overall and in relation to the normal population. Ongoing evaluation of the language performance of the child should be incorporated. Formal testing cannot be widely applied to children in this preschool group. Therefore, naturalistic sampling of the parent-child interaction is a most effective way of obtaining measures of communicative and language skills as they emerge. Guidelines charting normal development of play skills (Westby, 1980), pragmatic functions (Dore, 1974), syntactic development (Crystal, Fletcher, & Garman, 1976), and phonological development (Newman, Craighead, & Secord, 1985) will provide a broad framework within which the hearing-impaired child's emerging skills can be viewed and assessed.

Monitoring changes in the child's skills through this method will highlight any areas of development that should be emphasized by the parent or targeted through some formal intervention. For example, although language skills and pragmatic skills are developing well, some phonological processes may persist beyond the normal development period in the young child's connected speech. Some intensive auditory-based intervention to correct such errors may be most effective with this age group, as children at this age demonstrate a flexibility in altering speech production patterns more readily than older children.

It could be predicted that, as the quality of speech processing strategies improves even further, this naturalistic approach may apply to a larger percentage of very young implanted children. However, the current evidence suggests that for many children using implants, as with hearing aids, the signal alone is not sufficiently robust in the real world to allow for entirely natural development. These children need the steps toward meaningful listening behavior to be provided for them.

Research has shown that a range of speech perception performance occurs in any group of children using the cochlear implant (Boothroyd, 1991; Dawson et al., 1992; Dowell & Clark, 1994; Miyamoto et al., 1994; Staller et al., 1991). Whether these differences reflect cognitive variations or underlying learning or auditory processing problems warrants further research. However, based on what is currently known, the clinician needs to provide a program that is flexible, recognizes these varying needs, and provides for them on an individual basis.

COMPONENTS OF A POSTOPERATIVE HABILITATION PROGRAM

The following components of a postoperative habilitation program address the need to assist the auditory development of some children by introducing a hierarchy of auditory challenges. At each stage, auditory goals would also be incorporated as much as possible into the natural communicative environment of the child. All input would also be embedded in normal spoken phrases and ongoing conversational interaction.

Introducing the Hardware to the Child

The first issue to address with the young child approaching "start-up" of the device is how the parents will achieve full-time use of the device at home. This issue needs to be addressed in the preoperative phase to minimize future problems. All children should be encouraged to wear their hearing aids and tactaid (if applicable) full time prior to implantation. This should result in a routine for the child which includes putting on hardware every day in a consistent way. Substituting the speech processor for the hearing aids/tactaid should be straightforward if this routine is already familiar to the child. The clinician should also ensure that the parent is prepared prior to the day of "start-up" with an appropriate harness or pocket for the speech processor to fit into. Exposing the child to other children wearing the device or using a doll wearing a toy speech processor may also reduce the child's anxiety about the change.

Despite all of these preparations, some children do not initially cooperate with wearing the speech processor. Parents in this situation should be asked to record any amount of time the child wears the device so that small increases over time can be noted. The clinician should expect and reward wearing of the device in all clinical sessions and discuss behavior management strategies that the parent can use at home with the child. These strategies will vary due to individual differences among children and parenting styles but some broad suggestions can usually be made.

Always reward wearing of the device with an appropriate game or activity (e.g., getting a favorite toy, going to a favorite place, or eating a favorite food). Distract the child's attention as much as possible from the device and initially avoid frequent physical handling of the processor. Do not reward removal of the device with attention, take a short break to allow the incident to pass, and then firmly place the speech processor back on the child. Parents may sometimes need to use quite obvious tangible rewards initially to overcome rejection of the device. However, over time they should endeavor to phase this approach out as use of the device becomes habitual. Once the child begins to become aware of sound, the use of the device will become inherently rewarding and problems of rejection should decrease.

The clinician should always be aware of the child's current speech processor program when addressing problems of device rejection. In some circumstances, taking off the speech processor, particularly if it occurs suddenly, may indicate that further tuning of the speech processor is required.

The Use of Unisensory Input

Unisensory input can be defined as the deemphasis or exclusion of visual cues (lipreading) from spoken input provided to the child. The method may make use of a number of deliberate strategies to achieve this, ranging from naturalistic use of positioning (beside or behind the child) through the use of the hand or a screen covering the mouth to ensure a purely auditory signal. It has been suggested that unisensory input has a role to play in the habilitation program of the implanted child (Beebe,

Pearson, & Koch, 1984; Tye-Murray, 1992). Brown and Yaremko (1991, p. 27) went so far as to suggest that a habilitation program without a unisensory component is "useless." Although the authors will not suggest that the use of unisensory input to the total exclusion of all lipreading is appropriate for every implanted child, some key points regarding its role can be made.

The implant presents all of the sounds of speech covering the frequency range of 100 Hz to 6000 Hz (based on use of the Nucleus 22-channel device combined with a Spectra-22 speech processor). Detection of sounds in this range can be expected at the level of approximately 35–40 dBA. It can be assumed that the signal will be very different from anything the child has perceived before. In some cases it will be the first auditory signal ever perceived. In the case of the child who has developed other means of communication, utilizing visual or tactile information, some unisensory training will quickly demonstrate to the parents the new level of auditory awareness they can expect from the child. Some parents have developed a number of compensatory behaviors due to years of communicating with a partially hearing or totally deaf child. These behaviors may include tapping the child to get his or her attention, exaggerating lip patterns, or using excessive gestural cues. In demonstrating the child's awareness of sound through unisensory input, the clinician can encourage parents to raise their expectation of a response from the child. In general, the older the child and the more dependent the child has become on visual input, the more important some amount of unisensory input will be to draw attention to the new auditory percept.

In using unisensory input with a hearing-impaired child, it is desirable to use positioning as much as possible, rather than direct screening of the mouth. This ensures the best possible auditory transmission of the speech stimulus. However, some children may require the screening

method initially in order to develop a "listening attitude." This is a conscious response where the child attentively listens to a stimulus. Short activities using the screening method that target a level that is achievable for the child will increase self-confidence in the child's listening skills. The screening method should then not be needed as the child will become much less inclined to look for visual information, and will listen more readily.

Sound Detection

Detection of Environmental Sounds

During the first weeks of using the device, the parents may begin to notice the child responding to sounds in the environment. These responses may be evident by the child becoming still, looking around the environment, or showing an increased interest in noisy toys or the television. The clinician should encourage the parents to note these responses and report them as they are an early indication of the appropriateness of the program in the speech processor. The parents should also be observing for any signs of discomfort when the child is exposed to loud sounds.

A checklist of sounds that the child may hear can be provided to the parents as a guide to what to look for. However, clinicians should not encourage constant testing of the child using environmental sounds as he or she will be likely to respond inconsistently initially and the parents will be more effective if they interact as naturally as possible with the child.

Sound Detection Using Stimulus-Response Activities

The child using the cochlear implant can be expected to detect all of the sounds of speech in a quiet environment. At the beginning and end of all programming sessions the child should be encouraged to perform a sound detection task. This requires the child to place a peg in a board, push a candle into play-dough, or perform some other age-appropriate task in response to a sound. This task must be performed using audition alone to provide useful information regarding the functioning of the device and the appropriateness of the current "map." The adapted Ling sound test (1976) includes the phonemes /a/, /ɔ/, /u/, /i/, /s/, /ʃ/, and /m/. These sounds should elicit a consistent response from the implanted child at a distance of 1 meter, spoken at normal voice levels. In addition, other phonemes should also be audible to the child at this distance. These could include /t t t/, /p p p/, /tʃ tʃ tʃ/. That is, even the softest high frequency consonants should elicit a response.

Sound Detection in Play

The child might show awareness of sound during very simple and natural listening games that the parents can use. The stimulus used should be presented suddenly following a period of relative quiet. The stimulus may initially be linked to an action, such as peeking out from behind something, but after some exposure to the scenario the adult might produce the stimulus and watch for a looking response from the child to indicate awareness of the sound. Examples are listed here:

Activity	Speech Stimulus
Hiding behind a barrier	"peek-a-boo"
Pretending to be asleep	"wake up"
Holding a ball and waiting for a . . .	"go"

Sound Detection via Imitation

As soon as the child demonstrates a readiness to imitate speech sounds, this can be incorporated into the detection task. If the child is cooperative, detection and imitation can then become a daily activity for the parents to use to ensure that the speech processor is working properly. Correct imitation may not be possible initially, but the imitation of the correct pattern of presentation is sufficient to indicate detection. For example, if the parent produces /ʃ ʃ ʃ/ and the child produces /ɔ ɔ ɔ/, it can reasonably be assumed that detection of the sound has occurred even though the discrimination or speech production skills of the child may need to develop.

The parent should be trained to vary the timing and order of presentation, so that interpretation of the child's response is appropriate. This task might also indicate the child's awareness of broad loudness differences between sounds. The speaker might present a loud /a/ followed by a very soft /a/ and observe whether the child modifies his or her imitation in response to this change.

Sound Discrimination

The ability to discriminate between the acoustic features of speech sounds is a prerequisite to the ability to recognize a spoken word (Fry, 1979). It is easier to discriminate certain auditory cues than others (Boothroyd, 1991). Those that are easiest could be labeled as maximum auditory contrasts. These would include timing and intensity cues that make up the syllabic and prosodic patterns of speech. It is these features that hearing children naturally begin to imitate first in ongoing babble (Owens, 1992). It can be reasonably assumed from this that it is these cues that are most easily recognized first.

The natural awareness of parents of the role of maximum auditory contrasts in early communicative development of hearing children has been well recognized. The term "motherese" emerged in an attempt to label these behaviors, which appear to be universal as natural teaching tools for parents (Snow & Ferguson, 1977). The use of natural parental input with an awareness of the auditory cues available to the cochlear implant child will help facilitate maximum use of the device. Many of the ideas in this chapter for first steps in learning to listen are taken from the work of Judy Simser (1989) and the Auditory Verbal Programme (Romanik, 1990), which have been found to be effective clinical resources.

Discriminating Syllabic Cues

Syllabic information is represented by the vowel pulses of speech (Newman et al., 1985). There are a number of syllable shapes that may be used: vowel alone, vowel-consonant, consonant-vowel, consonant-vowel-consonant, and several others. In addition, repetitive consonants may be used in play to represent specific toys. For example, "t-t-t-t-t" for a watch ticking. The first awareness of syllabic patterns the child demonstrates is often the use of "phonetically consistent forms" (PCF) (Owens, 1992). PCFs are speech-like babble strings that are used meaningfully by the child to label objects or events, but are not adult word forms. Repeated consonant-vowel syllables are a common form of PCF. An example might be "brm brm" when the child pushes a car. It is semistructured vocal behavior that serves as a bridge between true babble and the first language-based words. PCFs can be encouraged and presented to the implanted child making use of syllabic pattern contrasts. The stimulus can be presented using simple phrases in association with a certain toy or activity. Examples are listed here:

Activity	Speech/Sound Contrast
Transport toys	"chug chug" (for the boat)
	"aaaarrrr" (for the plane)
	"ch ch ch", "tooooot" (for the train)
Putting doll to sleep	"sshh" "wake up"
Musical instruments	"bang bang bang" (for the drum)
	"too-da-loooooo" (for the trumpet)
Pushing cars on a mat	"round and round"
	"stop"
Blowing bubbles	"blooooow"
	"pop pop pop"
Making a house	"knock knock knock"
	"hello" or "hi"

The language used within this play should always consist of syntactically correct phrases; however, the key words may be repeated more often. For example:

> "*round and round and round . . . . . . .stop.*
> *. . . . . .there goes the car again. . . . . .*
> *round and round and round . . . . .stop*
> *. . . . . .he stopped at the light. . . . .off we*
> *go again. . . . .round and round and round*
> *. . . . . . stop . . . . . stop the car*"

The child is exposed to the ongoing exchange and plenty of pauses are left as opportunities for the child to respond, join in, babble, or imitate the pattern of vocal behavior being modeled by the parent. The syllabic pattern associated with the toy is often learned first as there is a high degree of auditory redundancy. The sound-toy association may then gradually be shaped toward the usual name for the toy by using both the object name (car) and its syllabic patterns association (round and round and round) equally. An example follows:

*"there's the car . . . . . . you drive the car
. . . . . round it goes . . . . round and round
. . . . . . oops the car stopped . . . . . that's
your car . . . . . . it stopped"*

Using the key words consistently and repeatedly will encourage the child to begin to identify the appropriate toy after hearing the adult refer to it and to spontaneously imitate the syllabic pattern to label it. This step alone indicates that the child has achieved some level of meaningful auditory processing. The parental input may then extend the child by highlighting more challenging (minimal) auditory contrasts.

Discriminating Spectral Cues

Discrimination on the basis of spectral cues requires that the child make use of information presented across the entire range of frequencies used in speech. Input may emphasize differences in vowel and consonant information, while maintaining a consistent syllabic pattern. As before, all contrasts are presented as key information embedded within normal ongoing language. However, increased repetition and association with a certain activity or toy will encourage development of auditory awareness.

Although individual children will react differently to apparently similar input and speech processing through the device, clinical experience and speech processing research suggest that certain auditory contrasts are more difficult to discriminate with the cochlear implant than others (Blamey et al., 1987). It makes sense from a developmental point of view to challenge the child with easier contrasts first and move gradually toward more difficult ones as the child demonstrates each skill. Using this step-like approach will also help the child gain confidence as he or she experiences success regularly and begins to regard himself or herself as a listener.

A hierarchy of auditory contrasts and examples follows, ordered from easy to more challenging spectral discriminations.

This hierarchy is adapted from the work of Romanik, as outlined in the Auditory Skills Programme for Students with Hearing Impairment (1990).

Sound Contrast	Example
vowels versus consonants	/a/ versus /ʃ/
vowel versus vowels with widely spaced formants	/i/ versus /ɔ/
vowels versus vowels/diphthongs with timing differences	/ʌ/ versus /a/ /i/ versus /ɑʊ/
vowels with close formant cues	/ɔ/ versus /u/
consonants varying in voicing/manner/ place cues	/pa/ versus /ba/ /ra/ versus /ma/ /pa/ versus /ta/ versus /ka/

All activities that highlight specific auditory contrasts should also take into account the appropriate language for the child. The clinician needs to consider the developmental order of acquisition of various semantic concepts, syntactic structures, and the development of auditory memory skills. The key contrast or word should be used in a variety of ways, in various positions at the phrase and sentence level, and in a variety of communicative situations. Thus, auditory goals should link with language and communicative goals as much as possible. The parent should be included in formulating overall communicative goals for the child and thinking of ways of promoting listening behavior at home.

Some suggested scenarios for developing spectral discrimination skills are listed here. Only the key words containing the contrast are listed but these should always be used embedded within natural phrases. The activities include those appropriate for the very young child and some that might be used with an older child who already has some language concepts.

Vowels Versus Consonants

This stage contrasts a single repeating consonant sound with a vowel or consonant-vowel syllable. It is often easier for the child initially to focus on highly contrasting features in the consonant such as high frequency information or frication. Contrasting the presence with the absence of a consonant at a word or syllable level will also draw the child's attention to consonant information.

Activity	Speech/Sound Contrast
Playing with a doll	"sshh" (going to sleep) "mmm" (feeding doll) "aarr" (cuddling doll)
Making a train	"ch ch ch" "toot toot toot"
Animal sounds	"moo" (for the cow) "hsss" (for the snake or cat)

Vowels Versus Vowels/Diphthongs with Timing Differences

This stage contrasts vowels that vary in length. The speaker should take care not to overly exaggerate the timing differences in the vowels used here or the contrast is made too easy and will not relate to timing differences in natural ongoing connected speech.

Activity	Speech/Sound Contrast
Making a swing	"up" "down" "up" "down"
Making traffic lights	"stop" "go" "stop" "go" "red" versus "green"

Playing dress-up	"hat" versus "shoe" "too big" versus "too small"

Vowels Versus Vowels with Widely Spaced Formant Cues

This section highlights vowels in which large differences in the formant frequencies within the speech spectrum are present. In this stage no length cues are available for discrimination. To highlight the spectral differences, continuous sounds that contrast vowel formants may be useful.

Activity	Speech/Sound Contrast
Pushing an ambulance	"ee" "or" "ee" "or"
Making play equipment	"see" "saw" "see" "saw"
Identifying people	"me" versus "you"
Drawing/looking at a face	"eye" versus "ear" "mouth" versus "nose"
Car play	"key" versus "car"

Vowels Versus Vowels with Close Formant Cues

This stage would use key words or phrases in which the pattern is consistent but the vowels vary with minimal formant contrasts. Vowels that are short in duration may also be used, as they provide less time in which to make the discrimination and therefore increase the difficulty of the task.

Activity	Speech/Sound Contrast
Farmhouse play	"clip" "clop" (for the horse) "quack" (for the duck) versus "hop" (for the rabbit) versus "woof" (for the dog)

Making a clock	"tick" "tock"
Hiding dolls/objects	"in" versus "on"
Coloring	"the pink one" versus "the black one"

Consonants Varying in Voicing or Manner or Place Cues

This would be considered the most difficult discrimination level to master and cochlear implant users achieve success in this category to varying degrees. Rhyming words that highlight consonant contrasts are very useful here. In general, children who can demonstrate some ability to discriminate consonants on the basis of these cues should be able to identify at least some speech or familiar words/phrases in their communicative environment.

Activity	Speech/Sound Contrast
Drawing body parts	"*toes*" versus "*nose*"
Making a snake	"sss" (slithering) versus "sshh" (asleep)
Counting out objects	"*four more*" "*two for you*" "*three for me*"
Using a switch toy	"turn it o*ff*" versus "turn it o*n*"
Coloring	"a *green tree*" "a p*ink* p*ig*" "a *purple turtle*"

If auditory cues alone are insufficient for a child to discriminate certain consonant cues, then the clinician may use visual or tactile cues to assist the child to recognize and produce the phoneme. However, the child should then be given the opportunity to listen to the contrast again to consolidate auditory awareness of the sound.

A discrimination activity may involve only drawing a picture, making a book, or exploring a doll house, but the parent and clinician, with a goal in mind, will be using the objects to repeat certain phrases that contrast consonant cues. The child might be asked to imitate the phrase on some occasions or to identify the referent to demonstrate discrimination and identification. The activity itself is of less importance, provided that it engages and maintains the child's interest. However, it should provide ample opportunities to model and practice with the child the particular auditory, speech production, or language goal identified as a target.

Achieving success in imitating, identifying, or comprehending the target in clinical sessions is only one step in the process of making listening a meaningful skill for the child. Carryover of newly learned skills into the home environment is the most important step of the process.

DEVELOPING AUDITORY COMPREHENSION AT HOME

Children learn language first by determining the meaning intended in communication, independent of the language forms. That is, they begin to recognize that the sound made when the adult speaks is meaningful and requires a reaction. The first "looking" response to a referent is often the earliest evidence of auditory processing. An example might be "Where's Daddy?" to which the child looks to the door or looks around. The child appears to understand that a response is required and takes his or her turn gesturally or with a head-turn response.

As soon as a program has been established in the speech processor, an expectation that the child can respond in this way should be established. Normal demands should be made on the child (e.g., "Where's Mummy?"). If the child does not respond the adult provides the answer or response (e.g., "There she is," pointing and looking, "There's Mummy"). The child soon learns the expected communicative routine, that is, when the adult speaks in this way, a response is required and rewarded. Many parents of profoundly deaf children have lost the habit of stimulating their children in this way after many failed attempts to elicit a response before diagnosis or even after the fitting of hearing aids. Demonstration and observation of responses in the clinical sessions will encourage the parent to try similar strategies at home.

Guidance for parents should include discussions of opportunities that will stimulate the child throughout the day, not just at specified play times. Regular daily living activities such as eating, dressing, walking, and going to bed provide many opportunities to challenge the child through audition, and the parents should take every opportunity to do so. Often throughout each day when the parent walks into a room, he or she could refer to an object and discuss it. The key element might highlight simple syllabic and suprasegmental features for the young child recently implanted (A), or other attributes for the older child with more language (B). Examples are listed here.

Activity	Language Prompt
Looking at the clock	"there's the clock . . . tick tock tick tock" (A)
	"there's the clock . . . what's the time? . . . it's three o"clock" (B)
Looking at a pet	"there's puss puss . . . mee-ow . . . mee-ow" (A)
	"there's the cat . . . she's hungry mee-ow . . . let's feed her now . . . she's hungry (B)

Looking at the light	"where's the light . . . up up up . . . it's up there" (A)
	"where's the light . . . up there . . . turn it off . . . turn it on" (B)

The child then begins to turn and point to these items as they are mentioned many times every day. Other common scenarios with young children will be greeting and parting rituals ("hello" or "hi" and "bye bye") and polite forms ("say thank you" or "say please"). Question forms used by the parent may become more complex and the child may start to imitate the question as well as the answer. Input that requires *auditory closure* may be introduced at this point to help develop a variety of response paradigms. This involves asking the child to process a question or incomplete phrase and fill in the final part. Examples are listed here.

Activity	Language Prompt
Looking at a book/pictures	"what does the cow say? . . . "
	"the cat says . . . "
Pushing cars	"ready . . . set . . . "
Singing a song	The adult starts singing, the child fills in a certain part or continues a line of the song

Once parents are confidently obtaining vocal responses from the child at home, they should then be encouraged to ensure that a variety of communicative experiences are provided for the child. Keeping in mind the level of auditory awareness demonstrated during activities in the clinical settings, the parent can gradually guide the child through the language associated with the daily and weekly routine of the family. Once the child has demonstrated that the skill of listening is developing, and some early language is emerging, the process has begun. A feedback loop is in place and the child is beginning to use it to communicate. The habilitation program at this point should allow numerous opportunities for the child to have a turn to speak and to practice his or her own expressive language skills and phonological self-monitoring. This ensures the child experiences the rewards of becoming an active and expressive communicator as well as a receptive one.

Postlingually Deaf Preschool Children

The rate of progress of any individual child in the acquisition of language will be highly influenced by a number of factors. Group data have identified the following factors as being predictive of a positive result with the cochlear implant: a short period of deafness, the presence of some usable preoperative residual hearing, and an oral educational setting (Dowell & Clark, 1994). Children who are postlingually deaf and implanted as preschoolers are among the best users of the implant and present a different picture in terms of the habilitation program. These children have the advantage of a partially developed linguistic system combined with the developmental readiness to absorb and make use of any new perceptual information available to them. For these children, habilitation becomes a combination of rehabilitation and normal teaching.

Parents of postlingually deafened children should be encouraged to return to normal communicative behavior as soon as possible. Preoperatively, the aim should be to conserve remaining oral language skills using any useful residual hearing available to the child. Using consistent communicative routines and repeating play scenarios that encourage familiar language will help maintain the child's exist-

ing receptive vocabulary and self-confidence as an oral communicator.

Postoperatively, the child should be immersed in aural language experience that is highly familiar. This will give the child the opportunity to relearn known language structures through the new auditory percept. Moving from closed-set listening activities (such as recognizing family names or identifying familiar nursery rhymes) to more open-set activities will allow for a gradual adjustment to the new perceptual information available to the child. In this way, the program may resemble the approach taken with postlingually deaf adults using the cochlear implant.

In addition, high level listening tasks such as talking on the telephone or listening to speech in noise will extend the skills of children who are postlingually deaf and prepare them for using the device in the classroom. Practice using the hearing provided through the implant to monitor and adjust speech production skills may also form a large part of the habilitation program for these children.

LANGUAGE ACQUISITION AND THE COCHLEAR IMPLANT

Boothroyd, Geers, and Moog (1991, p. 85) concluded that children with cochlear implants would "acquire spoken language skills more rapidly and effectively than would have been possible without the implant." This is encouraging but the challenge facing parents is to overcome the effects of the severe language delay present at the time of implantation that may persist for some years.

The patterns of normal language acquisition are well discussed and outlined in the literature (Dale, 1972; Owens, 1992). In most cases of early implantation, the expectation for language acquisition should be that it will follow the normal pattern. However, even a child implanted at

18 months of age has experienced a substantial delay in the commencement of the process of spoken language acquisition. Although parents may be able (through the strategies outlined) to facilitate their child's language acquisition, the overall rate of progress may not match that of hearing peers. The clinician must be aware of this aspect of the child's development to ensure that, through listening, the child is acquiring a sufficiently rich and sophisticated language system to allow for communication of a range of concepts with a range of people. As the child begins to acquire first words and combine them into phrases, it may be necessary to target certain semantic or syntactic structures through play activities. The parents may need to be provided with specific language goals as they are now trying to bring their child's language and communicative skills closer to his or her hearing peers. It is beyond the scope of this chapter to outline all the possible language goals and strategies that may be used to assist this problem. However, the following general areas should be considered.

Semantic Diversity

For the young child acquiring the first words in his or her language system, the clinician should ensure that a range of semantic intentions and vocabulary groups are included in the parental input. Words for objects, actions, attributes, feelings, greetings, and people must be modeled to provide a sufficiently wide range of words that the child will then combine into first phrases.

If the parents experience success initially with teaching object names to the child, they should also be aware of providing divergent semantic concepts related to the object. For example, if the child can imitate or label a doll as a "baby," the parents should make sure that they provide input that highlights other features related to the object. Examples include:

"wash/dry/feed/kiss the baby"
(action + object)

"the baby's dirty/wet/sore"
(object + attribute)

"there's no baby, that's not the baby"
(negative + object)

"the baby's here/there/in/under there"
(object + location)

"that's my/your/mummy's baby"
(possessive + object)

It should become habitual for the parent to model these expansions which contain diverse concepts for the child to access. Once the child begins to combine words, the parent must be aware of expanding via modeling the syntactic structure of the child's language at every opportunity.

Vocabulary

Using the *Peabody Picture Vocabulary Test* (PPVT), Dawson et al. (1995) found that most pediatric cochlear implant users showed considerable delay in vocabulary acquisition both pre- and postoperatively. However, significant group improvements were observed at varying postoperative intervals. Children who are relying on amplification for speech perception may experience difficulty in accessing ongoing vocabulary growth that occurs for hearing children by "overhearing" day to day conversational exchange in the home or kindergarten. The use of a radio frequency device may help overcome some of these problems. Parents should actively teach their child new words for known concepts and expect the child to learn and use these new words with them. The clinician should create opportunities during clinical sessions to model vocabulary expansion through play and discuss the importance of this with the parents. Some parents find that keeping a diary of new words and vocabulary used by the child helps them to identify areas needing expansion.

Speech Production

Many parents focus on this aspect of the child's communicative skills almost as soon as the first words begin to appear. The expectation of improvements in speech intelligibility is realistic in many cases of hearing-impaired children who are implanted when young (Grogan et al., 1995). However, the clinician has a role in guiding the parent to allow the natural processes that effect and influence phonological development and not encourage overt intervention in this area too soon. The child needs to hear a range of speech sounds with which to compare her or his own speech attempts, but this should occur naturally within any play or conversational exchange. The parent should reinforce and reward all speech attempts whether accurate or not and take opportunities to model correct productions back to the child. Constant feedback to the parent on the changes occurring in the child's productions and how these changes relate to overall development will help to reassure the parent that steps toward more normal speech are occurring. In many cases, some direct therapy may be required at a later stage if certain errors become entrenched in the child's speech, but the initial emphasis should be on diversifying language and conversational skills.

SUMMARY AND CONCLUSION

Children develop communicative competence in different ways with a variety of learning patterns, rates, and styles. Some children can use the auditory information provided by the implant to develop language through largely unmodified parental input and stimulation. Other children need the steps toward auditory discrimination of ongoing spoken language to be enhanced through habilitation in order to become confident, active listeners and communicators. The reason for these differences between children is an area requiring more research, and may become more evident as greater numbers of children are implanted.

The responsibility of the habilitationist is to monitor the child's hearing ability through vigilant technical management of the device. In addition, he or she must assist the parents in providing an auditory environment which is sufficiently rich and *accessible* to allow the child to begin the "search for meaning" through listening. An ongoing role in monitoring the acquisition of language and communication skills is vital in order to identify areas of the child's development in need of further intervention.

REFERENCES

Beebe, H. H., Pearson, H. R., & Koch, M. E. (1984). The Helen Beebe Speech and Hearing Center. In D. Ling (Ed.), *Early intervention for hearing-impaired children: Oral options* (pp. 15–63). San Diego: College-Hill Press.

Blamey, P. J., Dowell, R. C., Brown, A. M., Clark, G. M., & Seligman, P. M. (1987). Vowel and consonant recognition of cochlear implant patients using formant estimating speech processors. *Journal of the Acoustical Society of America, 82*(1), 48–57.

Bloom, L., & Lahey, M. (1978). *Language development and language disorders*. New York: John Wiley.

Boothroyd, A. (1991). Assessment of speech perception capacity in profoundly deaf children. *American Journal of Otology, 12*(Suppl.), 67–72.

Boothroyd, A., Geers, A. E., & Moog, J. S. (1991). Practical implications of cochlear implants in children. *Ear and Hearing, 12*(4), 81–89.

Brown, C., & Yaremko, R. (1991). Special considerations of cochlear implants in children. *Australian Journal of Human Communication Disorders, 19*(2), 25–30.

Bruner, J. (1975). The ontogenesis of speech acts. *Journal of Child Language, 2*, 1–19.

Clark, G. M, Dawson, P. W, Blamey, P. J, Dettman, S. J., Rowland, L. C, Brown, A. M, Dowell, R. C, Pyman, B. C., & Webb, R. L. (1991). Multiple-channel cochlear implants for children: The Melbourne Program. *Journal of the Otolaryngological Society of Australia, 6*, 348–353.

Cole, E. (1992). *Listening and talking: A guide to promoting spoken language in young hearing-impaired children.* New York: Alexander Graham Bell Association.

Cornett, R. O. (1974–1975). What is Cued Speech? *Gallaudet Today, 5*(2).

Crystal, D., Fletcher, P., & Garman, M. (1976). *The grammatical analysis of language disability: A procedure for assessment and remediation.* New York: Elsevier-North Holland.

Dale, P. S. (1972). *Language development structure and function.* Orlando, FL: Dryden Press.

Dawson, P. W., Blamey, P. J., Dettman, S. J., Barker, E. J., & Clark, G. M. (1995). A clinical report on receptive vocabulary skills in cochlear implant users. *Ear and Hearing, 16*(3), 287–294.

Dawson, P. W., Blamey, P. J., Rowland, L. C., Dettman, S. J., Clark, G. M., Busby, P. A., Brown, A. M., Dowell, R. C., & Rickards, F. W. (1992). Cochlear implants in children, adolescents and pre-linguistically deaf adults: Speech perception. *Journal of Speech and Hearing Research, 34*, 1–17.

Dettman, S. J., Barker, E. J., Rance, G., Dowell, R., Galvin, K., Sarant, J., Cowan, R., Skok, M., Hollow, R., Larratt, M., & Clark, G. M. (1996). Components of a rehabilitation programme for young children using the multichannel cochlear implant. In D. J. Allum (Ed.), *Cochlear implant rehabilitation in children and adults* (pp. 144–165). London, UK: Whurr.

Dore, J. (1974). A pragmatic description of early language development. *Journal of Psycholinguistic Research, 4*, 343–350.

Dowell, R. C., & Clark, G. M. (1994). Cochlear implants in children—Unlimited potential? *Australian Journal of Audiology, 15*, 10.

Fry, D. B. (1979). *The physics of speech.* Cambridge, UK: Cambridge University Press.

Grogan, M. L., Barker, E. J., Dettman, S. J., & Blamey, P. J. (1995). Phonetic and phonological changes in the connected speech of children using a cochlear implant. *Annals of Otology, Rhinology and Laryngology, 104*(Suppl. 104), 390–393.

Kaye, K., & Charney, R. (1981). Conversational asymmetry between mothers and children. *Journal of Child Language, 8*, 35–49.

Kuhl, P. K., Williams, K. A., Lacera, F., Stevens, K. N., & Linoblom, B. (1992). Linguistic experience alters phonetic perception in infants by six months of age. *Science, 31*, 606–608.

Ling, D. (1976). *Speech and the hearing impaired child: Theory and practice.* Washington, DC: Alexander Graham Bell Association for the Deaf.

Ling, D. (Ed). (1984). *Early intervention programs for hearing impaired children: A: oral options. B: total communication options.* San Diego: College-Hill Press.

Ling, D., & Ling, A. H. (1978). *Aural habilitation. The foundations of verbal learning in hearing-impaired children.* Washington, DC: The Alexander Graham Bell Association for the Deaf.

Miyamoto, R. T., Kirk, K. I., Todd, S. L., Robbins, A. M., & Osberger, M. J. (1994). Speech perception skills of children with multichannel cochlear implants or hearing aids. *Annals of Otology, Rhinology and Laryngology, 9*(Suppl. 4), 334–337.

Musselman, C. R., Lindsay, P. H., & Wilson, A. K. (1988). An evaluation of recent trends in preschool programming for hearing-impaired children. *Journal of Speech and Hearing Disorders, 53*, 71–88.

Newman, P. W., Craighead, N. A., & Secord, W. (1985). *Assessment and remediation of articulatory and phonological disorders.* New York: Charles E. Merrill.

Owens, R. E. (1992). *Language development: An introduction* (3rd ed.). New York: Charles E. Merrill.

Pollack, D. (1984). An acoupedic programme. In D. Ling (Ed.), *Early intervention for hearing-impaired children: Oral options* (pp. 181–253). San Diego: College-Hill Press.

Reid, J., & Lehnhardt, M. (1993). Post-operative speech perception results for 92 European children using the Nucleus mini system 22 cochlear implant. In B. Fraysse & O. Dequine (Eds.), *Cochlear implants: New perspectives. Advances in Otorhinolaryngology, 48*, 241–247.

Romanik, S. (1990). *Auditory skills programme for students with hearing impairment.* Sydney, Australia: NSW Department of School Education.

Schaffer, R. (1977). *Mothering.* London: Harvard University Press.

Simser, J. (1989). *Auditory verbal therapy.* Paper presented at Learning through Listening Conference, Melbourne, Australia.

Snow, C. E. (1972). Mother's speech to children learning language. *Child Development, 43,* 549–565.

Snow, C. E., & Ferguson, C. A. (Eds.). (1977). *Talking to children.* Cambridge, UK: Cambridge University Press.

Staller, S. J., Beiter, A. L., Brimmacombe, J. A., Mecklenburg, D. J., & Arnot, P. A. (1991). Paediatric performance with the Nucleus 22-channel cochlear implant system. *American Journal of Otology, 12*(Suppl.), 126–136.

Tait, D. M., & Lutman, M. E. (1996). The predictive value of measures of pre-verbal communicative behaviors in young deaf children with cochlear implants. *Proceedings from The Third European Symposium on Paediatric Cochlear Implantation,* Hannover, Germany.

Tait, M., & Wood, D. (1987). From communication to speech in deaf children. *Child Language Teaching and Therapy, 3,* 1–16.

Tomasello, M., & Todd, J. (1983). Joint attention and lexical acquisition style. *First Language, 4,* 197–212.

Tye-Murray, N. (Ed). (1992) *Cochlear implants and children: A handbook for parents, teachers and speech and hearing professionals.* Washington, DC: Alexander Graham Bell Association for the Deaf.

Westby, C. (1980). Language abilities through play. *Language, Speech and Hearing Services in Schools, 10,* 154–168.

11

HABILITATION:
SCHOOL-AGED CHILDREN

KARYN L. GALVIN
JULIA Z. SARANT
ROBERT S. C. COWAN

Although the school-aged population differs in many respects to the preschool population, the primary goal of habilitation remains the same: to facilitate the development of speech and language through audition by encouraging and developing maximal use of the cochlear implant. In the case of school-aged children, a further goal is to foster in the children a sense of responsibility for the use and care of their cochlear implant.

Hearing-impaired school-aged children are quite different from hearing-impaired preschool children, the fundamental difference being the large variation of communication skills in the population. Whereas preschool children are a relatively homogeneous group who have usually acquired little speech and language prior to implantation, the school-aged population includes children with a large range of ages and communicative, reading, writing, and cognitive skills. With preschool children, habilitation can usually follow a developmental model, promoting the acquisition of skills in the order attained by children with normal hearing. In contrast, a remedial model is often more appropriate for school-aged children, therefore habilitation with older children may include a

large component of filling in the gaps with knowledge that normally should have been acquired previously. In addition, due to the varying skills and needs of school-aged children, habilitation programs for this age group must be tailored individually to a greater extent than for preschool children. For example, a fully integrated, postlinguistically deafened teenager may require only technical and counseling support, while a newly implanted, congenitally hearing-impaired primary-school child will require weekly intervention, school liaison, and family support. These are extreme examples, however, they highlight the potential range of habilitation needs of school-aged children.

This chapter will discuss the need for habilitation, the individual habilitation session, counseling issues, and other issues relating to habilitation of school-aged children, particularly factors that contribute to the diversity of the population.

THE NEED FOR HABILITATION

The implantation of a cochlear prosthesis does not in itself ensure the development of speech and language. Despite the fact that implanted children have access to information across the speech frequency range, they are still considered to have a functional unaided hearing loss in the range of 80–110 dB (Boothroyd, 1993; Somers, 1991). It has been shown that there is a significant delay in speech and language acquisition between most children with a severe or profound hearing impairment and normally hearing children (Kretschmer & Kretschmer, 1986; Paul & Quigley, 1994). It is well documented that children with this level of hearing impairment have a slower rate of spoken and written language acquisition and that their overall competency with regard to use of pragmatics, syntax, and vocabulary is significantly poorer (Geers & Moog, 1995; Moores, 1987). Furthermore, although the implanted child can now access speech information across the frequency range, the quality of the auditory information received through the cochlear implant is very different from that received preoperatively through hearing aids. Intervention will always be required to aid and guide the child in learning to interpret and gain maximum benefit from the new auditory information received. In addition, families and teachers will require technical and counseling support if the use of the cochlear implant is to be integrated into the child's daily communication and the quality of auditory input is to be maximized at all times.

INDIVIDUAL HABILITATION SESSIONS

In planning habilitation programs for individual children, there are many characteristics of the child that the clinician should consider. The child's ability to use audition to gain meaningful information and whether or not he or she has developed confidence in, and relies on, listening skills are of prime importance. The language knowledge of

the child must be assessed so that the language goals for habilitation are appropriate for further developing the child's language skills. Educational materials from children's curricula should be incorporated, so that language development occurs in a meaningful and realistic context. Overall conversational competence must be evaluated, that is, does the child have an understanding of the rules and social conventions of communication? Furthermore, speech production abilities should be assessed so that specific activities for improving production and developing self-monitoring can be incorporated into habilitation sessions. It is also important to consider the child's age and cognitive skills, as these will influence the types of activities that may be suitable. This chapter does not attempt to describe in detail the content of individual habilitation sessions. However, we will comment briefly on aspects of habilitation with regard to school-aged children. These areas are outlined in Table 11–1.

Audition

Children with cochlear implants demonstrate a large range of listening skills depending, in part, on their auditory experience prior to implantation (Osberger et al., 1991; Staller, Beiter, Brimacombe, Mecklenburg, & Arndt, 1991). Whereas some newly implanted children may not be competent in their use of audition, others who have been implanted for some time, or who had developed auditory skills prior to implantation, may be quite adept at conducting conversations over the telephone. For other children, long-term use may be required before measurable improvements in speech perception skills are demonstrated. Therefore, a range of approaches is required in designing a program for maximizing the use children make of their audition.

For newly implanted school-aged children, experience in use of audition could

Table 11-1. Aims of habilitation.

Facilitation of speech and language development through audition:

- fostering a sense of responsibility for the cochlear implant
- encouraging maximal use of the cochlear implant
- encouraging reliance on and confidence in the information provided by the cochlear implant
- assessing language skills and providing language input at an appropriate level
- facilitating the acquisition of conversational skills
- improving speech intelligibility
- providing appropriate counseling for the child and his or her family

begin with identification of words and sentences that are already familiar to the child visually or through hearing aids (e.g., listening activities using family names). This will enable the child to experience early and functional success through listening. Some children may need an extended period of time at this level in order to become used to discriminating the new information. The detection of high frequency consonants is new perceptual information for most newly implanted children; therefore, working on these sounds would perhaps be more difficult for many children who heard mostly vowels through their hearing aids. However, discourse level materials should be included for even newly implanted children to facilitate the natural integration of new skills into functional use. Discourse activities also demonstrate to the child that listening is not purely an activity engaged in during a special session at school, but one that is valuable in daily communication. For most children, some part of each habilitation session could comprise audition-alone listening activities, as this encourages children to focus on the information provided by their implant, and success with these activities promotes confidence in perceptual abilities and further reliance on the cochlear implant. For children who have good audition-alone speech perception, telephone training can be an enjoyable and challeng-

ing activity that provides excellent opportunities to practice conversational skills and to learn a functional life skill.

Some children may need a period of gradual transition from using hearing aid input to reliance on the cochlear implant to minimize the disruption to their communication. This may mean coping initially with only a few hours' use of the cochlear implant each day, and slowly increasing this to full-time use. Conversely, other children will adjust to full-time use of their cochlear implant immediately. Children should always be encouraged to continue to wear their hearing aid in the unimplanted ear, as this gives them a degree of binaural hearing and therefore some ability to localize sounds. Wearing the hearing aid is not usually a problem for younger school-age children, who can often derive a sense of security from their old and familiar aid. However, some older children will refuse to wear their hearing aid because they feel it is either not very beneficial when compared with their cochlear implant or incompatible with the quality of sound provided by their cochlear implant. This is a difficult issue to deal with, as older children cannot and should not be forced to continue wearing their hearing aid. One option is to assess speech perception both with and without the hearing aid so that if there is an advantage it can be demonstrated objectively to the child. A second option is to arrange a contract with the child to wear the aid for a set period of time, over the course of which he or she may become accustomed to wearing the two devices together. There is considerable evidence to show that neural degeneration occurs with lack of auditory stimulation (Webster & Webster, 1977, 1979). Consideration must therefore be given to the fact that ceasing to wear the hearing aid may limit a child's options for further benefits from future advances in medical technology.

Language

Determining the level of language knowledge for each child is an essential requirement of any habilitation program, as teaching children to listen through their cochlear implant should not be the only goal for any habilitation session. Language assessment highlights areas of need in children's language development and enables clinicians to focus on these areas in habilitation and also to evaluate whether their teaching is effective. As a result of careful evaluation, habilitation activities can be tailored to the child's level of language knowledge to ensure that they are meaningful and relevant to the child and allow the child to achieve success.

Assessing language knowledge and identifying areas of deficit can be accomplished by administering formal language/ syntax and vocabulary tests. Although many tests are available for assessing normally hearing children, norms have not been established for many of these on the hearing-impaired population. Formal language tests have other inherent disadvantages in that they elicit only a restricted sample of responses based on the test stimuli, and therefore provide information on only a portion of children's knowledge. A further factor limiting the language sample obtained using some formal tests is that they require a baseline to be established before other areas of language knowledge on the test can be attempted. As the

language development of many hearing-impaired children is not only delayed but also deviant (i.e., they do not learn language in the normal developmental sequence), this may create false impressions of their overall abilities. Another unavoidable difficulty with formal tests is that children's knowledge of language is assessed in the absence of context, that is, without the aid of conversational or contextual cues. This factor has been shown to decrease scores for both hearing-impaired and normally hearing children (Kretschmer & Kretschmer, 1978; Muma, 1976). When using tests for which normative data are available for hearing-impaired children, it is important to check tests for the use of colloquial language that may affect the validity of test results. Furthermore, many tests have multiple-choice formats and children may become skilled at eliminating some options and then guessing their response correctly. Although formal language tests provide valuable information, these inherent disadvantages should be taken into account when interpreting results.

Natural language sampling on videotape is a comprehensive means of obtaining information about children's spontaneous expressive language, as the context in which the interaction occurred, including all nonverbal interactions, is preserved. Traditionally, only the child's utterances have been transcribed, but it is extremely useful to also record the contributions of the other participant, as this provides a measure not only of production but of comprehension. Language samples should be obtained in more than one environment, as it has been shown that the environment and the person with whom the child interacts elicit different types of language (Kramer, James, & Saxman, 1979). For example, a child will produce different language with a peer in the playground than with a teacher in the classroom, because the child will assume that the adult knows more than his or her peer and, therefore, will require less explanation. Kramer et al. (1979) found that the most accurate samples of language were obtained at home, next accurate at school, and least accurate in a clinic environment. Language samples for school-aged children should ideally be obtained across the styles of discourse that they require competence in at school and in their social environments. These styles are narration, description, explanation, and formal and informal (i.e., "chatting") conversation. When obtaining descriptive samples, more than one type of sample should be used. For example, describing an activity will elicit a predominance of verbs, describing an object will elicit mostly nouns, and describing what would happen in a hypothetical situation will elicit much more complex language than the two former activities. Written language sampling should also be included in a school-aged child's overall assessment, as written language differs from spoken language. Ideally, all of these types of language sampling should be used to gain an overall view of a child's strengths and areas of need.

The rate of language development may increase for some children after implantation simply because their access to language through their audition has improved. Conversely, deficits in language knowledge may significantly influence the amount of information a child perceives through audition. Clinicians may in fact underestimate the potential speech perception benefit from cochlear implants for children with very poor language skills, for whom speech perception testing may be simply an imitation task with little meaning. For example, if a child has never been expected to accurately express or respond to tense markers or plurals, he or she will be unlikely to identify those elements of speech as meaningful through listening. A pilot study by Sarant, Blamey, Cowan, and Clark (in press) showed that training syntactic knowledge and vocabulary with implanted children who had poor language skills significantly improved

their open-set speech perception scores. Therefore, it is important to establish the level of language knowledge children have and to take this into account when interpreting speech perception test results.

Conversational Skills

The ultimate measure of a hearing-impaired child's communicative competence is the ability to have a conversation. This involves integrating language, auditory, and speech production skills with knowledge of the social conventions of conversation. Although some school-aged children may have mastered many skills in these areas, it is likely they will be lacking much of the other knowledge necessary for engaging in a successful conversation. Conversely, it is not uncommon for hearing-impaired children in the early years of primary school to possess so few of these skills that they are unable to have a conversation. Whereas most normally hearing children absorb many of the social conventions associated with conversations through overhearing adult interactions, profoundly hearing-impaired children miss much of this natural modeling, and therefore usually need to be taught formally. Conversational skills include polite greetings, initiating and terminating a conversation, turn taking, topic maintenance, and providing appropriate nonverbal feedback to the speaker. Of particular importance for the hearing-impaired child are clarification techniques, as these facilitate the acquisition of information that may have been missed the first time it was provided, and therefore help to avoid conversation breakdown. Hearing-impaired children often try to avoid embarrassment by bluffing their way through a conversation with nods and smiles, not acknowledging that they have missed important information and are no longer understanding what the conversation is about. Many children, especially those in early primary school, are passive conversational partners and make no attempt to inform others that they do not understand what is being said. Building children's confidence in their ability to have successful conversations is extremely important, as it is through conversation that children naturally learn language, use their audition, and improve their speech production. Rewarding communication with others provides the motivation for children to continue to develop all these skills.

Speech

The potential for a child to spontaneously alter speech production due to improved auditory feedback from a cochlear implant varies greatly (Grogan, Barker, Dettman, & Blamey, 1995). Many children will have established deviant patterns of speech production and a reliance on visual and/or orosensory motor feedback at the articulatory level to compensate for the lack of auditory information through their aided residual hearing. As this feedback mechanism is used habitually and automatically, it is likely to remain stable without intervention. Although the speech of some children may not change significantly, it has been shown that improvements can be made with intensive work (Osberger, Johnstone, Swarts, & Levitt, 1978). The older the child, the more unrealistic it is to expect changes in their speech production unless particular areas are targeted. With younger children, effecting changes in speech with intervention may be easier. However, even for these children the development of intelligible speech is a great challenge. Developmental norms for acquisition of particular speech skills may apply only to the youngest of primary school children. It is important to remember that the development of intelligible speech in all profoundly hearing-impaired children is a long-term goal and in most cases will require many years of work.

Typical errors in the speech of severely to profoundly hearing-impaired children include prolongation of vowels, omissions, substitutions, and staccato errors (in which all syllables are stressed with intervening pauses) (Grogan et al., 1995; Osberger & Levitt, 1979). Although vowel errors are not as common as those with consonants, vowels convey information about the surrounding consonants through formant transitions. Therefore, a reasonable point at which to commence speech therapy is with vowel production. Once children are producing some vowels correctly, work can begin on consonants. For many children, additional cues through other modalities such as vision or the tactile sense may be necessary (McConkey Robbins, 1994). It is also important not to work on individual sounds in isolation, but to work on phonemes in context, in order to avoid creating a staccato effect (McGarr, 1987). A meaningful link to a language structure will also help the child to monitor his or her production at a sentence level. For example, if the speech target is the sound /z/, the language link can be plurals that follow a vowel (e.g., toes, trees). Maximal use of audition through the cochlear implant can be made by combining speech perception and production goals in the same activities, so that the relationship between listening and speaking is made obvious to the child (Ling, 1976). Integration of listening and speaking also facilitates the use of dialogue in speech teaching. This has the advantage of allowing the child to be more expressive and to assume both "teacher" and "student" roles, thereby practicing the production of target stimuli and listening to these stimuli presented by the clinician (McConkey Robbins, 1994). It is most important that once a child has attained a speech goal in a formal teaching session this ability be carried over into real-life communication. This is perhaps the greatest challenge with regard to speech teaching. Practices that facilitate this carryover include exercises that require children to produce a previously learned speech target after some time has elapsed since formal teaching of this target occurred. One of the most important things to remember with regard to the development of intelligible speech is that speech production skills do not develop in isolation; children must also have both the desire and the language ability to communicate with others.

Motivation is of prime importance with regard to changes in children's speech production. Encouragement and positive feedback regarding progress will help to maintain motivation, but the child must also be self-motivated if permanent changes in speech production are to occur. For children in a segregated school setting who usually interact with staff who are specialized in understanding relatively unintelligible speech, motivation can be a particular problem. As the school and home environments comprise most of a school-aged child's world, if the child can communicate with family, teachers, and peers, there is often no perceived need to improve speech production. In situations such as this, interactions with the world at large (e.g., going to the milk bar and asking for bread) may make the child more aware of his or her speech production and will also provide positive feedback when such improvements occur. It is also important to remember to balance children's need to communicate freely with their need for speech correction. Overcorrection of a multitude of errors is likely to serve to decrease their desire to communicate at all. It is therefore advisable to target and concentrate on only a few productions systematically, which should result in faster progress and less frustration on the part of the child.

COUNSELING

Issues such as etiology, the need for a cochlear implant, how a cochlear implant works, the postoperative program, the use of oral communication, and the influence of peers and the Deaf Community need to be discussed with the families of implant candidates. It is also important that the relevant issues are discussed with the child. This will require the clinician to make an assessment of the individual child's counseling needs and to ensure that the information given is presented at a level the child can understand. Counseling should continue in the postoperative period and the clinician can expand his or her explanations as the child's ability to understand increases. Although hearing-impaired children are likely to receive counseling and information from parents and teachers, it is the responsibility of the implant clinician to ensure that issues relating to the functioning and use of the cochlear implant are raised with the child.

The Cause of Deafness and the Need for a Cochlear Implant

The parents of children whose onset of deafness is congenital or prelingual are unable to explain to their children the etiology or consequences of their deafness at its onset. With passing years the deafness may become such an accepted fact that the families may not think to provide their children with an unsolicited explanation of their deafness. This situation may continue even when the children have developed the cognitive and language skills to question why they are deaf and to understand an explanation of the cause of their deafness. Hence, school-aged children may have no idea why they are deaf, or they may be under an incorrect impression as to the cause of their deafness. Also, these children may not necessarily think that their deafness is a permanent condition. For children who do not know any deaf adults, it is a reasonable misconception to expect to "grow out" of their hearing loss. All of these issues should be discussed with the families and the hearing-impaired children.

Preoperatively, it is important to discuss with children and their families how the cochlear implant functions and what auditory information it will provide that is not accessible through hearing aids. Postoperatively, it is worthwhile to continue to discuss this with the children as they become able to understand more detailed and complex explanations. A meaningful approach to this topic is to discuss with the children how the cochlear implant improves their quality of life. It is usually easiest for children to understand practical examples, such as being able to hear the doorbell, recognizing when someone is speaking, and being aware when their names are called. Discussing the experiences and feelings when the implant is not being worn, for example, in the bath, can help children to develop an understanding of the benefit provided by the cochlear implant.

The Postoperative Program and How the Cochlear Implant Works

Preoperatively, it is vital that families and children understand the requirements and value of the postoperative program. It is unlikely that the full potential of a cochlear implant could be realized if children or their families were not committed to the postoperative program. Postoperatively, if the clinician wishes children to be cooperative and motivated during habilitation, mapping, and evaluation, then he or she must explain why these activities are necessary. The aim is to develop in children a feeling that they have a stake in the whole process, such as is typically felt by adult implantees. This may not be as applicable to younger school-aged children, but is certainly important over the age of 10. All people, including children, like to feel a degree of control over their lives. This may be particularly so for deaf children, whose delayed development of communication will have caused them to often not understand what was happening to them. In discussing the meaning of the activities

and involving children as much as possible in their execution, clinicians can pass a degree of control across to children without compromising the activities being undertaken. An example of this approach is allowing the school-aged child, who will usually have learned to use computers at school, to actively participate in the mapping process. Explaining the next section of the task and allowing the child to manipulate the keyboard involves the child in the process and, at the very least, increases his or her level of concentration. In the long term, this approach can help the child to understand the functioning of the implant and the importance of mapping.

The Use of Oral Communication

As the aim of implantation is to provide improved auditory input, the use of oral communication and the role of signing will be significant issues for many families. It is ultimately the family's choice which mode of communication their child uses. The cochlear implant clinician should provide information regarding current thinking and experience on how to maximize the use of the auditory information provided by the cochlear implant and how to promote and develop the implanted child's use of oral communication.

Promotion of the use of oral communication will involve counseling school-aged children regarding the skills required to communicate successfully, specifically, auditory, speech production, language, and conversational skills. Particularly in the segregated school setting, but also in an integrated setting, it is likely that hearing-impaired children will develop, at best, a limited understanding of the wider implications of their communication difficulties. Unless the onset of hearing loss occurred in the teenage years, it can be expected that implanted children will be unable to identify with, or even fully understand, the ease with which their normally hearing peers communicate. They are also unlikely to recognize the implications of the difference between communicating with familiar adults and peers and communication with the wider community. It may have been beneficial with young hearing-impaired children not to continuously highlight deficiencies in their speech production, sentence construction, or use of vocabulary in order to encourage communication. However, the result may be school-aged children unaware of the difficulties others have in understanding their spoken messages. Also, they may not realize how much of the spoken message of their conversational partners they do not understand. The aim of discussing these issues is not to criticize the children, but rather to attempt to develop an understanding of the communication challenges they will face and how the habilitation sessions will promote the development of the skills they will need. These are unrealistic goals with many younger school-aged children, and can be very difficult to achieve even with older school-aged children.

Peers and the Deaf Community

The consistency of device use by the school-aged child at school and in social situations may be affected by peer pressure. This can occur regardless of the benefits to speech perception achieved by the child. Peer pressure is usually strongest during adolescence; however, even a younger child can be very aware of "looking different." The nature of peer pressure and a child's awareness of being different from his or her hearing peers can be partially dependent upon educational setting. These types of difficulties are likely to be greatest in the integrated setting, where hearing-impaired children will be different from their normally hearing peers. However, similar problems may also arise in the segregated setting, where the implanted child may want to be like the other children who wear hearing aids.

Adolescents in segregated settings may be subjected to further peer pressure directed at their decision to improve their hearing through use of a cochlear implant. Adolescents are the group of school-aged children most likely to have contact with the Deaf Community. As some members of the Deaf Community are active in their opposition to cochlear implantation, adolescents may encounter opposition and disapproval if they are considering an implant and an even stronger response if they proceed with implantation. It is not the role of the clinician to encourage children into a debate regarding the pros and cons of cochlear implantation. Rather, the clinician should ensure preoperatively that children understand that they may encounter opposition and encourage them to make their own choices and be prepared to persevere with those choices. This is a vital issue of preoperative and continued postoperative counseling, as adolescents are particularly prone to the effects of peer pressure. A lack of continuing postoperative support from the implant clinician can contribute to adolescents becoming nonusers of their cochlear implants. However, the provision of such support does not ensure that this outcome will not occur.

ISSUES IN HABILITATION OF THE SCHOOL-AGED POPULATION

The implant clinician needs to be aware of a number of issues specific to habilitation with school-aged children. The diversity of the population and the challenges of conducting habilitation in the school environment are discussed.

Diversity in the School-Aged Population

As mentioned previously, the school-aged population is very diverse, with many pre- and postoperative factors contributing to a wide variation in communication skills, cognitive skills, and management needs. Due to this great diversity, the planning and implementation of habilitation programs for these children requires careful assessment and tailoring for individual skills and needs.

The most obvious source of variation in the group is the wide age range of 5 to 18 years. As children grow, life experience, practice, and development will improve communication and cognitive skills, and therefore result in changing management needs. Other factors contributing to the diversity of this population are children's ages at the onset of profound hearing impairment and the period for which they were profoundly hearing-impaired prior to implantation. A later onset of profound hearing impairment is a positive predictor of success in using a cochlear implant (Boothroyd, 1993; Staller et al., 1991). The onset of a profound hearing loss before the development of spoken language will typically have a devastating effect on children's development of auditory, speech production, and language skills, and on their understanding of the communicative process. Children whose onset of hearing loss occurs later in childhood will have established auditory, speech production, and language skills. They therefore possess a framework of knowledge for use in interpreting the degraded auditory message they will receive. Given this established framework and appropriate intervention, these children are likely to continue, albeit at a slower rate, their development of oral communication. Therefore, postlinguistically deafened children will present as being very different from children with an earlier onset in terms of oral communication skills and management needs. Research has suggested that a shorter duration of profound deafness is correlated with an improved ability to make use of the auditory input through the cochlear implant (Boothroyd, 1993; Dowell, Blamey, & Clark, 1995; Staller et al., 1991). The age at onset of profound deafness will also interact with the duration of deafness. For example, the detri-

mental effect of 1 year of profound deafness between the ages of 1 and 2 years would be greater than the effect of 2 years of profound deafness between the ages of 14 and 16 years.

Of equal importance to children's oral communication skills at school age is the level and quality of their preoperative hearing. The more useful the residual hearing possessed by young children, the better the prognosis for the development of auditory, speech production, and language skills postoperatively. In an analysis of the speech perception results of 100 children from the implant clinics in Melbourne and Sydney, Dowell et al. (1995) found useful preimplant residual hearing to be associated with better perceptual performance.

A number of other important factors further contribute to the varying management needs and communication skills of school-aged children. The provision of signed English input in Total Communication (use of signed English and spoken English in combination) appears to promote the development of signed language, and perhaps written and spoken language, for some children. However, for children using Total Communication, the ease of communicating using sign may make them less reliant on the auditory information they receive (Quittner & Steck, 1991). The children may therefore make less use of this auditory information. It has been suggested that children using oral communication are dependent on the auditory information they receive and have more opportunity to practice their listening and speech production skills (Quittner & Steck, 1991). This variation between school environments will impact on the development of oral communication and the management requirements of individual children. Even in comparing different oral programs, or teachers within a program, there will be differences in listening opportunities, speech production, and language intervention provided.

If any member of a family is hearing-impaired, a great deal of extra stress is placed on all family members. In particular, a hearing-impaired child will place extra demands on the time, emotional energy, and skills of the parents. Just as each hearing-impaired child is an individual, so are parents individuals, with their own capacities, skills, and personalities. Therefore, each parent will deal differently with a hearing-impaired child and will be able to play a different role in the child's development of auditory, speech production, and language skills. The role and contribution of the parent, both earlier in the child's life and when he or she is school aged, is a critical factor in the development of the child's oral communication skills and his or her management needs. Some parents are able to act as an interaction partner on a very intensive basis and can provide their child with quality input and guidance to maximize the development of oral communication. If this occurs, the child's oral communication skills at school age are likely to be superior to those of children with a similar hearing and educational history who did not receive the same level of parental contribution. These children and their families are also likely to require less support than some other children. Other parents may not have developed the skills, or may lack the time or capacity to provide the same level of input and guidance for their children. In these cases the child is not likely to be as skilled in oral communication, and the child and family will require significantly more professional support in terms of habilitation, technical information, and counseling.

The professional intervention received, both earlier in life and at school age, is also critical. An early intervention center should support the family and provide appropriate parental guidance with regard to maximizing communication development. The quantity and, more importantly, the quality of this early intervention will greatly influence the oral communication and management needs of the child at school age.

Not only environmental factors significantly affect the oral communication skills and management needs of an implanted child at school age. Although no two children are ever identical, two implanted children with similar hearing histories and environmental backgrounds may make very different progress in their development of oral communication. In some cases, children's ability to detect and discriminate phonemes using their implants may not correspond with their relatively poor levels of speech understanding and language development. It is possible that children who do not appear to make maximum use of the auditory input provided by the cochlear implant have difficulty processing the information they are receiving. As it is not fully understood how auditory information is processed, it is difficult to evaluate the possible processing difficulties of these children. For some children who also exhibit other problems, such as limited academic progress, more than one factor may be contributing to their slow rate of progress in oral communication development. It should also be kept in mind that some causes of severe or profound deafness, for example meningitis (Peloquin & Davidson, 1988), may have other neurological and psychological effects.

When the rate of progress in development of oral communication is slower than expected, children should be referred to other professionals for evaluation of other capabilities, such as nonverbal intelligence, memory capacity, and visual skills. The decision to refer children for further assessment should be made after careful consideration of their progress. Continued, unnecessary assessments are not to the advantage of the child or to the parents, whose time, money, energy, and peace of mind can be wasted in the pursuit of an "answer." On the other hand, if additional difficulties remain unidentified, the effect on the child's long-term development may be severe. Even if there is no solution for the problem, knowledge of limitations on the child's capabilities can help the clinician to appropriately tailor the habilitation program, and to counsel the family regarding the child's likely progress. The same knowledge can also help the teacher and the parents in their approach with the child.

For children who use an oral communication mode, lack of progress may suggest that a change to Total Communication would be beneficial. Parents who have chosen oral communication for their children usually consider it to be the best approach for developing listening, speech production, and language skills. It may therefore be difficult for them to consider changing this approach. In some of these cases, a change to a Total Communication approach may benefit the child's academic progress and overall communication. However, clinical experience also suggests that it may be quite a number of years postimplantation before some children make significant progress in their development of oral communication (Gantz, Tyler, Woodworth, Tye-Murray, & Fryauf-Bertschy, 1994; Miyamoto, Osberger, Robbins, Myres, & Kessler, 1993). The implant clinician may be asked for his or her advice regarding a child's potential for improvement in the current communication mode and likely response to a change of mode.

Challenges of Habilitation in the School Environment

As the school-aged child is now in the formal learning environment of the classroom, the clinician must be aware of a number of new issues relevant to habilitation, such as balancing the child's need for habilitation and mastering the curriculum, integration, and the limited time available to the child, the family, and the teacher.

As children progress through school they will be expected to complete the curriculum of their school (see Figure 11–1). Inevitably, a hearing impairment will make this task more time-consuming and demanding for implanted children than for their normally hearing peers. Therefore, consideration must be given to each child's needs so that an appropriate balance can be found between habilitation and curriculum demands. An alternative to individual habilitation sessions during school time is to utilize homework tasks that the child may complete alone or with his or her parents. Further difficulties arise here as both parents and child have demands on their time after school. Children must complete school-assigned homework tasks, with the amount of homework increasing as the child gets older. In many families both parents work and there is limited time for them to spend on homework tasks. The availability of free play time for the child must also be considered. It is reasonable to expect that a hearing-impaired child who must concentrate all day on communication would need free play time after school, during which he or she can relax from the stress of continually striving to understand and be understood.

Teachers often have limited time for consultation with other professionals due to their teaching commitments. Particularly in the integrated setting, where the hearing-impaired child may be one of 30 or 35 children, it can be difficult for the child's teacher to organize free time. However, liaison with the child's teacher and inservicing of school staff are important functions for which time needs to be found. If possible, teacher involvement in habilitation activities, such as one-on-one sessions and mapping, can benefit both the teacher's and the clinician's knowledge of the child.

CONCLUSION

A severe-to-profound hearing impairment is an enormous barrier to the development of speech and language through audition.

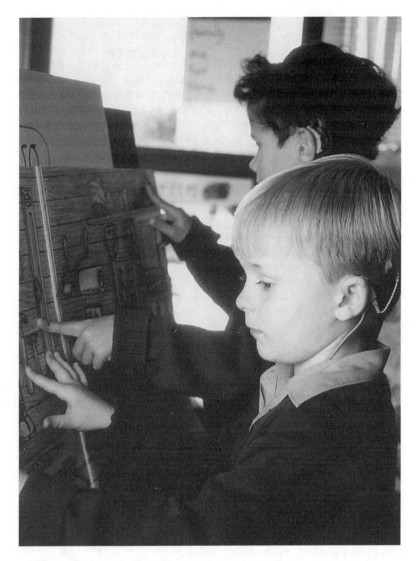

FIGURE 11-1. An implanted child in a classroom setting enjoys listening activities that are integrated into the curriculum.

For children with cochlear implants, however, it is not an insurmountable difficulty. The steps that are taken by habilitationists are significant in determining the degree of success each child achieves.

ACKNOWLEDGMENTS

We thank Dr Peter Blamey for his valuable comments on the chapter. We also thank St Mary's School for Children with Impaired Hearing for their kind permission to reproduce Figure 11–1.

REFERENCES

Boothroyd, A. (1993). Profound deafness. In R. S. Tyler (Ed.), *Cochlear implants: Audiological foundations.* (pp. 1–33) San Diego: Singular Publishing Group.

Dowell, R. C., Blamey, P. J., & Clark, G. M. (1995). Potential and limitations of cochlear implants in children. *Annals of Otology, Rhinology and Laryngology, 104*, 324–327.

Gantz, B. J., Tyler, R. S., Woodworth, G. G., Tye-Murray, N., & Fryauf-Bertschy, H. (1994). Results of multichannel cochlear implants in congenital and acquired prelingual deafness in children: Five-year follow-up. *American Journal of Otology, 15*(Suppl. 2), 1–7.

Geers, A., & Moog, J. (1995). Spoken language results: Vocabulary, syntax, and communication. *Volta Review Monograph, 96,* 131–148.

Grogan, M. L., Barker, E. J., Dettman, S. J., & Blamey, P. J. (1995). Phonetic and phonologic changes in the connected speech of children using a cochlear implant. *Annals of Otology, Rhinology and Laryngology, 104*(Suppl. 166), 390–393.

Kramer, C, James, S, & Saxmann, J. (1979). A comparison of language samples elicited at home and in the clinic. *Journal of Speech and Hearing Disorders, 44,* 321–330

Kretschmer, R. R., & Kretschmer, L. W. (1978). *Language development and intervention with the hearing-impaired.* Baltimore, MD: University Park.

Kretschmer, R. R., & Kretschmer, L. W. (1986). Language in perspective. In D. M. Luterman (Ed.), *Deafness in perspective.* San Diego: College-Hill Press.

Ling, D. (1976). *Speech and the hearing-impaired child: Theory and practice.* Washington, DC: Alexander Graham Bell Association for the Deaf.

McConkey Robbins, A. (1994). Guidelines for developing oral communication skills in children with cochlear implants. *The Volta Review, 96,* 75–82.

McGarr, N. (1987). Communication skills of hearing-impaired children in schools for the deaf. *American Speech and Hearing Association Monographs, 26,* 91–107.

Mecklenburg, D. J. (1988). Cochlear implants in children: Nonmedical considerations. *American Journal of Otology, 9,* 163–168.

Miyamoto, R. T., Osberger, M. J., Robbins, A. M., Myres, W. A., & Kessler, K. (1993). Prelingually deafened children's performance with the Nucleus multichannel cochlear implant. *American Journal of Otology, 14,* 437–445.

Moores, D. F. (1987). *Educating the deaf: Principles and practices.* Boston: Houghton Mifflin.

Muma, J. (1986). *Language acquisition: A functionalistic perspective.* Austin, TX: Pro-Ed.

Osberger, M. J., Johnstone, A., Swarts, E., & Levitt, H. (1978). The evaluation of a model speech training program for deaf children. *Journal of Communication Disorders, 11,* 293–313.

Osberger, M. J., & Levitt, H. (1979). The effect of timing errors on the intelligibility of deaf children's speech. *Journal of the Acoustical Society of America, 66,* 1316–1324.

Osberger, M. J., Maso, M., & Sam, L. K. (1993). Speech intelligibility of children with cochlear implants, tactile aids, or hearing aids. *Journal of Speech and Hearing Research, 36,* 186–203.

Osberger, M. J., Miyamoto, R. T., Zimmerman-Phillips, S., Lemink, J. L., Stroer, B. S., Firszt, J. B., & Novak, M. A. (1991). Independent evaluation of the speech perception abilities of children with the Nucleus 22-channel cochlear implant system. *Ear and Hearing, 12*(Suppl.), 66–80.

Paul, P. V., & Quigley, S. P. (1994). *Language and deafness.* San Diego: Singular Publishing Group.

Peloquin, L. J., & Davidson, P. W. (1988). Psychological sequelae of pediatric infectious diseases. In D. K. Roth (Ed.), *Handbook of pediatric psychology.* New York: Guilford Press.

Quittner, A. L., & Steck, J. T. (1991). Predictors of cochlear implant use in children. *American Journal of Otology, 12*(Suppl.), 89–94.

Sarant, J. Z., Blamey, P. J., Cowan, R. S. C., & Clark, G. M. (in press). The effects of language knowledge on speech perception; What are we really assessing? *American Journal of Otology.*

Somers, M. N. (1991). Speech perception abilities in children with cochlear implants or hearing aids. *American Journal of Otology, 12*(Suppl.), 174–178.

Staller, S. J., Beiter, A. L., Brimacombe, J. A., Mecklenburg, D. J., & Arndt, P. A. (1991). Pediatric performance with the Nucleus 22-channel cochlear implant system. *American Journal of Otology, 12*(Suppl.), 126–136.

Staller, S. J., Dowell, R. C., Beiter, A. L., & Brimacombe, J. A. (1991). Perceptual abilities of children with the Nucleus 22-channel cochlear implant. *Ear and Hearing, 12,* 34S–47S.

Webster, D. B., & Webster, M. (1977). Neonatal sound deprivation affects brain stem auditory nuclei. *Archives of Otolaryngology, 103,* 392–396.

Webster, D. B., & Webster, M. (1979). Effects of neonatal conductive hearing loss on brain stem auditory nuclei. *Annals of Otology, Rhinology and Laryngology, 88,* 684–688.

12

EVALUATION OF BENEFIT: INFANTS AND CHILDREN

RICHARD C. DOWELL
ROBERT S. C. COWAN

This chapter discusses the importance of evaluating benefits in a cochlear implant program for children, outlines the problems encountered in assessing outcomes in young children, provides an integrated approach to some of these problems, and reviews the currently available results. This discussion emphasizes the need to obtain reliable information about the auditory skills of children as these are the skills that a cochlear implant attempts to restore or improve.

IMPORTANCE OF SPEECH PERCEPTION

The desired outcomes for children using cochlear implants relate to improved speech production and auditory language development, in addition to speech perception ability. The success of cochlear implants for children will rest on providing significant improvements in these areas. On the other hand, the first step in this process must be to improve auditory skills, in particular to provide detection, discrimination, recognition, and comprehension of speech. The integration of these abilities into auditory language skills and improved speech intel-

ligibility will depend on many factors, some of which are discussed later in this chapter. The contribution of the cochlear implant to these aspects of communication, however, is best determined from assessment of speech perception.

TYPES OF SPEECH PERCEPTION ASSESSMENT

The investigation of speech perception abilities in hearing-impaired adults and children, and in particular, cochlear implant users, has spawned a vast array of measurement tools. The reader is referred to Boothroyd (1995), Dillon and Ching (1995), and Plant (1995) for a comprehensive review of currently available speech perception tests. It can be confusing for audiologists new to this area to sort out which tests may be suitable for a particular situation. It is possible, however, to simplify this field as there are only a limited number of skills that these tests attempt to quantify.

Open-Set Tests

Open-set assessments present meaningful speech material without providing a list of alternatives, contextual clues, or other information to help identify the material. Most standard speech perception assessments used in clinical audiology are open-set word (AB words, Boothroyd, 1968; CNC words, Peterson & Lehiste, 1962) or sentence tests (CID Everyday Sentences, Davis & Silverman, 1970; BKB sentences, Bench & Bamford, 1979). The use of these tests allows direct comparison with a wealth of data for hearing-impaired adults and children. These assessments also provide measures relevant to everyday communication, as the ability to understand words and sentences in an open-set context can be related to real life communication skills. Some disadvantages of open-set tests are the need for multiple test lists, as there are learning effects if material is presented more than once. In addition, the open-set tests may provide a measure of overall speech perception benefit but give little information about how subjects are achieving this performance. For instance, it cannot be easily deduced from results of open-set sentence testing whether the implant is providing specific acoustic phonetic information.

Closed-Set Tests

Closed-set testing provides a more controlled assessment in which subjects choose from a list of possible alternatives. The alternatives can be arranged such that any aspect of the discrimination of speech is assessed. As an example, the NU-CHIPS test (Elliott & Katz, 1980), commonly presented to children with implants, has a set of four pictures for each item. These pictures correspond to rhyming words differing in the initial or final consonant such as "coat/boat/goat/note." One of the words is presented and subjects point to the one they hear. If the child scores significantly above chance, it can be concluded that he or she can discriminate some consonants using audition. Many

different tests have been developed that assess speech feature discriminations in this way (Dillon & Ching, 1995). The advantage of such tests is their ability to provide such specific information. Their disadvantage is the difficulty of relating scores to the perception of connected speech used for communication. The discrimination of particular features of speech in isolation does not guarantee the processing of the 10 or so phonemes per second encountered in connected speech.

In using any test of speech perception, it is important to understand the purpose of the test and the appropriate statistical interpretation of scores. This is particularly important in some closed-set tests where scores as high as 65% may be achieved by chance.

Speech Perception Abilities

In most cases, tests of speech perception can be classified in one of four categories:

1. Suprasegmental discrimination tasks
2. Segmental discrimination tasks
3. Open set word recognition
4. Open-set recognition of connected speech

The first type includes assessments generated in early cochlear implant and tactile aid work where speech perception performance was limited. These assessments use closed-set formats with pitch, amplitude, or rhythm differences between the alternatives. As such, they assess gross auditory discrimination skills and do not provide a great deal of information about speech perception. The tests in the second class isolate acoustic phonetic features of speech and measure their discriminability using closed-set tasks. Such tests cover a wide range of difficulty as they may involve fine or gross phonetic contrasts. The ability to discriminate such contrasts is a prerequisite for understanding connected speech.

The open-set recognition tasks assess actual perception of speech and can be related to aspects of communication performance. Tests using connected speech, as opposed to isolated words, are influenced more by language skills (in particular, the use of semantic and syntactic context) as well as auditory ability. This must be taken into account in applying these assessments to children with hearing impairment and delayed language development.

PROBLEMS OF SPEECH PERCEPTION MEASUREMENT IN CHILDREN

Limitations of Language Ability

In both hearing and hearing-impaired children, speech production and language ability is developing in the first 5 years of life. In many children with profound hearing impairment, these abilities are significantly delayed or even absent. The tests used to assess the performance of adult implant users, such as open-set sentences, rely on a knowledge of the vocabulary used and the structure of the language. Even for tests designed specifically for children, there is a limitation on the age range due to the lack of vocabulary skills in very young implant users. In attempting to provide some information about these young children, tests must rely on using imitated nonsense syllables (Dettman et al., 1995).

Limitations of Speech Production Ability

In recording responses to speech perception testing, adult subjects will either write or repeat their responses, which can then be scored by the tester. Many of the children using implants cannot yet write and have poor speech production skills. A child's auditory abilities may be underestimated due to imitated responses that cannot be deciphered by the tester.

Task-related Issues

The tasks involved in some speech perception tests may not be understood by very young children. For instance, 3-year-olds, presented with a picture pointing, closed-set assessment may point to their favorite picture repeatedly rather than relating auditory input to the choice of picture. Young children will also struggle to maintain concentration and motivation for speech perception tasks and this can have a significant effect on results.

Suggested Approaches

Despite some of the problems detailed here, it is possible to obtain useful speech perception information on most children using cochlear implants. A battery of tests is needed to provide suitable assessments for both younger and older children and to give appropriate measurement across the wide range of speech perception abilities. Testing must take into account the language skills and speech production ability of the child. In particular, knowledge of the vocabulary used in any test must be confirmed. As soon as possible, open-set testing should be included in the assessment battery as this provides the most appropriate measure of benefit. This can begin with open-set word testing as soon as the child is able to imitate on demand (see Chapter 10), leading to sentence recognition when language skills have reached an appropriate level.

OVERVIEW OF SPEECH PERCEPTION RESULTS

Categorical Treatment of Speech Perception Results

One approach to dealing with the variety of test results and the wide variation in speech perception ability in implanted children is to define a number of categories of performance related to tasks of increasing difficulty. From available results and a knowledge of the tests used, children can be placed into these categories and an overall perspective on speech perception performance can be obtained. It should be kept in mind that in categorizing test scores in this way some information from the original results is lost. On the other hand, an advantage of this treatment is the ability to compare a large number of children and show trends in performance related to pre- and postoperative individual factors.

Performance in a Clinical Population

One such study reviewed the speech perception results for children using cochlear implants in Melbourne and Sydney (Dowell, Blamey, & Clark, 1995). Results for 100 unselected children and adolescents were categorized based on the level of ability demonstrated in formal tests. The scale used was based on other categorical scales proposed for hearing-impaired children (Geers & Moog, 1987) and cochlear implant users (Staller et al., 1991) with additional levels of performance for children scoring well on open-set tests. The categories were defined as follows:

1. Detection of speech sounds only
2. Discrimination of suprasegmental aspects of speech in addition to 1.
3. Discrimination and recognition of vowels in addition to 1 and 2.
4. Discrimination and recognition of consonants in addition to 1–3.
5. Minimal open-set speech perception in addition to 1–4.
6. Open-set speech perception (>20% phoneme score for PBK words)
7. Good open-set speech perception (>50% phoneme score for PBK words)

A summary of the results of this categorical analysis is shown in Figure 12–1.

This indicates that approximately 60% of children in this group achieve significant open-set speech recognition, and approximately 30% of the group recognize over half of the phonemes in an open-set monosyllabic word test. For these children it is reasonable to conclude that they are capable of using audition alone for interactive communication.

Predictive Factors for Speech Perception Performance

Statistical analysis of these results showed that the duration of profound hearing loss had a significant ($p < 0.001$) negative association with speech perception performance. Children with onset of profound hearing loss after the age of 4 years (postlinguistic hearing loss) performed better ($p < 0.01$) as did those with useful preimplant residual hearing ($p < 0.001$). Experience with the implant also showed a significant ($p < 0.001$) positive association with good perceptual performance, as did an oral/aural educational placement ($p < 0.05$). These five variables accounted for 37% of the variance in the categorical speech perception results.

There was no significant difference between the results for children with congenital hearing losses and those with acquired losses. Age at implantation was not a significant factor for those with an acquired hearing loss, although it was important for the children with congenital profound hearing loss. Various additional parameters such as mode and dynamic range for electrical stimulation were not found to be significant in this analysis.

The results obtained from this analysis can be interpreted in the following way. On average, a profoundly deaf child or adolescent will be expected to have some closed-set discrimination of segmental aspects of speech immediately after implantation, but open-set speech perception may take some years to develop. If an im-

Categorical speech perception results for 100 implanted children

Number of children

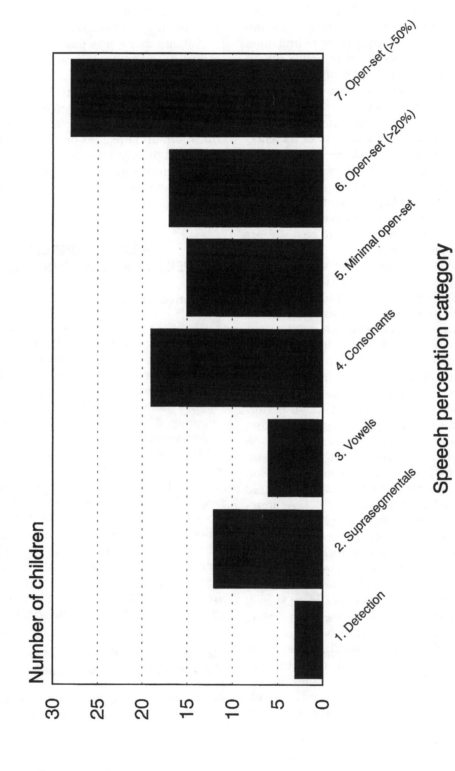

Speech perception category

FIGURE 12–1. Summary of categorical speech perception performance for 100 children and adolescents using the Nucleus-22 cochlear implant in Australia.

planted child has been profoundly deaf for a considerable time, initial speech perception ability may be reduced and long-term potential more limited. If a child has had a postlinguistic profound hearing loss or has useful residual hearing prior to implantation, open-set speech performance may be achieved relatively quickly after surgery. In addition, children in an auditory/oral educational program may have a better chance of achieving significant open-set speech perception. As an illustration of the effect of experience on speech perception skills, mean categorical speech perception performance versus implant experience is shown for the group of 100 children in Figure 12–2. Note that, on average, results continue to improve until at least 4 years after implantation.

Having proposed an interpretation of the categorical results, it is important to note that the significant factors account for less than 40% of the variance in the categorical speech perception data. This implies that speech perception in children with cochlear implants is inherently unpredictable and/or there are factors not included in this analysis that have significant effects on speech perception performance. Clinical experience suggests that at least one of these factors may be the child's home environment. It is well established that this plays an important role in educational progress for hearing-impaired children (Geers & Moog, 1987). As long-term implant experience plays a role in achieving good speech perception, it is likely that children who receive intermittent auditory input after implantation will be disadvantaged. This can occur simply because of poor maintenance of the speech processor or inconsistent use of the device. Another major factor may be the effect of additional handicaps, which are relatively common among profoundly deaf children. Between 15% and 20% of children implanted in Melbourne have significant additional disabilities in conjunction with

profound hearing loss. The possible effect of such problems on performance with a cochlear implant must be reviewed on an individual basis and will depend on the type and degree of disability.

In summary, it is possible to demonstrate a number of significant factors associated with good speech perception performance in implanted children. These can be divided into those related to prior auditory experience, such as residual hearing, duration, and onset of profound hearing loss, and those related to learning to use the auditory input provided by the implant, such as postoperative experience and educational placement.

OPEN-SET SPEECH PERCEPTION IN CHILDREN

Sentence Recognition

Figure 12–3 shows results for 38 children and adolescents implanted in Melbourne on the open-set BKB sentence test using audition alone. This includes all children with appropriate language ability and response skills to complete the task. This generally means that the children were at least 6 years of age although some completed the test earlier. Twenty-one of the 38 children (55%) had congenital profound hearing losses and 15 (42%) were over 10 years of age when implanted. Results were obtained during 1994 using the MSP-Multipeak speech processor. All children had at least 12 months of experience with the device, with an average of 4.1 years. The mean score for this group was 32% with a range from 0% to 94%. Eighty-five percent of the group performed significantly on this task.

Comparison with Results for Postlinguistically Deaf Adults

It is interesting to compare these results to those obtained for postlinguistically deaf

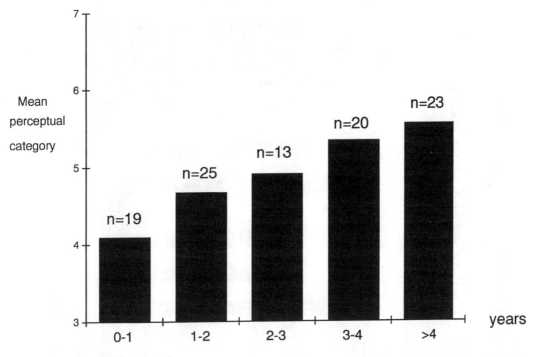

FIGURE 12–2. Mean categorical speech perception performance as a function of implant experience in years for 100 children and adolescents using the Nucleus-22 cochlear implant in Australia.

adults on similar tests. Results for adults implanted in Melbourne using the MSP-Multipeak speech processor on the CID Everyday Sentence Test show a mean score of 59.1% (Hollow et al., 1995). The mean result for the group of children compares favorably with the adult results, particularly when the proportion of congenital losses and late implants is considered. When the children implanted under the age of 5 years are analyzed as a separate group, the mean score rises to 49% (*n* = 19).

Significant Factors in Sentence Recognition

These results were subjected to a stepwise multiple regression analysis to assess the influence of possible predictive factors.

Duration of profound hearing loss, postlinguistic onset of profound deafness, and educational placement were found to be highly significant factors associated with open-set sentence perception. These results are consistent with the analysis of the categorical speech perception data on the larger group of children described previously. Figure 12–4 shows the sentence results sorted on the basis of the child's postoperative educational setting. Inspection of these data shows that scores vary widely in both groups but only within the oral/aural group are scores greater than 40% encountered. This type of evidence suggests that parents of implanted children should be encouraged to aim for an oral/aural or mainstreamed educational environment wherever possible.

212

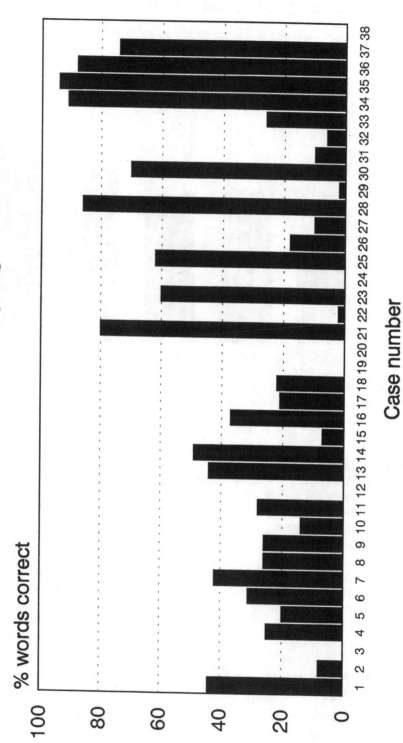

FIGURE 12–3. Results for open-set sentence recognition using audition alone for 38 children and adolescents in Melbourne.

Speech perception and educational placement

BKB open-set sentence scores

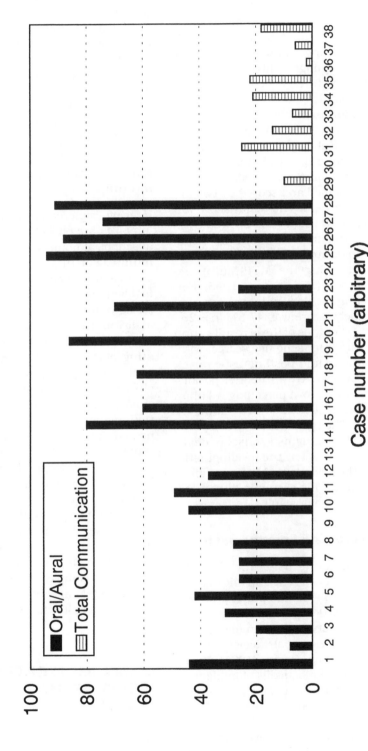

FIGURE 12–4. Results for open-set sentence recognition for 38 children and adolescents implanted in Melbourne sorted into two groups based on the educational environment of the child following implantation.

Monosyllabic Word Recognition

The described open-set sentence results provide useful information on school-aged children, but younger implanted children without the language skills for this task are also of interest. The PBK open-set word test can be completed in younger children as an imitation task. Results have been collected on all children implanted in Melbourne with the ability to complete this assessment. Due to the speech production limitations of many of the children, the tests are videotaped and scored by two independent listeners. The mean score for this group was 38.9% ($n = 47$, SD = 23.8%), again comparing favorably with the mean score for implanted adults of 47.9% on similar tests using the MSP-Multipeak speech processor (Hollow et al., 1995). For the children implanted under the age of 5 years, the mean score was 47.3% ($n = 26$, SD = 23.9%). Analysis of these results support the findings for sentence scores, with shorter duration and postlinguistic onset of deafness associated with better performance. The scores as a percentage of phonemes correctly identified are shown in Figure 12–5. The results have been sorted into pre- and postlinguistic onset of deafness groups, and for the prelinguistic group, into those implanted before or after 10 years of age. This grouping illustrates the effect of the major significant factors.

Speech Processing Improvements

The ability of adults using the Nucleus multiple channel cochlear implant to benefit from developments in speech processing has been well documented (Clark 1995). However, the ability of children to adapt to new speech processing strategies has received less attention. Cowan (1995) evaluated speech perception skills of implanted children aged 6 to 14 years who changed from the Multipeak to the SPEAK speech processing strategy.

Seven children were followed for a period of 18 months following change over to SPEAK. The results (see Figure 12–6) showed that, for six of the seven children, scores were significantly better when using the SPEAK speech processing strategy, particularly in the test situation with background noise (+15 dB signal-to-noise ratio). This supports the results of studies with adults and shows that children are also able to benefit from additional information provided by new signal coding developments.

Assessment of Speech Perception in Competing Noise

Hearing-impaired children using cochlear implants are often in noisy environments at school, at home, and in the general community. For this reason, it was of interest to assess whether specific habilitation involving speech perception in controlled background noise could improve the child's ability to use the cochlear implant in noisy environments. A preliminary study evaluating perception of open-set words and sentences in background noise for four children has been completed. Each of the children was assessed over a 6-month period, using repeated assessments of connected discourse tracking and word and sentence perception scores.

During the 6-month period, each child had weekly habilitation sessions, which included specific perceptual training in controlled background noise. Preliminary results (see Figure 12–7) showed post-training scores on open-set words to be significantly higher than pretraining when testing was completed in background noise. No similar significant increase was evident in quiet, despite the training received by each child.

COMPARISON OF BENEFITS FROM COCHLEAR IMPLANTS, HEARING AIDS, AND TACTILE DEVICES

The communication benefits available from cochlear implants have now been docu-

PBK phoneme scores - all children

Results sorted by age at implantation and onset of deafness

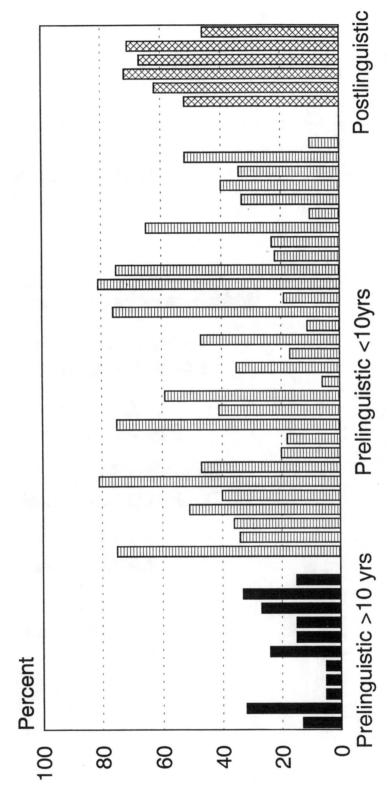

FIGURE 12-5. Results for open-set monosyllabic word recognition scored by percentage of phonemes correct for 47 children and adolescents implanted in Melbourne.

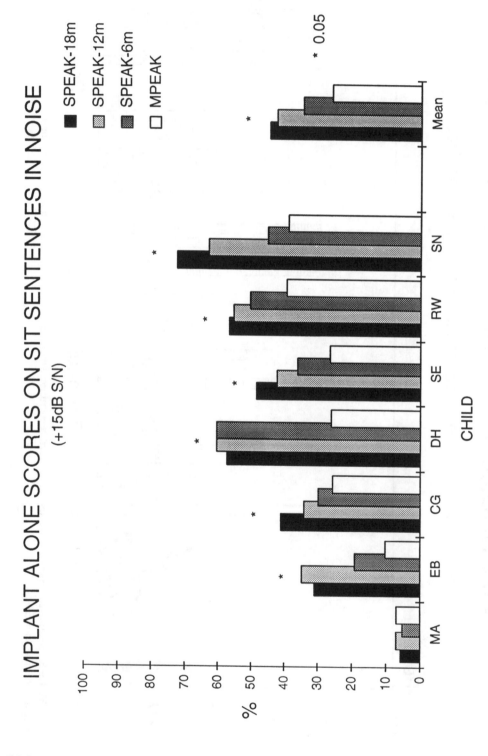

FIGURE 12-6. Speech perception scores on SIT sentences in noise for seven children using Multipeak and SPEAK speech processing strategies after 6, 12, and 18 months experience.

CNC Phoneme Scores

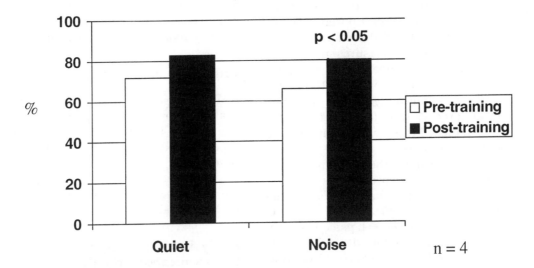

FIGURE 12–7. CNC phoneme scores for four implanted children tested in quiet and in +15 dB signal-to-noise ratio before and after completion of training in competing noise.

mented in a number of studies specifically evaluating children (Dawson, Blamey, Dettman, Barker et al., 1995; Dawson, Blamey, Dettman, Rowland et al., 1995; Dowell et al., 1995; Geers & Moog, 1994; Osberger, Maso, & Sam, 1993; Osberger et al., 1991). Studies have also assessed the benefits from cochlear implant for specific groups of users, such as congenitally deaf adolescents (Sarant, Cowan et al., 1996).

For some implant candidates, it has been suggested that trials with tactile aids should be incorporated into preoperative programs, particularly for children who do not receive benefit from hearing aids. Two recent studies have evaluated benefits for matched groups of children using cochlear implants, tactile devices, and hearing aids. Geers and Moog (1994) reported results on comparative assessments of speech perception, speech production, and language acquisition for children enrolled at the Central Institute for the Deaf in St Louis, Missouri. Results of that long-term study

showed that the children using cochlear implants achieved higher speech perception scores than the children using a multichannel vibrotactile device and scores similar to hearing aid users with 90–100 dB HL pure tone average thresholds. However, the children using implants showed significantly faster speech and language acquisition than the children using hearing aids. Even after intensive training directed toward discrimination of speech features, the vibrotactile device did not provide sufficient information to allow the children to recognize recorded words based on vowel or consonant differences or to significantly enhance lipreading.

Kirk et al. (1995) also compared performance of children with cochlear implants, tactile aids, and hearing aids. Results showed that children using the cochlear implant improved significantly between the preimplant and postimplant intervals on closed-set tests of phoneme and word recognition and on open-set tests of phrase recognition. In contrast, the scores for the tactile aid group showed little change with additional device use with the exception of closed-set word recognition. The scores for the cochlear implant group were also significantly higher than those for the vibrotactile group on all measures in the post-device period. In comparison with hearing aid users, the performance of the tactile group was significantly poorer. No significant differences were found between the performance of the cochlear implant and hearing aid groups.

To some extent, these results should be interpreted to be specific to the comparison of the multiple-channel Nucleus implant and vibrotactile Tactaid VII. Sarant et al. (1996) evaluated speech perception benefits for three congenitally deaf adolescents who received the Nucleus 22-channel cochlear implant following a period of preoperative assessment using the electrotactile "Tickle Talker" (Blamey & Clark, 1985).

For all of the children, the postoperative scores with the cochlear implant were significantly higher than preoperative scores with hearing aids. For two of the three patients, significant audition alone scores were obtained when using the cochlear implant. To date, this level of benefit has not been possible with any tactile device (Cowan et al., 1995).

These studies suggest that multiple channel cochlear implants provide greater potential for the development of speech perception skills than available tactile aids. Tactile aids should be considered an option for profoundly hearing-impaired children who are not suitable candidates for cochlear implantation.

ASSESSMENT OF SPEECH PRODUCTION AND LANGUAGE

Evaluation of Articulation

A range of formal speech production measures can be used in assessing articulation and speech production (see Busby et al., 1990). Such assessments provide quantification of the elicited phonetic repertoire of a child at a word level. This can be useful to track the acquisition of new phonemes but does not indicate whether they are used appropriately in conversational speech.

Evaluation of Language

A number of formal language tests are available for hearing-impaired children. Selection of the appropriate materials is dependent on the age and linguistic knowledge of the child. Details of many of the language assessments appropriate for children using cochlear implants can be found in Busby et al. (1990).

Analysis of Videotaped Communication Samples

Videotaped samples of conversation can be useful in the evaluation of speech production, language, and pragmatics. They allow for repeated viewing of the interaction for analysis and provide a more complete picture of communication than formal testing. Research has indicated that the use of meaningful contexts, familiar settings, non-contrived situations, and age-appropriate, motivating activities will result in more representative communication samples.

Recently, a computer-assisted speech and language analysis (CASALA) software program was developed by Blamey (1994), which allows for the automated analysis of videotaped samples collected over time. The CASALA program provides phonetic inventory, phonological process analysis, and a mean length of utterance calculation. Results can also be used to measure the acquisition of specific phonemes, providing information valuable to habilitation management, or for research.

Results of Speech and Language Analysis for Implanted Children

Results from CASALA evaluating the phonetic inventories of 20 children before and after implantation (Grogan et al., 1995) showed that phonemes were acquired in an order similar to that of normally hearing children. The most common phonological processes affecting vowels were elongation, nasalization, and monophthongization. For consonants, the most common processes were deletion, voicing, stopping, and cluster reduction. A more detailed study of nine children over a 4-year period (Serry, Blamey, & Grogan, 1996) showed that individual phonemes take about 2 months to progress from the stage where they are first produced accurately (either in words or babble) to the stage where they are used in meaningful words with 50% or greater accuracy. These studies confirm previous speech production data based on articulation tests (Dawson et al., 1995; Tobey et al., 1991) and language samples (Osberger et al., 1991).

The CASALA analysis also indicated steady growth in the mean length of utterance (MLU) over a 4-year period, at a mean rate of 0.65 morphemes per year in the postoperative period. The mean MLU observed 48 months postoperatively for a group of nine implant users who were all implanted at age 5 or less was 3.91 morphemes. The observed rate of increase in MLU was less than the rate of about 1.2 morphemes per year for normally hearing children at ages 1–4 years (Miller & Chapman, 1981). However, all children showed a significant improvement in both speech production and language skills in their spontaneous interactions postoperatively. These mean improvements are shown in Figure 12–8.

CONCLUSION AND IMPLICATIONS FOR THE FUTURE

We have reviewed the evaluation of the benefits of cochlear implants in children

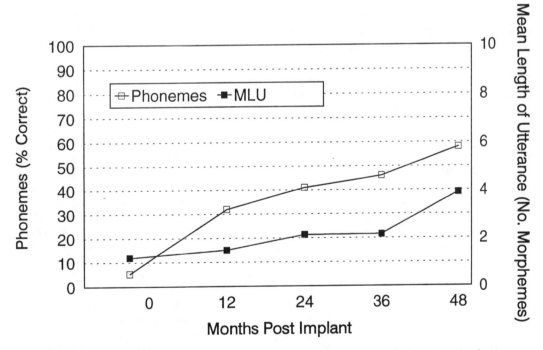

FIGURE 12–8. Mean values for the percentage of phonemes correct and mean length of utterance (MLU) for nine children implanted at age 5 or younger. Values were derived from conversational language samples analyzed with the help of the CASALA program.

with an emphasis on speech perception assessment. Such assessments provide direct information about the children's auditory input from the device and how they use this information. The development of speech production and language skills in implanted children is of paramount importance and will depend on speech perception ability as well as other factors, some of which have been discussed here.

Long-term speech perception results show that a majority of children with multiple channel implants develop open-set speech perception ability. The results also suggest that children implanted younger, or soon after the onset of profound deafness, have the best chance of developing such skills. As cochlear implantation becomes more common in young children and infants, the majority of profoundly hearing-impaired children will have the opportunity to develop good open-set speech perception, with the consequent benefits in speech and language development under the right conditions. Variation in performance will still occur in individual cases and long-term follow-up from a medical, audiological, and habilitation perspective appears to be crucial to success. The results already obtained, however, provide a strong foundation for continued improvement in performance of young children using cochlear implants.

REFERENCES

Blamey, P. J., & Clark, G. M. (1985). A wearable multiple-electrode electrotactile speech processor for the profoundly deaf. *Journal of the Acoustical Society of America, 77,* 1619.

Blamey, P. J., Dawson, S. J., Dettman, S. J., Rowland, L. C., Brown, A. M., Busby, P. A., Dowell, R. C., Rickards, F. W., & Clark, G. M. (1992). Speech perception, production and language results in a group of children using the 22-electrode cochlear implant. *Australian Journal of Otolaryngology, 1,* 105–109.

Blamey, P. J. (1994). Computer-Assisted Speech and Language Analysis (CASALA) Software.

Melbourne: Human Communication Research Centre Annual Report.

Bench, J., & Bamford J. (Eds.). (1979). *Speech-hearing tests and the spoken language of hearing-impaired children.* London: Academic Press.

Boothroyd, A. (1968). Developments in speech audiometry. *Sound, 2,* 3–10.

Boothroyd, A., (1995). Speech perception tests and hearing-impaired children. In G. Plant & K.-E. Spens (Eds.), *Profound deafness and speech communication* (pp. 345–371). London: Whurr Publishers.

Busby P. A., Dettman, S. J., Altidis, P. M., Blamey, P. J., & Roberts S. A. (1990). Assessment of communication skills in implanted deaf children. In G. M. Clark, Y. C. Tong, & J. F. Patrick (Eds.), *Cochlear prostheses* (pp. 223–236). Edinburgh: Churchill Livingstone.

Clark, G. M. (1995). Historical perspectives. In G. Plant & K.-E. Spens (Eds.), *Profound deafness and speech communication* (165–218). London: Whurr.

Clark, G. M. (1995). Cochlear implants: Future research directions. *Annals of Otology, Rhinology and Laryngology 104*(Suppl. 166), 22–27.

Cowan, R. S. C., Galvin, K. L., Sarant, J. Z., Blamey, P. J., & Clark, G. M. (1995). Issues in the development of multichannel tactile devices for hearing-impaired adults and children. In D. K. Oller (Ed.), *Tactile aids for the hearing impaired. Seminars in Hearing, 16,* 356–369.

Cowan, R. S. C., Brown, C., Whitford, L. A., Galvin, K. L., Sarant, J. Z., Barker, E. J., Shaw, S., King, A., Skok, M., Seligman, P. M., Dowell, R. C., Everingham, C., Gibson, W. P. R., & Clark, G. M. (1995). Speech perception in children using the advanced Speak speech-processing strategy. In G. M. Clark & R. S. C. Cowan (Eds.), *International Cochlear Implant, Speech and Hearing Symposium 1994. Annals of Otology, Rhinology and Laryngology, 104*(Suppl. 166), 318–321.

Cowan, R. S. C., Deldot, J., Barker, E. J., Sarant, J. Z., Dettman, S. J., Pegg, P., Galvin, K. L., Rance, G., Larratt, M., Hollow, R., Herridge, S., Skok, M., Dowell, R. C., Pyman, B., Gibson, W. P. R., & Clark, G. M. (6 June 1996). *Speech perception for children with different levels of preoperative residual hearing.* Paper presented at the Third European Symposium on Paediatric Cochlear Implantation, Hannover, Germany.

Davis, H., & Silverman, R. (1970). *Hearing and deafness*. New York: Holt, Rinehart, & Winston.

Dawson, P. W. (1992). *Vowel Imitation Test*. Melbourne: Human Communication Research Centre Annual Report.

Dawson, P. W., Blamey, P. J., Rowland, L. C., Dettman, S. J., Clark, G. M., Busby, P. A., Brown, A. M., Dowell, R. C., & Rickards, F. W. (1992). Cochlear implants in children, adolescents, and prelinguistically deafened adults: Speech perception. *Journal of Speech and Hearing Research, 35,* 401–417.

Dawson, P. W., Blamey, P. J., Dettman, S. J., Barker, E. J., & Clark, G.M. (1995). A clinical report on receptive vocabulary skills in cochlear implant users. *Ear and Hearing, 16,* 287–294.

Dawson, P. W., Blamey, P. J., Dettman, S. J., Rowland, L. C., Barker, E. J., Tobey, E. A., Busby, P. A., Cowan, R. C., & Clark, G. M. (1995). A clinical report on speech production of cochlear implant users. *Ear and Hearing, 16,* 551–561.

Dettman, S. J., Barker, E. J., Dowell, R. C., Dawson, P. W., Blamey, P. J., & Clark, G. M. (1995). Vowel imitation task: Results over time for 28 cochlear implant children under the age of eight years. In G. M. Clark & R. S. C. Cowan (Eds.), *International Cochlear Implant, Speech and Hearing Symposium 1994. Annals of Otology, Rhinology and Laryngology, 104*(Suppl. 166), 321–324.

Dillon, H.,& Ching, T. (1995). What makes a good speech test? In G. Plant & K.-E. Spens (Eds.), *Profound deafness and speech communication* (pp. 305–344) London: Whurr Publishers.

Dowell, R. C., Blamey, P. J., & Clark, G. M. (1995). Potential and limitations of cochlear implants in children. In G. M. Clark & R. S. C. Cowan (Eds.), *International Cochlear Implant, Speech and Hearing Symposium 1994. Annals of Otology, Rhinology and Laryngology, 104*(Suppl. 166), 324–327.

Dowell, R. C., Dawson, P. W., Dettman, S. J., Shepherd, R. K., Whitford, L. A., Seligman, P. M., & Clark, G. M. (1991). Multichannel cochlear implantation in children: A summary of current work at the University of Melbourne. *American Journal of Otology, 12*(Suppl.), 137–143.

Elliott, L. L, & Katz, D. R. (1980) *Northwestern University Children's Perception of Speech (NU-CHIPS)*. St Louis: Auditec.

Geers, A. E, & Moog, J. S. (1987). Predicting spoken language acquisition of profoundly hearing-impaired children. *Journal of Speech and Hearing Disorders, 52,* 84–94.

Geers, A. E., & Moog, J. S. (Eds.). (1994). Effectiveness of cochlear implants and tactile aids for deaf children. *The Volta Review, 96,* 1–231.

Grogan, M. L., Barker, E. J., Dettman, S. J., & Blamey, P. J. (1995). Phonetic and phonologic changes in the connected speech of children using a cochlear implant. In G. Plant & K.-E. Spens (Eds.), *Profound deafness and speech communication* (pp. 390–393) London: Whurr Publishers.

Hollow, R. D., Dowell R. C., Cowan R. S. C, Skok, M. C., Pyman B. C., & Clark G. M. (1995). Continuing improvements in speech processing for adult cochlear implant patients. In G. M. Clark & R. S. C. Cowan, (Eds.), *International Cochlear Implant, Speech and Hearing Symposium 1994. Annals of Otology, Rhinology and Laryngology, 104* (Suppl. 166), 292–294.

Kirk, K. I., Osberger, M. J., McConkey-Robbins, A., Allyson, I. R., Todd, S. L., & Miyamoto, R. T. (1995). Performance of children with cochlear implants, tactile aids and hearing aids. In D. K. Oller, (Ed.), *Tactile aids for the hearing impaired. Seminars in Hearing, 16,* 370–381.

Miller, J., & Chapman, R. (1981). The relationship between age and mean length of utterance in morphemes. *Journal of Speech and Hearing Research, 24,* 154–161.

Osberger, M., Robbins, A., Berry, S., Todd, S., Hesketh, L., & Sedey, A. (1991). Analysis of the spontaneous speech samples of children with a cochlear implant or tactile aid. *American Journal of Otology, 12*(Suppl.), 151–164.

Osberger, M. J., Maso, M., & Sam, L. K. (1993). Speech intelligibility of children with cochlear implants, tactile aids, or hearing aids. *Journal of Speech and Hearing Research, 36,* 186–203.

Peterson, G. E., & Lehiste, I. (1962) Revised CNC lists for auditory tests. *Journal of Speech and Hearing Disorders, 27,* 62–70.

Plant, G. (1995) Speech perception tests for use with Australian children. In G. Plant and K.-E. Spens (Eds.), *Profound deafness and speech communication* (pp. 372-392). London: Whurr.

Sarant, J., Cowan, R., Blamey P., Galvin K., & Clark, G. (1996). Within-subject comparison of speech perception benefits for congenitally deaf adolescents with an electrotactile speech processor and cochlear implant. *Journal of the American Academy of Audiology, 7,* 63–70.

Serry, T., Blamey, P. J., & Grogan, M. (6–8 June 1996). *Phoneme acquisition in the first four years of implant use.* Paper presented at The Third European Symposium on Paediatric Cochlear Implantation, Hannover, Germany.

Staller, S. J., Beiter, A. L., Brimacombe, J. A., Mecklenburg, D. J., & Arndt, P. (1991). Pediatric performance with the Nucleus 22-channel cochlear implant system. *American Journal of Otology, 12*(Suppl.), 126–136.

Tobey E., Angelette S., Murchison C., Nicosia J., Sprague S., Staller S., Brimacombe J., & Beiter, A. (1991). Speech production in children receiving a multichannel cochlear implant. *American Journal of Otology, 12*(Suppl.), 164–172.

Tobey, E. A., & Hasenstab, M. S. (1991). Effects of a Nucleus multichannel cochlear implant upon speech production in children. *Ear and Hearing, 12*(Suppl.), 48S–54S.

13

Socioeconomic
and Educational
Management Issues

ROBERT S. C. COWAN

The presence of severe to profound hearing loss significantly reduces a child's ability to perceive spoken language. As a consequence, the child may develop articulation patterns that deviate significantly from those of the general community. Although these two factors in themselves create enormous barriers to the child's ability to interact with society, the impact of the hearing disability on acquisition of oral and written language places the greatest limitations on the child's educational and life choices (Bamford & Saunders, 1991). For this reason, the evaluation of benefits from use of the cochlear implant has focused on the changes in speech perception, speech production, and, in children, development of linguistic competence that occur over time and with added experience in using the device.

The effectiveness of the multiple-channel cochlear implant in enhancing the acquisition of auditory skills and improving speech perception and speech production has been well documented (Blamey et al., 1992; Cowan et al., 1995; Dawson et al., 1992; Dawson et al., 1995; Dowell et al.,

1995; Geers & Moog, 1994; Kirk et al., 1995; Miyamoto et al., 1992; Staller et al., 1991; Tobey & Hasenstab, 1991; Tye-Murray et al., 1995). However, the impact of improved auditory skills on enhancing language development and educational outcomes in implanted children has received more limited investigation (Geers & Moog, 1994; Hasenstab & Tobey, 1991). In reviewing current data on the effects of cochlear implants on language development in children, the National Institutes of Health (NIH) Consensus Statement on Cochlear Implants in Adults and Children (1995) reported that, on the basis of available evidence, "implantation in conjunction with education and habilitation leads to advances in oral language acquisition" (p. 10).

However, benefit from the cochlear implant should be considered not only in relation to the auditory and linguistic function of the child, but also in terms of how the child interacts as a member of a family and the wider community. The consideration of benefits that accrue to the society as a result of the child's improved auditory and linguistic function

223

introduces the concept of socioeconomic analysis of benefit, which assesses the interrelationship between social and economic factors. Such analysis considers both the benefits and the costs of providing them which accrue to the individual and society. An important issue in the analysis is ensuring that funding provided by health authorities for a particular treatment is in practice the most effective means of obtaining identified benefits both for the child and the society. The relevance of socioeconomic analysis of cochlear implants was noted in the NIH Consensus Statement (1995), which stated that the assessment of medical and surgical interventions should be based not only on establishment of efficacy and safety, but should also assess cost-effectiveness.

APPLICATION OF ECONOMIC ANALYSIS TO MEDICAL INTERVENTION

Economic evaluation measures the long-term benefit and cost of an intervention and establishes whether the treatment represents "value for money" when compared to other competing uses of public health resources. The benefits that accrue to the individual patient through direct amelioration of the disability or disease are an important component to be measured. For example, the placement of a cardiac pacemaker has a direct benefit in prolonging the patient's life. Benefits can also accrue to the patient from the indirect consequences flowing from the treatment. In our example, the patient may be able to resume pleasurable social pastimes or return to employment as an indirect consequence of restored health. Benefits that accrue to the society as a result of the intervention are also measured in economic evaluation. These may result from a restored or resumed ability of the individual to make a contribution to the

society, for example, through employment or public office. Benefits may also accrue to the society through cost savings as a result of eliminating the need to implement an alternative care or treatment for the patient. Put simply, savings may result from the difference in cost between two treatments or programs of intervention. Again, in our example, if the fitting of the cardiac pacemaker decreases the risk that the patient will require high-cost intensive emergency care or long-term nursing care that might arise if he suffered recurrent cardiac insults, then the pacemaker technology represents "value for money," in that it prolongs the patient's life and is less costly to the society than the alternative treatment option.

There are a number of different approaches to economic analysis as applied to medical intervention. Each of these approaches measures the costs of the procedure in monetary terms. What differentiates the approaches is the manner in which outcomes are measured and valued.

Cost-effectiveness analysis measures outcomes in terms of natural units, for example, the number of life-years added or disability saved. Benefits can be directly measured for individuals or groups of patients. In the case of cochlear implants, speech perception scores resulting from use of the implant could be compared with those that were obtained preoperatively using hearing aids or other sensory devices. A number of studies have directly compared benefits to speech perception, speech production, and acquisition of language skills arising through use of cochlear implants, tactile devices and hearing aids (Geers & Moog, 1994; Kirk et al., 1995; Osberger et al., 1993). These studies suggest that the direct benefits available to individuals from use of cochlear implants were signficantly higher than those from either hearing aids or tactile devices. Despite the higher cost of the implant technology, it delivers benefits that are unavailable from other technologies. However, this analysis does not consider indirect benefits that may accrue to the individual or the society resulting from long-term use of the device or easily allow comparisons between medical procedures with differing health outcomes.

Cost-benefit analysis measures outcomes directly in monetary terms. The benefits to the individual are considered in relation to the savings to the society in future monetary outlays for care or support. In the case of cochlear implants for children, cost-benefit analysis could value the savings to the society arising from implanted children being mainstreamed into the community school system, as compared with the costs that would have accrued had the child required education in a special segregated school for hearing-impaired children. Chute and Nevins (1994) reported the growing trend for children using cochlear implants to move from self-contained facilities or classrooms to more mainstream settings. Mainstreaming can result in significant savings to the society, particularly as special education facilities have higher costs due to lower teacher-student ratios. Wyatt and Niparko (1996) estimated a cost-benefit ratio for childhood implantation that suggested a savings of U.S. $152,000 in educational costs and a net present-value-of-implant of U.S. $99,501 for each child implanted at age 4 years (assuming 50% mainstreaming at 3 years postimplant and 90% partial mainstreaming by 6 years postimplant).

Cost-utility analysis measures outcomes in terms of the changes to the individual's quality of life and life expectancy relative to the costs of the intervention. Because hearing loss is not in general a life-threatening disability (except in cases of acoustic neuroma or brainstem lesions), the cochlear implant procedure itself has little direct impact on life expectancy. However, cochlear implantation does improve the patient's quality of life, through restoring or allowing acquisition of auditory skills, improving articulation, and enhancing the development of language comprehension, including reading and writing skills in children. "Indirect" benefits flowing from improved communication in implant patients are a major contributor to the improvement in quality of life experienced (Lea, 1991). Because it allows assessment of the impact of both direct and indirect benefits, cost-utility analysis has advantages in the economic evaluation of cochlear implants in adults and children.

The measure of outcome used in cost-utility analysis is the improvement in quality of life arising from the intervention, where the health-related quality of life is represented by the quality adjusted life year (QALY). The QALY is a numerical health-utility factor ranging in value from 0 (representing death) to 1 (representing perfect health). The value of the QALY represents the benefits to either life-expectancy or quality of life that accrue from the medical treatment. For example, a treatment that prolongs the life of the patient represents a significant increase in QALY (a value of 1.0). In contrast, a treatment that improves the patient's general health and ability to resume normal life is represented as a proportional increase in QALY (a value between 0.1 and 0.9). The QALY values both the prevention of morbidity or life improvement and the duration over which this is maintained. The cost per QALY can be calculated through establishing all relevant costs of the treatment, and this monetary figure provides a measure of the value of the treatment to the individual and the economic costs and impact on the health authority or society in general. The calculation of cost per QALY allows direct comparison of the cost-effectiveness of different medical treatments, as the measure can evaluate both changes to life expectancy and quality of life. Thus, cost-effectiveness for cochlear implantation, which improves quality of life but has little impact on life expectancy, can be directly compared with interventions such as cardiac surgery, which prolong the patient's life expectancy. From the standpoint of the health authority, this direct comparison allows for objective assessment of the outcomes achieved for each dollar spent on competing medical technologies.

Before reviewing the results of economic evaluation studies, it is relevant to consider a number of background factors that are of importance in specifically establishing and valuing the benefits and costs of cochlear implants for children. These factors include indirect benefits from the cochlear implant procedure, educational management issues, medical and surgical issues, and device design and reliability issues in long-term use of cochlear implants.

INDIRECT BENEFITS FROM COCHLEAR IMPLANTS

Clickener (1989) provided a personal patient perspective on the value of indirect benefits for adult cochlear implant users. She noted that improvements in speech perception, voice quality, and the ability to achieve telephone communication had an immediate impact on her quality of life. However, the reduction in stress resulting from increased awareness of environmental sounds and the need for less concentration in lipreading were regarded as major benefits. As a result of improved ability to communicate at work and in social and family settings, the implant also allowed an enhancement of self-image and confidence.

Difficulties in communication experienced by deaf persons may impact directly on employment opportunities. Lea (1991) reported that 78.8% of deaf persons regis-

tered for Commonwealth Employment Services (CES) in Australia had been unemployed for periods in excess of 12 months, as compared with a figure of only 30.4% for the total CES population. Vernon and LaFalce-Landers (1993) also reported low employment rates among congenitally deaf adults. A survey profiling employment and education within the deaf community in New South Wales (Deaf Society of New South Wales, 1989) reported that the majority of deaf adults were employed within the manual, construction, materials handling, and tertiary services sectors. The report suggested that hearing-impaired persons were disadvantaged economically primarily due to a reduced access to education and vocational training resulting from their communication disability. The survey reported that 42% of hearing-impaired job seekers had the equivalent of a school certificate, whereas only 1.6% possessed high school graduation levels. Comparable figures for the general population show that 55% of adults possess at least high school graduation or have tertiary qualifications. Allen (1986) reported mean reading comprehension among 15-year-old hearing-impaired students in the United States to be at a 3rd-grade level, as compared to a mean 10th-grade ability for normally hearing 15-year-old students.

Improved communication resulting from use of the cochlear implant may have a direct influence on employment prospects. Dinner et al. (1989) reported on a U.S. survey of adult cochlear implant patients (four different cochlear implant systems were used) which assessed the impact of use of the device in the patient's workplace. A significant majority of implant users noted increased job satisfaction and feelings of success as a result of the improved communication resulting from cochlear implant use. In addition, enhanced pay, increased activities and duties, access to on-the-job training opportunities, and enhanced employer-employee relationships were also noted as important benefits.

The indirect benefits of cochlear implants may not be predictable on the basis of traditional measures of outcome such as speech perception. For example, Zwolan et al. (1996) reported on a study of 12 prelingually deaf adults that contrasted performance on speech recognition tests with satisfaction from implant use. All 12 patients surveyed had shown little or no improvement on speech recognition tests as measured at 12 months postimplant. However, all of the patients surveyed were regular device users, all expressed satisfaction with their device as a communication aid, and all felt that they had improved their expressive and receptive communication skills. Bouse (1987) provided a parent's perspective, noting that use of the cochlear implant by her teenage son had resulted in better control of voice volume and articulation through use of auditory feedback. This allowed enhanced communication between her son and family members, resulting in improved self-confidence and motivation to use the implant. Capelli et al. (1995) reported on the psychosocial functioning of 23 hearing-impaired children using sociometric assessments and self-report measures. The children were assessed on measures of social anxiety, knowledge, and self-competence. Children with hearing impairment were more likely to experience lower social acceptance, particularly in the case of younger children. Surprisingly, results from this study suggest that these children were more likely to be rejected by their hearing-impaired peers than by normally hearing children. The results suggest the need for intervention at the earliest age to develop social skills and highlight the need to consider the impact of early implantation on the child's social development when assessing benefits.

EDUCATIONAL ISSUES

Although the benefits to acquisition of auditory skills, articulation, and development of language resulting from use of cochlear implants are now clearly established (NIH, 1995), establishing the cost-effectiveness of cochlear implants in children has several difficulties. Although it is assumed that improved speech perception and language will result in enhanced reading and writing skills, and improved spoken language, these skills may take many years to develop. Moog and Geers (1994) noted that the cochlear implant provides sufficient access to sound for the teaching of spoken language to many prelingually deaf children, but that this may not be successfully accomplished without intensive speech instruction. The effectiveness of the habilitation and educational management of the implanted child are important factors that affect the extent to which improved communication results in enhanced employment prospects and broader career and life opportunities. Although intensive habilitation increases the costs of cochlear implantation, in the case of young children, there is a greater potential for offsetting cumulative gains as compared to adults (Lutman et al., 1996). This is a direct consequence of the intervention occurring at a critical formative time in the development of spoken language and the potential long-term impact of the implant on educational placement over the school-life of the implanted child. If the decision to provide a child with a cochlear implant at a younger age does enable the child to more rapidly acquire the linguistic competence necessary for mainstream education, then savings will accrue from the reduced need for or time spent in special education facilities.

A full discussion of the educational management of implanted children is beyond the scope of this chapter (educational management issues are comprehensively discussed by Chute et al., 1996, and Moog and Geers, 1995. However, in considering the relevance of educational management to cost-utility analysis, it is important to review a number of points.

Need for an Interdisciplinary Team

First, as discussed in Chapter 4, cochlear implantation in children requires an interdisciplinary team involving strong collaboration between the otologist, audiologist, speech-language pathologist, and educator. The need for an educator, and for cross training of team professionals in the development of language and the effects of hearing impairment on that process, are critical. Hearing-impaired children are at risk of delayed or reduced educational outcomes because their sensorineural hearing impairment impedes the natural developmental processes for learning language. Language is first acquired in the child as a means of achieving communicative functions, which develop initially in the nonverbal context, and then progress to verbal context through the input and interaction of parents with their child. The hearing impairment delays crucial aspects of the early learning process and disrupts the natural interactions between parents and their child. Although the cochlear implant can restore the auditory channel through which input is received by the child, habilitation is necessary to restore or, in the case of infants, to start the developmental process for acquiring language. To provide the necessary habilitation, professionals require a sound knowledge of developmental principles of language acquisition and teaching techniques that can be successfully used with hearing-impaired children. The educator on the cochlear implant team provides important input regarding the appropriateness of placement, the curriculum, and the communication mode used by the implanted child. Decisions on these issues play a criti-

cal part in ensuring that the child's opportunities for improved speech perception, speech production, and language development are maximized. The educator also plays a critical role in cross training of the otologist and other clinic team members in principles of language development. Funding of an interdisciplinary team and cross education of expertise among the cochlear implant team should be viewed as a critical element that must be included in cost-effectiveness evaluations.

Need for Agreement on Goals and Responsibility

The educational management of the child requires agreement on diverse goals. For example, the parents may wish their child to be mainstreamed, and see this goal as a measure of successful outcome. The clinic team may wish to stress the effective use of the implant in the classroom and the use of one-to-one habilitation sessions to ensure the acquisition of auditory and articulation skills. The educator on the team may wish to ensure that the acquired auditory skills in young children are effectively used to develop linguistic competence and resultant reading and writing skills. The classroom teacher also has a responsibility to ensure that, to the greatest possible extent, the hearing-impaired child masters the same curriculum as his or her normally hearing peers. The key to effective educational outcomes is the successful merging of these varying goals and shared responsibility between the child, parents, clinic team, and educators.

Fryauf-Bertschy and Kirk (1992) suggested that educational goals for deaf children should include (a) helping the child to develop language and communication skills to his or her maximum potential and (b) using these skills to master curriculum. Although the cochlear implant facilitates achieving these goals, the teacher must combine communication and educational goals within the school day, incorporating auditory training and speech-reading training into academic subjects and materials. However, particularly in the case of young children, the development of spoken language skills must be seen as a priority. The inclusion of instruction in speech and listening skills incorporated into school subjects and activities should be supplemented by specific lessons aimed at improving vocabulary, syntax, speech, and listening skills (Moog & Geers, 1994). This will accelerate the rate of acquisition of spoken language, increasing the impact of the cochlear implant on educational outcomes.

Although there is general agreement that the cochlear implant clinic team and school share a joint responsibility for maximizing outcomes for implanted children, there are various approaches in practice (Chute et al., 1996). In some instances, funding is provided only for rehabilitation within the implant center, and there is little direct interaction with the child's classroom teacher. A different approach is for the cochlear implant clinic to employ educators, audiologists, or speech pathologists who act as an interface with the school system, working with the classroom teacher. A third approach is the establishment of an educational facility that directly incorporates a cochlear implant center. Each of these approaches can be efficiently implemented, however, in each case there is a very different cost structure that must be measured for cost-utility analysis.

Mainstreaming of Children with Cochlear Implants

Given effective educational management of children with cochlear implants, it is reasonable to have higher expectations for the development of auditory skills and the development of intelligible speech and improved voice quality. In addition, these factors should increase expectations that the child will acquire the spoken language and academic skills necessary to allow mainstreaming to occur at the earliest stage, and with greater success. Waltzman et al. (1994) reported a long-term study of 14 children who were implanted with the Nucleus multiple-channel cochlear implant before the age of 3 years. Results showed a continuous improvement over 2–5 years in auditory perceptual skills. All of the children demonstrated open-set speech recognition using electrical stimulation alone, all used oral/aural communication, and all attended age-appropriate nursery or mainstream schools.

The mainstreaming of higher numbers of hearing-impaired children using cochlear implants, and at an earlier age, has significant cost-saving potential through reducing the use of special education facilities. Cost-utility analysis of cochlear implants in children should include these cost-savings in establishing true valuation of the long-term benefits.

MEDICAL AND SURGICAL ISSUES

Medical and surgical issues in the management of children with cochlear implants have been discussed in previous chapters. Surgical procedures have been developed that ensure the safe placement of the receiver-stimulator package and electrode array during surgery. Webb et al. (1991) and Cohen and Hoffman (1993) reviewed complications arising from the cochlear implant procedure and noted that complications with the Nucleus multiple-channel implant system were relatively rare and, in most cases, could be resolved without the need for explanting the device. In reviewing the current status of surgical issues, the NIH Consensus Statement on Cochlear Implants in Adults and Children (1995) noted that "cochlear implantation entails risks common to most surgical procedures, as well as unique risks that are influenced by device design, individual anatomy and pathology and surgical technique" (p. 14). The report noted that the postoperative complication rate was approximately 5% in 1993, and that the complication rate in pediatric implantation was currently less than that reported for adults. On the basis of these findings, costs of complications need not be considered as a major factor in cost-utility analysis.

DEVICE DESIGN AND RELIABILITY ISSUES

The initial cost of the device and associated upgrades are obvious factors in cost-utility analysis. Device design issues have also been discussed in detail in Chapter 8. Multiple-channel cochlear implants are a high-cost technology in comparison to hearing aids or tactile devices. However, the higher initial costs of the cochlear implant can be justified if they provide benefits that cannot be gained from other alternative sensory devices.

Boothroyd (1993) reviewed the inherent engineering limitations of conventional hearing aids in providing sufficient acoustic input for remediating profound deafness. A number of problems were identified. The upper frequency limit of hearing aid transducers is approximately 3.5 kHz. This limits the user's access to important speech information required for consonant recognition, which is spread across the speech spectrum from 2–6 kHz. In addition, significant levels of amplification are required to provide an acoustic signal within the profoundly hearing-impaired child's auditory thresholds. This can result in acoustic feedback problems due to limitations in earmold technology and materials, in particular for the higher frequencies. The child's use of conventional hearing aids may also be limited by toler-

ance problems, resulting from the need to supply the broadest possible bandwidth at a very high power output. This may limit the child's dynamic range, restricting the transmission of important speech amplitude information.

In contrast, the cochlear implant presents its sound input to the child through a pattern of direct electrical stimulation of the sensory elements, bypassing the normal auditory conductive pathway (Clark, 1995). As a result, the engineering design of the cochlear implant inherently overcomes the technical barriers described for conventional amplification. The difficulties in providing an appropriate dynamic range are addressed through the mapping of the speech processor, which adjusts the electrical stimulus levels to ensure that the full range of speech amplitude information is presented at levels between threshold and a maximum comfortable level. The cochlear implant can also provide access to the full spectrum of speech sounds, at a comfortable loudness without the risk of feedback. Although developments in digital hearing aids are addressing these problems, at present they remain as significant barriers to the effectiveness of hearing aids in the management of severe and profound deafness. Tactile aids are also not currently a viable alternative to cochlear implants. Although they are less costly, as discussed in Chapter 12 and in a number of research reports, the benefits available to speech perception, articulation, and language development are more limited (Geers & Moog, 1994; Kirk et al., 1995; Sarant et al., 1996).

Cost-utility analysis also assumes that there is a useful life for the device, after which it must be replaced or upgraded. The reliability of the Nucleus multiple channel cochlear implant in terms of the cumulative experience has been reported previously (VonWallenberg & Brinch, 1995), and is discussed in detail in Chapter 8. Figure 13–1

COCHLEAR CI-22M Implant Reliability

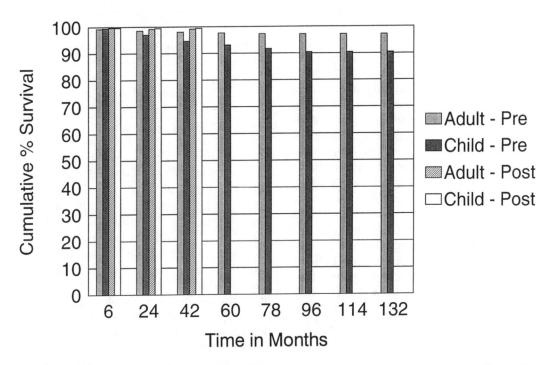

FIGURE 13–1. Cochlear CI-22M implant reliability (data show percentage cumulative survival for adults and children both prior to and after the 1993 design change to the antenna feedthrough connection).

shows reliability data for the Cochlear CI-22M implant for both adult and children both before and after a design change, introduced in late 1993, which improved the mechanical robustness of the connection for the antenna feedthrough. As shown, over 97% of the implants were working after 3 years of operation, over 96% after 5 years, and over 95% of Nucleus 22-channel implants were functioning after 132 months of use. Cumulative experience prior to the design change showed that there was a flat trend after 5 years of implant use. Following the design change, reliability has been improved, with 98.9% of the devices in operation after 3.5 years of operation. On the basis of these results, it is evident that the cochlear implant is highly reliable, and that it is reasonable to assume for the purposes of cost-utility analysis a minimum useful life of the cochlear implant in children to be more than 10 years.

COST-UTILITY ANALYSIS OF COCHLEAR IMPLANTS

Review of Adults Studies

A number of studies have applied cost-utility analysis to cochlear implants, primarily in adult users (Evans et al., 1995; Lea, 1991; Summerfield & Marshall, 1994; Summerfield et al., 1995; Wyatt et al. 1995a, 1995b; Wyatt & Niparko, 1996).

Lea (1991) reported a preliminary Australian study which showed a 10% increase in QALY resulting from the cochlear implant procedure, with an associated cost per QALY between $14,000 and $22,000. Wyatt et al. (1995a) analyzed adult Nucleus cochlear implant users in the United States, using U.S.-sourced cost variables and a decision model based on data derived from a review of the literature on performance, manufacturer's data on device reliability, data collected from otologists and audiologists as well as from profoundly deaf patients. The calculated cost-utility estimates were U.S. $15,600 per QALY. Sensitivity analysis, which modeled the effect on these cost estimates of revising factors such as the health utility index of benefit, the patient's life expectancy, device initial costs, costs of surgery, follow-up management costs, rehabilitation costs, and factors relating to complications and medical issues, provided a range in the cost per QALY of U.S. $12,000 to $30,000. Wyatt et al. (1995b) reported a further study that estimated the health utility change through surveys of 229 Nucleus implant users. The patients considered their health status, and how their health affected their quality of life both for the current situation in which they used their cochlear implant, and for a hypothetical situation in which they could no longer use their implant. Results from this study suggested a cost per QALY of approximately $9,325 (sensitivity analysis suggested range of $7,988–$11,201). These results suggest that changes in the measurement of the health utility outcome may have a high impact on the calculated cost-effectiveness. Wyatt and Niparko (1996) reported a further analysis conducted from survey data from profoundly deaf implant users and candidates awaiting implantation. Results of cost-utility calculations, which used the Ontario Health Utilities Index to measure attributes (hearing, speech, vision, emotion, pain, ambulation, dexterity, cognition and self-care), showed a cost per QALY of U.S. $15,928.

Similar studies have been reported by Summerfield and Marshall (1994) and Summerfield et al. (1995) for adult cochlear implant users in the United Kingdom. The first of these studies reported a health utility improvement for adults of 23% in quality of life as measured using a visual-analogue scale and retrospective survey of 208 implant patients. Accumulating this improvement over the average remaining lifetime of adults in the U.K. study showed a gain of 2.99 QALYs if the benefits were discounted at 6% per annum. The cost utility was calculated at £11,440 per QALY. Summerfield and Marshall (1995b) also used a theoretical mapping approach, using the EuroQol instrument, which estimated a cost per QALY for multichannel cochlear implants in adults as between £8,624 and £25,871, which placed adult cochlear implantation in the middle of the range for U.K. cost-utility ratios for health technologies. However, the authors noted that costs in the United Kingdom were influenced for the Nucleus 22-channel system by the materially higher maintenance costs arising from the practice of purchasing maintenance contracts and processor upgrades.

The NIH Consensus Statement (1995) summarizing these studies of available cost-effectiveness research findings, primarily in adult cochlear implant users, suggested that cochlear implants in adults compared favorably with other commonly used medical procedures. However, the need for special studies considering the cost-effectiveness of cochlear implants in children was stressed. Because the parent gives the consent for the procedure, rather than the child making an informed independent decision, it is vital that the benefits and costs be objectively and independently analyzed. In addition, because rehabilitation outcomes in children require a strong commitment in time and resources from both the family, and health and education professionals, it is important that economic analysis consider broader issues such as differing approaches to clinical management and education in valuing the benefits and costs of cochlear implants.

Economic Evaluation of the Cochlear Implant in Children

Given the potential for children with cochlear implants to acquire sufficient language skills to enable education in a mainstream setting, a simple method of estimating cost benefit is to compare the overall educational costs for hearing-impaired children in various settings. Cullen and Brown (1992) reported that the costs for educating nondisabled students in regular government schools in Australia were $4,420 per primary student and $6,461 per secondary student. The average cost for students in special schools (i.e., vision or hearing impairment) was $25,039. Over the 12 years of Australian schooling, this amounts to $65,286 for a nondisabled student, as compared with $300,468 for a special school student. For a similar 12-year period, the cost for a semi-integrated setting (i.e., a hearing unit attached to a mainstream school) are estimated at $13,317 per year or a total of $159,804 per student through secondary school (Review of the Provision of Education to Catholic Deaf Children in the Archdiocese of Melbourne, 1995). If we consider these costs for a child implanted at age 2 years, and fully mainstreamed at age 5 (3 years postimplant), then the total savings in educational costs might be between $94,518 and $235,182. The net present-value of the implant procedure is then calculated as between $49,518 and $190,182 (given costs of $45,000 for the device, surgical procedure, and clinic-based rehabilitation program). Obviously, cost savings would be reduced if implanted children were not fully mainstreamed for all or a part of their education. However, this simple model suggests that significant savings may be available to government in the costs of provding education to hearing-impaired children

who receive cochlear implants at an early age, thus allowing mainstream education.

A more detailed economic evaluation which considered indirect benefits resulting from cochlear implants has been completed for adults and children using the Nucleus multiple-channel cochlear implant in Australia (Carter & Hailey, 1995). Although the study produced an estimate of costs per QALY for cochlear implants in adults which was in broad agreement with those reported by Wyatt and Niparko (1996), we will concentrate on reporting the methodology and outcomes of the analysis for implanted children.

The evaluation measured quality of life using the Sintonen HRQOL-15D (Sintonen & Pekurinen, 1993), a health-related quality of life instrument that has a specific hearing dimension, plus a range of functional consequences relevant to hearing disability, including measures of speech, usual activities, and distress. The dimensions included in the instrument and their relevance to cochlear implantation are shown in Table 13–1.

In this initial study, the ratings for before and after the procedure were obtained by interviewing the health professionals involved in the management of the implanted child. In each case, two assessors, one otologist and one nonmedical member of the cochlear implant clinic team, were used to provide pre- and postimplantation values for each dimension. Results of the outcomes measures for children are shown in Table 13–2. Both a low value (including only four dimensions) and a high value of index (including all 10 dimensions) were calculated. As shown, the total change in QALY ranged from a low value of 17% to a high value of 38%. Direct amelioration of the hearing disability accounted for between 4–5% of the change, whereas the functional consequences from the change in hearing resulted in a further 13–32% QALY improvement. It is evident that, as measured on

Table 13-1. Basis for decisions on score selection from HRQOL-15D scale.

Attribute	Relevance to Cochlear Implantation in Children
Mobility	Improved awareness of environment and safety
Vision	Relevant to reading skill improvements
Hearing	Significant improvement for most children
Breathing	Not relevant
Sleeping	Decreased tinnitus and feelings of increased security
Eating	Not relevant
Speech	Assistance in development of speech
Elimination	Not relevant
Usual Activities	Improved group communication and activities, both in family and wider social settings
Mental Function	Improvements in cognition
Discomfort	Dizziness usually transitory, not applicable
Depression	Issue for children and families
Distress	Can be significant for young children and parents
Vitality	Improvements through reduction in need for concentration
Sexual Activity	Not relevant in children

Note: Modified with permission from *Economic Evaluation of the Cochlear Implant* by R. Carter and D. Hailey, 1995. Victoria, Australia: Centre for Health Program Evaluation.

this index, the variability in outcome measure is primarily due to the valuation on indirect benefits consequential to the changes in hearing directly.

Calculation of costs of the cochlear implant procedure were based on a number of assumptions arising from the decision model:

■ cohorts were followed over 10, 15, and 20 years of device lifetime;
■ costs of all procedures were identified and costed on public hospital scales;
■ ongoing costs were discounted at a rate of 5% for both costs and life years;
■ it was assumed that 70% of children assessed were suitable for surgery;
■ a 3-day bed stay was associated with the surgery;

■ a 5% complication rate was incorporated within the first year costs;
■ 145 hours of rehabilitation were costed in the first year postimplantation; 75 hours in years 2 and 3, and 50 hours in the fourth and subsequent years up to 15 years;
■ potential cost savings from mainstreaming of implanted children were not commenced until 18 months following implantation; mainstreaming was applied to 65% of the children in each cohort (a savings figure of $7,978 per child was derived from public school costs);
■ savings in secondary school assumed a 100% retention rate in years 10–12;
■ a tertiary education entrance rate of 20% was included in the 20-year model

TABLE 13–2. Outcome measures for children on the Sintonen HRQOL 15D.

Dimensions	Low Value	High Value
Mobility		0.0264
Vision (Reading)		0.0209
Hearing	0.0434	0.0484
Sleeping		0.0304
Speech	0.0387	0.0508
Usual activities	0.0623	0.0712
Mental function		0.0407
Depression		0.0108
Distress	0.0284	0.0284
Vitality		0.0517
Total Change in Score	**0.1728**	**0.3797**
QOL Improvement (Hearing Disability)	4%	5%
QOL Improvement (Consequences)	13%	32%

Note: Modified with permission from *Economic Evaluation of the Cochlear Implant* by R. Carter and D. Hailey, 1995. Victoria, Australia: Centre for Health Program Evaluation.

for children, and savings included were derived from Commonwealth figures for education of persons with disabilities (Andrews & Smith, 1993);

■ processor upgrades were costed for 100% of implanted children on a 5-year cycle, at a cost of $4,378 per user;

■ ongoing maintenance costs for the device were $400 per year, commencing in the second year.

Figure 13–2 summarises cost per QALY calculations from the study, as shown over 10, 15 or 20 years for the low and high values of health-related QALY improvements. As shown, costs ranged from $3,465 to $13,020 for the low values, and $1,580 to $5,940 for the high values. Results of the sensitivity analysis are shown in Figure 13–3. Variations were made to the discount rate (increasing to 7.5% or 19%) and the cost of the device (increasing to $22,500) and costs of speech processor upgrades (increasing to $6,000). In addition, variations were made to the rate of long-term rehabilitation, first by increasing the year 1 rehabilitation to 200 hours, and second by increasing year 1 to 200 hours, years 2 and 3 to 100 hours, and year 4 to 75 hours. Finally, the effect of decreasing the proportion of mainstream schooling to 50% was evaluated in respect of the estimates for children. These results showed that, although the estimates were relatively insensitive to cost of the device and upgrades, they were moderately sensitive to changes in discount rate. The rates of long-term rehabilitation and proportion of implantees who were able to attend normal schools were main

Cost per Quality Adjusted Life Year (QALY) for Children

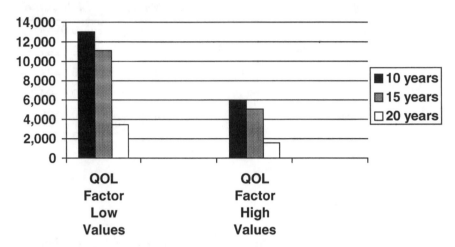

FIGURE 13–2. Cost per quality adjusted life year for implanted children (measured over 10, 15, and 20 years using low and high values for estimates of quality of life improvements). (Based on data from *Economic Evaluation of the Cochlear Implant* by R. Carter and D. Hailey, 1995. Victoria, Australia: Centre for Health Program Evaluation.)

Sensitivity Testing for Estimates of Costs per QALY for Deaf Children (over 15 years)

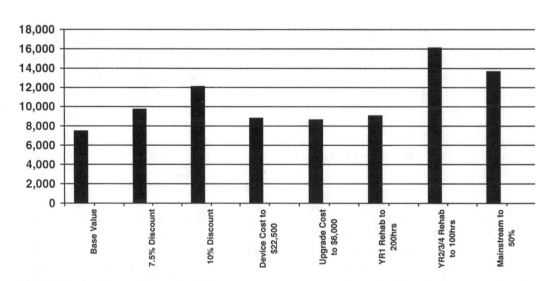

FIGURE 13–3. Sensitivity testing for estimates of costs per QALY for deaf children (all values are measured over 15 years, using average of high and low values for costing, $7,480 per QALY). (Based on data from *Economic Evaluation of the Cochlear Implant* by R. Carter and D. Hailey, 1995. Victoria, Australia: Centre for Health Program Evaluation.)

factors affecting the cost of the procedure as identified by the sensitivity analysis.

Figure 13–4 shows the comparison of the cost-utility analysis of cochlear implants with that of other available medical procedures in Australian-valued prices. As shown, comparison of cost per QALY shows that cochlear implantation provides good "value for money" as compared with other technologies. This was particularly evident in the case of profoundly deaf children. The sensitivity of these estimates to changes in the rate of long-term rehabilitation and to the proportion of children who are able to attend normal schools gives an indication of the importance of rehabilitation support post-implantation.

An important limitation of the study is that the improvements in quality of life dimensions reported were obtained from professionals expert in the field of cochlear implantation. The difficulty in obtaining valid quality of life measures for children has been noted by other researchers (Wyatt & Niparko, 1996), who addressed the issue of cost-effectiveness in children by calculating a cost-benefit ratio for U.S. children. Further study will be required in which health outcome measures are obtained from pediatric implantees and their families, and more detailed analyses are made of the effects of intensive early rehabilitation and educational outcomes.

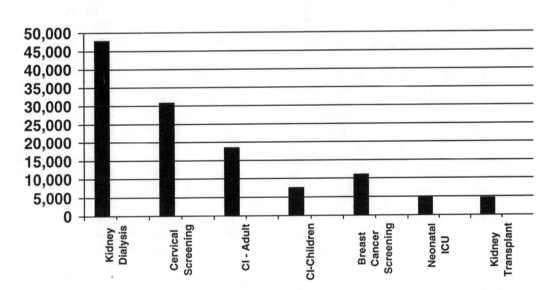

Cost Utility/Cost Effectiveness of Selected Medical Procedures (Adjusted Cost Per Life Year or QALY)

FIGURE 13–4. Cost-utility of selected medical procedures (all estimates are in Australian funds, using Australian valuations for hospital practice). (Based on data from *Economic Evaluation of the Cochlear Implant* by R. Carter and D. Hailey, 1995. Victoria, Australia: Centre for Health Program Evaluation.)

ACKNOWLEDGMENTS

We acknowledge the assistance of Cochlear Limited, in particular, Mr. Johan Brinch and Mr. Andrew Evans, who kindly provided data on reliability of the Nucleus CI-22M implant. We thank Professor Field Rickards for his contribution to the discussion of educational management. We are also grateful to Mr. Rob Carter and Dr. David Hailey, Health Economics Unit, Centre for Health Program Evaluation, Victoria, Australia, for their generosity in allowing citation and use of data from their *Economic Evaluation of the Cochlear Implant.*

REFERENCES

Allen, T. (1986). Patterns of academic achievement among hearing-impaired students: 1974 and 1983. In A. Schridroth, M. Karchman. (Eds.), *Deaf children in America.* San Diego: College-Hill Press.

Andrews, R., & Smith, J. (1993). *Additional costs of education and training for people with disabilities.* Canberra: Australian Government Publishing Service.

Bamford, J. M., & Saunders, J. C. (1991). *Hearing impairment, auditory perception and language disability.* San Diego: Singular Publishing Group.

Blamey, P. J., Dawson, S. J., Dettman, S. J., Rowland, L. C., Brown, A. M., Busby, P. A., Dowell, R. C., Rickards, F. W., & Clark, G. M. (1992). Speech perception, production and language results in a group of children using the 22-electrode cochlear implant. *Australian Journal of Otolaryngology, 1,* 105–109.

Boothroyd, A. (1993). Profound deafness. In R. S. Tyler (Ed.), *Cochlear implants: Audiological foundations* (pp. 1–32). San Diego: Singular Publishing Group.

Bouse, C. (1987, September). Impact of a cochlear implant on a teenager's quality of life: A parent's perspective. *The Hearing Journal, 40,* 1–4.

Capelli, M., Daniels, T., Durieux-Smith, A., McGrath, P. J., & Neuss, D. (1995). Social development of children with hearing aids who are integrated into general education classrooms. *Volta Review, 97,* 197–208.

Carter, R., & Hailey, D. (1995). *Economic evaluation of the cochlear implant.* Working Paper 44. Victoria, Australia: Centre for Health Program Evaluation.

Chute, P. M., & Nevins, M. E. (1994, May). *Educational placements of children with multichannel cochlear implants.* Paper presented at European Symposium on Paediatric Cochlear Implantation, Montepellier, France,

Chute, P. M., Nevins, M. E., & Parisier, S. C. (1996). Managing educational issues through the process of implantation. In D. J. Allum (Ed.), *Cochlear implant rehabilitation in children and adults* (pp. 119–130). London: Whurr.

Clark, G. M. (1995). Historical perspectives. In G. Plant & K.-E. Spens (Eds.), *Profound deafness and speech communication.* (pp. 165–218). London: Whurr.

Clickener, P. A. (1989). The life enhancements of a cochlear implant. *The Hearing Journal, 42,* 40–42.

Cohen, N. L., & Hoffman, R. A. (1993). Surgical complications of multichannel cochlear implants in North America. *Advances in Otorhinolaryngology, 48,* 70–74.

Cowan, R. S. C., Brown, C., Whitford, L. A., Galvin, K. L., Sarant, J. Z., Barker, E. J., Shaw, S., King, A., Skok, M., Seligman, P. M., Dowell, R. C., Everingham, C., Gibson, W. P. R., & Clark, G. M. (1995). Speech perception in children using the advanced Speak speech-processing strategy. In G. M. Clark & R. S. C. Cowan (Eds.), *International Cochlear Implant, Speech and Hearing Symposium 1994. Annals of Otology, Rhinology and Laryngology, 104*(Suppl. 166), 318–321.

Cullen, R. B., & Brown, N. F. (1992). *Integration and special education in Victorian schools: A program effectiveness review.* Melbourne: Department of School Education.

Dawson, P. W., Blamey, P. J., Rowland, L. C., Dettman, S. J., Clark, G. M., Busby, P. A., Brown, A. M., Dowell, R. C., & Rickards, F. W. (1992). Cochlear implants in children, adolescents, and prelinguistically deafened adults: Speech perception. *Journal of Speech and Hearing Research, 35,* 401–417.

Dawson, P. W., Blamey, P. J., Dettman, S. J., Barker, E. J., & Clark, G. M. (1995). A clinical report on receptive vocabulary skills in cochlear implant users. *Ear and Hearing, 16,* 287-294.

Dawson, P. W., Blamey, P. J., Dettman, S. J., Rowland, L. C., Barker, E. J., Tobey, E. A., Busby, P. A., Cowan, R. C., & Clark, G. M. (1995). A clinical report on speech production of cochlear implant users. *Ear and Hearing, 16,* 551–561.

Deaf Society of New South Wales. (1989). *Project Knock Knock: A profile of the deaf community of NSW 1989.* New South Wales, Australia: Deaf Society of NSW.

Dinner, M. B., Ackley, R. S., Lubinski, D. J., Balkany, T. J., Reeder, P., & Genert, L. (1989). Cochlear implants in the workplace: A nationwide survey. *Journal of the American Deafness and Rehabilitation Association, 22,* 41–47.

Dowell, R. C., Blamey, P. J., & Clark, G. M. (1995). Potential and limitations of cochlear implants in children. In G. M. Clark & R. S. C. Cowan (Eds.), *International Cochlear Implant, Speech and Hearing Symposium 1994. Annals of Otology, Rhinology and Laryngology, 104*(Suppl. 166), 324–327.

Evans, A. R., Seeger, T., & Lehnhardt, M. (1995). Cost-utility analysis of cochlear implants. In G. M. Clark & R. S. C. Cowan (Eds.), *International Cochlear Implant, Speech and Hearing Symposium 1994. Annals of Otology, Rhinology and Laryngology, 104*(Suppl. 166), 239–230.

Fryauf-Bertschy, H., & Kirk, K. I. (1992). The implanted child at school. In N. Tye-Murray (Ed.), *Cochlear implants and children: A handbook for parents, teachers and speech and hearing professionals.* (pp. 25–40). Washington, DC: Alexander Graham Bell Association.

Geers, A. E., & Moog, J. S. (Eds.). (1994). Effectiveness of cochlear implants and tactile aids for deaf children. *The Volta Review, 96,* 1–231.

Hasenstab, M. S., & Tobey, E. A. (1991). Language development in children receiving Nucleus multichannel cochlear implants. *Ear and Hearing, 12,* 55S–65S.

Kirk, K. I., Osberger, M. J., McConkey-Robbins, A., Allyson, I. R., Todd, S. L., & Miyamoto, R. T. (1995). Performance of children with cochlear implants, tactile aids and hearing aids. In D. K. Oller. (Ed.), *Tactile aids for the hearing impaired. Seminars in Hearing, 16,* 370–381.

Lea, A. R. (1991). Cochlear implants. (Australian Institute of Health: Health Care Technology Series 6). Canberra: Australian Government Printing.

Lutman, M. E., Archbold, S., Gibbon, K. P., McCormick, B., & O'Donaghue, G. M. (1996). Monitoring progress in young children with cochlear implants. In D. J. Allum (Ed.), *Cochlear implant rehabilitation in children and adults* (pp. 31–51). London: Whurr.

Miyamoto, R. T., Osberger, M. J., Robbins, A. M., Myres, W. A., Kessler, K., & Pope, M. L. (1992). Longitudinal evaluation of communication skills of children with single- or multichannel cochlear implants. *American Journal of Otology, 13,* 215–222.

Moog, J. S., & Geers, A. E. (1994). Cochlear implants: What should be expected. In J. M. Barnes, D. Franz, & W. Bruce (Eds.), *Pediatric cochlear implants: An overview of the alternatives in education and rehabilitation.* (pp. 1–21). Washington, DC: Alexander Graham Bell Association.

Moog, J. S., & Geers, A. E. (1995). Impact of the cochlear implant on the educational setting. In A. S. Uziel & M. Mondain, (Eds.), *Cochlear implants in children. Advances in Otorhinolaryngology, 50,* 174–186.

National Institutes of Health. (1995). *Cochlear implants in adults and children.* (NIH consensus statement 13 [2]).

Osberger, M. J., Maso, M, & Sam, L. K. (1993). Speech intelligibility of children with cochlear implants, tactile aids, or hearing aids. *Journal of Speech and Hearing Research, 36,* 186–203.

Sarant, J. Z., Cowan, R., Blamey, P., Galvin, K., & Clark, G. (1996). Within-subject comparison of speech perception benefits for congenitally deaf adolescents with an electrotactile speech processor and cochlear implant. *Journal of the American Academy of Audiology, 7,* 63–70.

Sintonen, H., & Pekurinen, M. (1993). A fifteen-dimensional measure of health-related quality of life (15D) and its applications. In S. R. Walker & R. M. Rosser (Eds.), *Quality of life assessment—Key issues in the 1990s.* Dordrecht: Kluwer Academic Publishers.

Staller, S. J., Beiter, A. L., Brimacombe, J. A., Mecklenburg, D. J., & Arndt, P. (1991). Pediatric performance with the Nucleus 22-channel cochlear implant system. *American Journal of Otology, 12*(Suppl.), 126–136.

Summerfield, A. Q., & Marshall, D. H. (1994). *Cochlear implantation in the UK 1990–1994.* MRC Institute of Hearing Research Main Report.

Summerfield, A. Q., Marshall, D. H., & Davis, A. C. (1995). Cochlear implantation: Demand, costs and utility. In G. M. Clark & R. S. C. Cowan (Eds.), *International Cochlear Implant, Speech and Hearing Symposium 1994. Annals of Otology, Rhinology and Laryngology, 104*(Suppl. 166), 245–248.

Tobey, E. A., & Hasenstab, M. S. (1991). Effects of a Nucleus multichannel cochlear implant upon speech production in children. *Ear and Hearing, 12*(Suppl.), 48S–54S.

Tye-Murray, N., Spencer, L., & Gilbert-Bedia, E. (1995). Relationship between speech production and speech perception skills in young cochlear implant users. *Journal of the Acoustical Society of America, 98,* 2454–2460.

Vernon, M., & LaFalce-Landers, E. (1993). A longitudinal study of intellectually gifted deaf and hard of hearing people. Educational, psychological and career outcomes. *American Annals of the Deaf, 138,* 427–434.

VonWallenberg, E. L., & Brinch, J. M. (1995). Cochlear implant reliability. In G. M. Clark & R. S. C. Cowan (Eds.), *International Cochlear Implant, Speech and Hearing Symposium 1994. Annals of Otology, Rhinology and Laryngology, 104*(Suppl. 166), 441–443.

Waltzman, S. B., Cohen, N. L., Gomolin, R. H., Shapiro, W. H., Ozdamar, S. R., & Hoffman, R. A. (1994). Long-term results of early cochlear implantation in congenitally and pre-lingually deafened children. *American Journal of Otology, 15*(Suppl.), 9–13.

Webb, R. L., Lehnhardt, E., Clark, G. M., Laszig, R., Pyman, B. C., & Franz, B. K.-H. (1991). Surgical complications with the Cochlear multiple-channel intracochlear implant: Experience at Hannover and Melbourne. *Annals of Otology, Rhinology and Laryngology, 100,* 131–136.

Wyatt, J. R., & Niparko, J. K. (1996). Evaluation of the benefit of the multichannel cochlear implant in relation to its cost. In D. J. Allum (Ed.), *Cochlear implant rehabilitation in children and adults* (pp. 22–30). London: Whurr.

Wyatt, J. R., Niparko, J. K., Rothman, M. L., & DeLissovoy, G. V. (1995a). Cost effectiveness of the multichannel cochlear implant. *The American Journal of Otology, 16,* 52–62.

Wyatt, J. R., Niparko, J. K., Rothman, M. L., & DeLissovoy, G. V. (1995b). Cost-effectiveness of the multichannel cochlear implant. In G. M. Clark & R. S. C. Cowan (Eds.), *International Cochlear Implant, Speech and Hearing Symposium 1994. Annals of Otology, Rhinology and Laryngology, 104*(Suppl. 166), 248–250.

Zwolan, T. A., Kileny, P. R., & Telian, S. A. (1996). Self-report of cochlear implant use and satisfaction by prelingually deafened adults. *Ear and Hearing, 17,* 198–210.

14

ETHICAL ISSUES

GRAEME M. CLARK
ROBERT S. C. COWAN
RICHARD C. DOWELL

The ethics of cochlear implantation in infants and children is an important issue which has received a lot of attention, in particular from the signing deaf community and their advocates. Many of the issues raised by the signing deaf community are in regard to human experimentation and are therefore ethical in nature. Others are concerned with whether it is natural to have a hearing loss, and this goes beyond the realm of ethics. This chapter examines cochlear implantation in children in light of generally accepted ethical principles.

Ethics is a general term referring to both morality and ethical theory. In considering whether cochlear implantation in infants and children is morally acceptable we need to also consider morality. Morality in general refers to social conventions about right and wrong human conduct which are widely shared by members of the community. Common morality refers to socially approved norms of human conduct. In particular, it highlights acceptable and nonacceptable conduct we refer to in discussing "human rights." It is also important to consider moral theology, which provides a perspective on moral issues from a theological or religious point of view.

In considering the ethics or morality of cochlear implants in infants and children at this point in time, we must consider to what extent the benefits outweigh the risks, and to what extent it is an accepted clinical procedure and not primarily research. In considering these issues we need to view the procedure against its background and history.

The first single-channel implant was placed in a child in the early 1980s (Luxford et al., 1987) and the first Nucleus multiple-channel implant in 1985 (Clark et al., 1987; see Chapter 2). At the time, although the devices had previously been implanted in adults, implantation in children was looked on as clearly research. However multicenter studies of the Nucleus multiple-channel system showed that, for the Nucleus-22 system, the benefits outweighed the risks and the U.S. Food and Drug Administration (FDA) became the first health regulatory body in the world to approve of a cochlear implant for use in children, on June 27, 1990. The Nucleus-22 system was considered safe and effective for children from 2 to 18 years of age. Nevertheless, it is desirable to continue to appraise the continued use of the cochlear implant in children when used either on a regular clinical basis or in further research studies. In both cases, this should be on the basis of ethically acceptable practices for research as laid down in the Helsinki Declaration on Biomedical Research involving human subjects adopted by the 18th World Medical Assembly, Finland 1969, and revised by the 29th World Medical Assembly, Tokyo 1975, and in accordance with the Convention on the Rights of the Child, adopted by the General Assembly of the United Nations, November 20, 1989.

The basic principles of the Helsinki Declaration are reproduced here.

1. Biomedical research involving human subjects must conform to generally accepted scientific principles and should be based on adequately performed laboratory and animal experimentation and on a thorough knowledge of the scientific literature.

Comment: The biomedical cochlear implant research on children has always been preceded by extensive work with deaf adults. Our research in this area was based on a body of knowledge in auditory physiology, speech science, and other disciplines. It was also undertaken after adequate laboratory and animal experimentation as outlined in Chapters 2 and 3.

2. The design and performance of each experimental procedure involving human subjects should be clearly formulated in an experimental protocol which should be transmitted to a specially appointed independent committee for consideration, comment and guidance.

Comment: The findings from cochlear implant research studies on children published in international journals with a high standard of peer review can in general be accepted as reliable information having been based on clearly formulated and achievable experimental protocols. The same review has been made by agencies funding the cochlear implant research, for example, the U.S. National Institutes of Health and the National Health and Medical Research Council of Australia. The FDA has

also carefully reviewed the experimental protocols for any studies reported to it.

3. Biomedical research involving human subjects should be conducted only by scientifically qualified persons and under the supervision of a clinically competent medical person. The responsibility for the human subject must always rest with a medically qualified person and never rest on the subject of the research, even though the subject has given his or her consent.

Comment: The research in Melbourne has always been undertaken under the control of the Cochlear Implant Clinic of the Royal Victorian Eye and Ear Hospital. The Head of the Clinic must be an appropriately qualified medical person who is responsible to the Board of the Hospital and the University.

4. Biomedical research involving human subjects cannot legitimately be carried out unless the importance of the objective is in proportion to the inherent risk to the subject.

Comment: The successful outcomes of implantation in adults and children with severe-to-profound hearing loss are now well documented in properly controlled studies reported in international journals with a high standard of peer review. The outcomes, complications, and cost-effectiveness of cochlear implants for cochlear implantation in the U.K. from 1990–1994 have been documented in detail by Summerfield and Marshall (1994) from the MRC Institute of Hearing Research, University of Nottingham. A major study funded by the U.S. National Institute of Deafness and Other Communication Disorders was undertaken at the Central Institute for the Deaf (CID) where a group of profoundly deaf children were managed with either hearing aids, tactile aids, or cochlear implants. The speech perception and production results from this study were reported by Geers, and Brenner (1994) and Tobey, Geers, and Brenner (1994).

The study was a longitudinal study of 39 children with prelingual profound deafness, who were evaluated over a 3-year period while enrolled in the auditory-oral education program at Central Institute for the Deaf in St. Louis, Missouri. The 39 children were matched in triads, 13 using cochlear implants (CI), 13 tactile aids (TA), and 13 conventional hearing aids (HA). The primary focus of the study was to document differences, if any, in the rate of acquisition in speech perception, speech production, and spoken language with use of these sensory devices. The study used a stringent measure of benefit, requiring not only improvement in children compared to themselves, but also compared to similar orally educated children using hearing aids.

Initial scores on a battery of speech perception tests were similar for all three groups. After 36 months, there was a significant difference between the performance of the children using cochlear implants and the other two groups. With speech perception, the cochlear implant group moved from a median category 1 (detection only) to category 5 (consonant perception). In contrast, the tactile group moved from category 1 to category 2 (pattern perception), whereas the hearing aid group remained at category 2 over the entire 36 months of the study. In addition, statistical analysis showed that feature perception for the three groups was significantly different after 36 months of habilitation. Although there were no significant differences between the TA and HA groups, the CI group scored significantly higher than the TA or HA group on pitch perception (95% versus 65% and 84%), vowel perception (84% versus 35% and 42%), and consonant place perception (36% versus 16% and 21%). The CI group also moved on the MATRIX phrase perception task from being the lowest of the three groups to the highest. Finally, after only 12 months, the lipreading enhancement scores of the CI group were found to exceed those of children using either hearing aids or tacile aids.

The CI group also demonstrated significantly greater scores than either the TA or HA groups in production of vowels and consonants in their spontaneous speech. Children who used the cochlear implant for 3 years performed at a comparable level to children using hearing aids with a PTA of 90–100 dB HL. The children in the CI group were also significantly more accurate on their production of the less visible place and complex manner features and on some voicing features, as compared to the TA and HA groups.

In terms of spoken language, the CI group exhibited faster acquisition of all language and communication skills measured. The mean scores for the CI group were signficantly higher than the TA or HA groups in the areas of expressive vocabulary, receptive syntax, and everyday use of sensory aid (Geers, & Moog, 1994).

Furthermore, a U.S. National Institute of Health (NIH) Consensus Statement, Vol 13(2), Cochlear Implants in Adults and Children was issued in 1995. This statement concluded that, using tests commonly applied to children and adults with hearing impairments, perceptual performance increases on average with each succeeding year postimplantation. Over time, performance may improve to match that of children who have residual hearing and are highly successful hearing aid users. Children implanted at younger ages are on average more accurate in their production of consonants, vowels, intonation, and rhythm than older children. Speech produced by children with implants is more accurate than speech produced by children with comparable hearing losses using vibrotactile devices or hearing aids. One year after implantation, speech intelligibility is twice that typically reported for children with profound hearing impairments, and continues to improve. Oral-aural communication training appears to result in substantially greater speech intelligibility than manually based total communication. The nature and pace of language acquisition may be influenced by the age of onset, age at implantation, nature and intensity of habilitation, and mode of communication.

Oral language development in deaf children, including those with cochlear implants, remains a slow, training-intensive process and results typically are delayed in comparison with normally hearing peers.

The risks of implantation have been reported by a number of surgeons and are referred to in Chapter 7. A total of 6,084 children had received the Nucleus multiple-channel cochlear implant worldwide by September 1996.

5. Every biomedical research project involving human subjects should be preceded by careful assessment of predictable risks in comparison with foreseeable benefits to the subject or to others. Concern for the interests of the subject must always prevail over the interests of science and society.

Comment: The rehabilitation of the first two adult patients operated on by the University of Melbourne team in 1978 and 1979 was a requirement of the program and has continued to be the case. Rehabilitation and habilitation have always been the first priority even when there was a need to do speech and psychophysical research studies. With the study on children for the FDA, training and assessment preceded any research investigation.

6. The right of the research subject to safeguard his or her integrity must always be respected. Every precaution should be taken to respect the privacy of the subject and to minimize the impact of the study on the subject's physical and mental integrity and on the personality of the subject.

Comment: As outlined in Chapters 4 and 11, it is our practice to minimize the impact of the implant on the child's physical and mental integrity and his or her personality by providing guidance to parents in their management at home and at school. Regular meetings are held with parents and the child's teacher of the deaf is involved to ensure that all aspects of the child's welfare are considered. This includes guidance on how to deal with interest from children in a mainstream school and help on how to cope with any tensions created by signing deaf peers. Later, as teenagers, they need assistance in coping with any self-consciousness about being different in using the device.

7. Physicians should abstain from engaging in research projects involving human subjects unless they are satisfied that the hazards involved are believed to be predictable. Physicians should cease any investigation if the hazards are found to outweigh the potential benefits.

Comment: The hazards in carrying out cochlear implantation on children can in general be predicted on the basis of experience with adults. In the case of infants and young children there are special biological safety issues, and these are the effects of implantation on head growth, the effects of head growth on the lead wire assembly, the effects of implantation and electrical stimulation on tissue in the young animal, the effects of explantation and reimplantation if a replacement electrode is required some years later, and the likelihood of labyrinthitis postimplantation, as infants are prone to episodes of otitis media. These special issues have been studied under an NIH contract No.1-N5-7-2342 and the results are outlined in Chapter 3.

Furthermore, it is assumed that the physician in charge has the responsibility of ensuring that the procedure will stop if the hazards outweigh the benefits. At each stage of our program, a multidisciplinary team assesses the benefits for each individual child, and the results are discussed with the parents.

> 8. In publication of the results of his or her research, the physician is obliged to preserve the accuracy of the results. Reports of experimentation not in accordance with the principles laid down in this Declaration should not be accepted for publication.

Comment: The published results from Melbourne and other centers in the cochlear implant field have been validated by other multicenter studies. We have also endeavored to report the findings in scientific journals and meetings regardless of how well they fitted expectations, and it has been a requirement of the FDA that Cochlear Limited and other firms report any faults or problems to them.

> 9. In any research on human beings, each potential subject must be adequately informed of the aims, methods, anticipated benefits and potential hazards of the study and the discomfort it may entail. He or she should be informed that he or she is at liberty to abstain from participation in the study and that he or she is free to withdraw his or her consent to participation at any time. The physician should then obtain the subject's freely-given informed consent, preferably in writing.

Comment: All our patients have been informed of the aims, methods, anticipated benefits, and potential hazards of implantation. This has been done by the surgeon and audiologist, first by discussion and then by presenting the information in writing when further discussion and explanation ensue. This also takes the form of a plain language statement that can be readily understood. This is accompanied by a consent form and the parents' written consent is obtained.

To ensure that the information has been understood, it is now our procedure to require another person, for example, an independent doctor, to ask simple questions of the parent and child such as, "What do you expect to get out of the procedure, and what are the risks?"

It is accepted that parents act on behalf of their children when the child is not of an age to understand the risk/benefits or able to make an informed decision. This is not the case with older children, in which case both child and parents are involved in making the decision.

> 10. When obtaining informed consent for the research project the physician should be particularly cautious if the subject is in a dependent relationship to him or her or may consent under duress. In that case the informed consent should be obtained by a physician who is not engaged in the investigation and who is completely independent of this official relationship.

Comment: It has been our practice to require the consent form to be discussed with the patient by both a surgeon on the team as well as independently by a noninvolved medical practitioner or lawyer. This now applies only for new research projects that may involve greater risk.

> 11. In case of legal incompetence, informed consent should be obtained from the legal guardian in accordance with national legislation. Where physical or mental incapacity makes it impossible to obtain informed consent, or when the subject is a minor, permission from the responsible relative replaces that of the subject in accordance with national legislation.

Comment: It is our practice for older children with mental or severe physical handicaps to consult psychological, psychiatric, or pediatric specialists to help determine the child's ability to give informed consent. With young children, it is the parents' responsibility to give consent as it is a therapeutic procedure.

> 12. The research protocol should always contain a statement of the ethical considerations involved and should indicate that the principles enunciated in the present Declaration are complied with.

The patients' consent forms in use in the Melbourne Cochlear Implant Clinic include a Statement of Patient Rights, based on the requirements of the National Health and Medical Research Council of Australia. This statement is consistent with the Helsinki Declaration. In all cases, the individual rights of patients to the highest quality of health care are paramount in the considerations of the Royal Victorian Eye and Ear Hospital Ethics Committee.

The rights of the child having a cochlear implant should also be considered in relation to the Convention on the Rights of the Child adopted by the General Assembly of the United Nations on 20 November 1989. Specific articles of direct relevance to the ethics of cochlear implantation in the child are discussed and quoted as follows:

> Article 3.1: In all actions concerning children, whether undertaken by public or private social welfare institutions, courts of law, administrative authorities or legislative bodies, the best interests of the child shall be a primary consideration.

Comment: The best interests of the child are served by a careful evaluation by the interdisciplinary cochlear implant team as outlined in Chapter 4. Discussions with the parents and consultation with the teachers of the deaf are an important component in ensuring that the best interests of the child are paramount.

> Article 5: State Parties shall respect the responsibilities, rights and duties of parents or, where applicable, the members of the extended family or community as provided for by local custom, legal guardians or other persons legally responsible for the child, to provide, in a manner consistent with the evolving capacities of the child, appropriate direction and guidance in the exercise by the child of the rights recognized in the present Convention.

Comment: The rights of parents to decide what is best for their child is accepted if it is a therapeutic procedure such as a cochlear implant. Also, in accord with the world view embodied in the U.N. Universal Declaration of Rights, the child is involved in the decision-making process from the earliest possible stage.

> Article 12.1: State Parties shall assure to the child who is capable of forming his or her own views the right to express those views freely in all matters affecting the child, the views of the child being given due weight in accordance with the age and maturity of the child.

Comment: The older the child the more responsibility he or she needs to be given in deciding whether to have a cochlear implant. This is especially important as the results of cochlear implantation are not as good and are more variable in older children who have had a longer duration of deafness. A full and free discussion should be undertaken. It is, however, a complex matter in assessing the competence of the child to make decisions.

> Article 18.1: State Parties shall use their best efforts to ensure recognition of the principle that both parents have common responsibilities for the upbringing and development of the child. Parents or, as the case may be, legal guardians, have the primary responsibility for the upbringing and development of the child. The best interests of the child will be their basic concern.

Comment: Not only is it important to recognize that parents have the right to decide the care needed for their child on the basis of the future needs of the child to fit into society, but also the communication needed at home. Parents with hearing will usually prefer their children to be able to communicate with them in an auditory/oral mode. Approximately 85–90% of deaf children are in families with normally hearing parents. On the other hand, if two deaf parents have a deaf or hearing child there may be a need for the child to learn to sign. In both cases the two educational modes should not be initially exclusive, providing the cochlear implant is carried out at an early age during the child's critical period for speech and language development.

Article 23.1: State Parties recognize that a mentally or physically disabled child should enjoy a full and decent life, in conditions which ensure dignity, promote self-reliance, and facilitate the child's active participation in the community.

Article 23.2: States Parties recognize the right of the disabled child to special care and shall encourage and ensure the extension, subject to available resources, to the eligible child and those responsible for his or her care, of assistance for which application is made and which is appropriate to the child's condition and to the circumstances of the parents or others caring for the child.

Article 23.3: Recognizing the special needs of a disabled child, assistance extended in accordance with paragraph 2 of the present article shall be provided free of charge, whenever possible, taking into account the financial resources of the parents or others caring for the child, and shall be designed to ensure that the disabled child has effective access to and receives education, training, health care services, rehabilitation services, preparation for employment and recreation opportunities in a manner con-

ducive to the child's achieving the fullest possible social integration and individual development, including his or her cultural and spiritual development.

Comment: If a child receives a cochlear implant then the clinic should attempt to ensure that there are adequate educational, rehabilitation, and other resources to support the child. It is also important that industry act in such a way that there is continuity in patient support should there be sales or takeovers. In this latter situation, Cochlear Limited has provided continuity in the case of implant patients when they acquired control of 3M and Ineraid.

Article 24.1: State Parties recognize the right of the child to the enjoyment of the highest attainable standard of health and to facilities for the treatment of illness and rehabilitation of health. State Parties shall strive to ensure that no child is deprived of his or her right of access to such health care services.

Comment: The highest standard of help for the child and parents is best achieved through the support of a team or clinic rather than a single clinician. The clinic should be hospital-based with strong links to the educational authority. The clinical team should also be able to provide considerable support to the home or school. The support services provided by the firm manufacturing the device are also an important consideration.

Article 28.1: State Parties recognize the right of the child to education, and with a view to achieving this right progressively and on the basis of equal opportunity, they shall, in particular: (a) Make primary education compulsory and available free to all; (b) Encourage the development of different forms of secondary education, including general and vocational education, make them available and accessible to every child, and take appropriate measures such as the introduction of free education and offering financial assistance in case of need; (c) Make higher education accessible to all on the basis of capacity by every appropriate means; (d) Make educational and vocational information and guidance available and accessible to all children; (e) Take measures to encourage regular attendance at schools and the reduction of drop-out rates.

Comment: It has been shown in a number of studies (e.g., Walker & Rickards, 1992) that the language development of severely to profoundly deaf children lags behind their normal hearing peers as illustrated in Figure, 14–1. In addition, fewer deaf children succeed at secondary or tertiary education especially when using sign language of the deaf. Cochlear implants offer the possibility for more children to utilize their educational potential.

Article 29.1: State Parties agree that the education of the child shall be directed to: (a) The development of the child's personality, talents and mental and physical abilities to their fullest potential; (b) The development of respect for human rights and fundamental freedoms, and for the principles enshrined in the Charter of the United Nations; (c) The development of respect for the child's parents, his or her own cultural identity, language and values, for the national values of the country in which the child is living, the country from which he or she may originate, and for civilizations different from his or her own; (d) The preparation of the child for

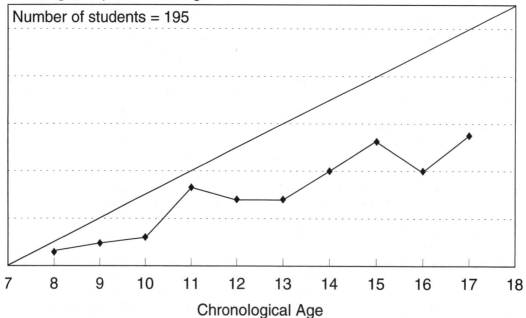

Reading Comprehension of Profoundly Hearing Impaired Students in Victoria (Prelinguistically Deafened)

Reading Comprehension Age

Number of students = 195

Chronological Age

FIGURE 14–1. Reading comprehension age of profoundly hearing impaired students in Victoria (prelinguistically deafened) versus chronological age. n = 195 (Walker and Rickards, 1992).

responsible life in a free society, in the spirit of understanding, peace, tolerance, equality of sexes, and friendship among all peoples, ethnic, national and religious groups and persons of indigenous origin; (e) The development of respect for the natural environment.

Comment: The cochlear implant must ultimately help the child to be a well rounded mature individual capable of living with self-reliance in society. Developing competence in language will help achieve this goal. There is also no reason why a child with an implant and auditory/oral communication should not be able to communicate with and have friends in the deaf signing community.

ACKNOWLEDGMENTS

We thank Dr. Nicholas Tonti-Philippini for helpful comments and Mrs. Carole Smith, Mrs. Sue Davine, and Ms. Jacky Gray for the typing and Mr. Trevor Carter for the figures.

REFERENCES

Clark, G. M. Blamey, P. J., Brown, A. M., Busby, P. A., Dowell, R. C., Franz, B. K.-G., Pyman, B. C., Shepherd, R. K., Tong, Y. C., Webb, R. L., Hirshorn, M. S., Kuzma, J., Mecklenburg, D. J., Money, D. K., Patrick, J. F., & Seligman, P. M. (1987). The University of Melbourne—Nucleus Multi-Electrode Cochlear Implant. *In Advances in Oto-Rhino-Laryngology, 38.* Basel.

Convention on the Rights of the Child General Assembly of the United Nations. 20 November 1989.

Declaration of Helsinki. Recommendations guiding physicians in biomedical research involving human subjects. Adopted by the 18th World Medical Assembly, Helsinki, Finland, June 1964, amended by the 29th World Medical Assembly, Tokyo, Japan, October 1975, and the 35th World Medical Assembly, Venice, Italy, October 1983.

Geers, A. E., & Brenner, C. (1994) Speech perception results: Audition and lipreading enhancement. In A. E. Geers & J. S. Moog (Eds.), *Effectiveness of cochlear implants and tactile aids study at Central Institute for the Deaf* (pp. 97–108) *The Volta Review, 96*(5).

Geers, A. E., & Moog, J. S. (1994). Spoken language results: Vocabulary, syntax, and communication. In A. E. Geers & J. S. Moog (Eds.), *Effectiveness of cochlear implants and tactile aids for deaf children. The Volta Review, 96*(5), 131–148.

Luxford, W. M., Berliner, K. I., Eisenberg, M. A., & House, W. F. (1987). Cochlear implants in children. *Annals of Otology, Rhinology and Laryngology, 96*, 136–38.

Summerfield, A. Q., & Marshall, D. H. (1994). *Cochlear implantation in the UK 1990–1994.* Report by the MRC Institute of Hearing Research on the Evaluation of the National Cochlear Implant Program. Nottingham, UK: MRC Institute of Hearing Research, University of Nottingham.

Tobey, E., Geers, A., & Brenner, C. (1994) Speech production results: Speech feature acquisitions. In A. E. Geers & J. S. Moog (Eds.), *Effectiveness of cochlear implants and tactile aids for deaf children. The Volta Review, 96*(5), 109–129.

Walker, L. M., & Rickards, F. W. (1992). Reading comprehension levels of profoundly, prelingually deaf students in Victoria. *The Australian Teacher of the Deaf, 3*, 32–47.

EPILOGUE

GRAEME M. CLARK

Cochlear implantation in children has made considerable progress in the last decade, and it is now an established clinical procedure. Together with cochlear implants for adults, it could be said to have reached the stage of being a subdiscipline in otology. It is truly an interdisciplinary field where surgery, audiology, speech-language pathology, education, engineering, and the biological sciences continue to make essential contributions. Like any interdisciplinary field, the best patient management and future progress will occur when there is maximal exchange of information and expertise between these disciplines.

To retain effective communication among cochlear implant disciplines, it is important that the specialists in each discipline have a good knowledge of the other disciplines. This will be achieved by ensuring that future otological training programs require considerably more experience in audiology and speech science and especially in the pediatric field. Second, there is a need to increase the training in cochlear implantation in the disciplines of audiology, speech science, and education of the deaf. This will break down the lines of demarcation relevant to cochlear implants in these disciplines. This should then lead to the development of a subspecialty for cochlear implant communication. It is hoped this book,

with its emphasis on diagnosis, selection, surgery, management, habilitation, and evaluation, will form a basis for the training of the specialist.

Cochlear implantation has influenced a number of disciplines. Prior to its origins in the mid 1970s there was, for example, little interest in audiological tests for people with a profound hearing loss, as not a great deal could be done to help them audiologically. Furthermore, there was only marginal interest in speech science and its application to the management of a hearing loss. Implants, however, have required the application of a number of tests to assess communication abilities. In addition, with an increasing emphasis on cochlear implantation in children and its extension to infants, there is a need for more research on the development of speech perception and production and the acquisition of receptive and expressive language. This is particularly important as there is great variability in the performance of children, and we have limited understanding of the factors predicting communication skills postoperatively.

Not only is there a need to study areas of importance in the development of speech and language in implanted children, but further research is required to improve the quality of the signal that children and adults receive. Cochlear implants

251

derived their inspiration from auditory neurophysiology and an understanding of the coding of sound. On the other hand, physiological and psychophysical research on electrical stimulation of the auditory pathways over the years has contributed to our understanding of the coding of sound. To further improve the transmission of auditory information through the "electroneural bottleneck" existing between the external world and electrical stimulation of the central auditory neural pathways, there is a need to understand how electrical stimulation can better reproduce the temporospatial responses to sound occurring normally in the auditory nerve. Cochlear implant speech processing has

also contributed to our understanding of speech perception and similarly there is a need for further research in speech science and its application to electrical stimulation at the auditory nerve in order to maximize the information transmitted through the electroneural bottleneck.

Finally, it has been remarkable how quickly technological advances have been incorporated into the development of cochlear implants. With speech processing engineering for cochlear implants it has only taken from 1978 until 1996 for a behind-the-ear speech processor to be developed following the initial realization of a wearable device needing to be carried in a bag. Further advances can be expected.

INDEX

....

253